Munro Kerr's
OPERATIVE
OBSTETRICS

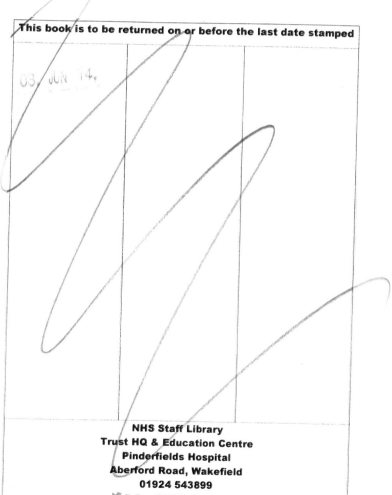

Cover illustration: The tenth table. 'Front view of twins in utero', from William Smellie's, *A Sett of Anatomical Tables With Explanation and an Abridgement of the Practice of Midwifery*. London: D. Wilson, 1754. Smellie employed the Dutch artist, Jan van Rymsdyk, who made coloured crayon drawings directly from the anatomical dissections, followed by engraved copper plates from which the tables were produced.

For Elsevier
Content Strategist: *Pauline Graham*
Content Development Specialist: *Helen Leng*
Project Manager: *Vinod Kumar*
Designer/Design Direction: *Christian Bilbow*
Illustration Manager: *Jennifer Rose*

Munro Kerr's

OPERATIVE OBSTETRICS

TWELFTH EDITION

Edited by
Thomas F. Baskett
MB BCh BAO(The Queen's University of Belfast)
FRCS(C) FRCS(Ed) FRCOG FACOG DHMSA
Professor Emeritus, Department of Obstetrics and Gynaecology,
Dalhousie University, Halifax,
Nova Scotia, Canada

Andrew A. Calder
MB BCh, MD(University of Glasgow)
FRCS(Ed) FRCP(Glas) FRCP(Ed) FRCOG HonFCOG(SA)
Professor Emeritus, Department of Obstetrics and Gynaecology,
University of Edinburgh, UK

Sabaratnam Arulkumaran
KB MB BS(University of Ceylon)
MD PhD FRCS(Ed) FRCOG FACOG HonFCOG(SA)
Professor Emeritus, Department of Obstetrics & Gynaecology, St George's
University Medical School,
London, UK

Illustrations by Ian Ramsden

SAUNDERS
ELSEVIER

Edinburgh London New York Oxford Philadelphia
St Louis Sydney Toronto 2014

SAUNDERS
ELSEVIER

First published 1908 as *Operative Midwifery* by J. Munro Kerr
Second edition 1911
Third edition 1916
Fourth edition 1937 as *Operative Obstetrics* by J. Munro Kerr, D. McIntyre and D. Fyfe Anderson
Fifth edition 1949 by J. Munro Kerr and J. Chassar Moir
Sixth edition 1956 and Seventh edition 1964 as *Munro Kerr's Operative Obstetrics* by J. Chassar Moir
Eighth edition 1971 by J. Chassar Moir and P. R. Myerscough
Ninth edition 1977 and Tenth edition 1982 by P. R. Myerscough
Eleventh (Centenary) edition 2007 by T. F. Baskett, A.A. Calder and S. Arulkumaran
Twelfth edition 2014

ISBN 9780702051852

British Library Cataloguing in Publication Data
A catalogue record for this book is available from the British Library

Library of Congress Cataloguing in Publication Data
A catalogue record for this book is available from the Library of Congress

ELSEVIER your source for books, journals and multimedia in the health sciences

www.elsevierhealth.com

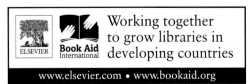

Working together to grow libraries in developing countries

www.elsevier.com • www.bookaid.org

The publisher's policy is to use paper manufactured from sustainable forests

Printed in China

CONTENTS

PREFACE, vii
CONTRIBUTORS, ix

1 HUMAN BIRTH, 1
AA Calder

2 RISK MANAGEMENT IN LABOUR
AND DELIVERY, 7
LC Edozien

3 AUDIT AND STANDARDS OF INTRAPARTUM
CARE, 15
MS Robson

4 COMPETENCE AND SKILLS TRAINING, 22
TJ Draycott

5 ASSESSMENT AND MANAGEMENT OF
LABOUR, 31
MS Robson

6 FETAL SURVEILLANCE IN LABOUR, 41
S Arulkumaran

7 FETAL ASPHYXIA, 57
S Arulkumaran

8 INDUCTION OF LABOUR, 71
SJ Stock • AA Calder

9 PRETERM LABOUR, 80
JE Norman

10 ASSISTED VAGINAL DELIVERY, 88
TF Baskett

11 MALPRESENTATIONS, 116
TF Baskett • AA Calder

12 SHOULDER DYSTOCIA, 123
JF Crofts

13 CAESAREAN SECTION, 132
TF Baskett • AA Calder

14 VAGINAL BIRTH AFTER CAESAREAN
SECTION, 145
VM Allen • TF Baskett

15 UTERINE RUPTURE, 152
MJ Turner

16 BREECH DELIVERY, 157
TF Baskett

17 TWIN AND TRIPLET DELIVERY, 169
JFR Barrett

18 CORD PROLAPSE, 174
TF Baskett

19 ANTEPARTUM HAEMORRHAGE, 178
JCP Kingdom

20 POSTPARTUM HAEMORRHAGE, 198
TF Baskett

21 RETAINED PLACENTA, 207
AD Weeks

22 ACUTE UTERINE INVERSION, 211
TF Baskett

23 LOWER GENITAL TRACT TRAUMA, 217
AH Sultan • R Thakar

24 HAEMORRHAGIC SHOCK, 225
TF Baskett • VS Talaulikar

25 DISSEMINATED INTRAVASCULAR
COAGULATION, 230
TF Baskett • VS Talaulikar

26 AMNIOTIC FLUID EMBOLISM, 234
DJ Tuffnell

27 ANALGESIA AND ANAESTHESIA, 236
A Addei • TF Baskett

28 PROCEDURES AND TECHNIQUES, 242
a. Cervical cerclage (AA Calder)
b. Acute tocolysis (TF Baskett and S Arulkumaran)
c. Version (TF Baskett)
d. Uterine and vaginal tamponade (TF Baskett and S Arulkumaran)
e. Uterine compression sutures (TF Baskett and S Arulkumaran)
f. Pelvic vessel ligation and embolization (TF Baskett)
g. Obstetric hysterectomy (TF Baskett)
h. Symphysiotomy (TF Baskett and RC Pattinson)
i. Destructive operations on the fetus (TF Baskett and RC Pattinson)

INDEX, 283

It must be acknowledged that all errors of practice do not proceed from ignorance of the art. Some of them may justly be imputed to our entertaining too much confidence in our own dexterity, or too little dependence on the natural efforts and resources of the constitution... The abuse of art produces more and greater evils than are occasioned by the imperfections of Nature.

Thomas Denman, 1795

PREFACE

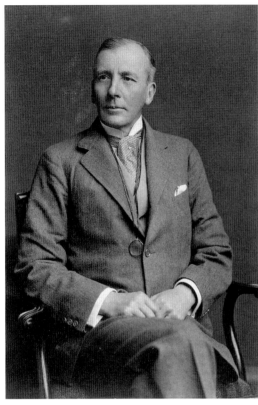

Munro Kerr

An obstetric text which has evolved through twelve editions and across more than a hundred years must inevitably have reflected profound changes and progress in many aspects. When Munro Kerr took up his pen to write the first edition (1908) the maternal mortality in Britain was around four per thousand and the perinatal death rate about 80 per thousand. The intervening years have witnessed such dramatic medical and social changes that only one in eight such babies and one in 40 such mothers are lost nowadays. In many developing countries, however, the picture remains as bad as or even worse than that observed by the founding father of this textbook. Clearly those less fortunate parts of the world lack the equipment, personnel, educational and training levels which we are privileged to enjoy. As well as lack of investment

and motivation, however, a major obstacle to improvements is frequently the low status of women in communities and cultures where a low priority is given to their health and wellbeing. Regardless of those humbling disparities though, it must be recognized that outcomes can be optimized within all settings by the application of the sound clinical, obstetrical and surgical techniques and principles which have been embodied in that first and every subsequent edition of *Munro Kerr*.

Some aspects of obstetric care have hardly changed across those decades while others would be unrecognizable to the obstetrician of the early 20th century. There has been a substantial swing from a climate within which the safety and survival of the mother inevitably took precedence, to one in which more and more attention is directed to the fetus. The most obvious change in operative obstetrics has been the ever greater employment of caesarean section, which has changed from a procedure of last resort to what begins to look like the answer to every obstetric complication. Nevertheless, the imperative to strive for a safe outcome for both the mother and her baby continues to depend on tried and tested principles of high-quality clinical care. As important as the skill to perform operations is the judgement to decide when it is appropriate to do so, a maxim which applies across the whole spectrum of Operative Obstetrics.

As this text has progressed through successive editions the nature of its authorship has changed. The first three were monographs written by 'MK' himself. For the fourth he was assisted by two colleagues from his own Glasgow hospital and for the fifth he collaborated with Chassar Moir, Foundation Nuffield Professor at the University of Oxford. By 1956 Munro Kerr had ceased his involvement and Moir continued to produce the next two. For the eighth edition Moir collaborated with Philip Myerscough of Edinburgh, who continued as sole author for the ninth and tenth. His proposal to collaborate with his Edinburgh colleague Andrew Calder was delayed while a new publisher was found and by then he felt he was too remote to remain involved.

In due course with Saunders (Elsevier) agreeing to publish the eleventh (Centenary) edition it was felt appropriate to have a more international authorship and so Calder was joined by Tom Baskett and Sabaratnam Arulkumaran. The current edition sees the biggest change. While the authors of the previous edition have continued to provide the bulk of the text we have recruited seventeen younger experts to contribute or share in joint authorship of the new chapters. This reflects the trend in modern obstetrics for clinicians to become prominent authorities in different facets of our discipline.

Despite broadening the authorship we have striven to retain the essential flavour which has characterized this textbook for more than a century with emphasis on a practical, common sense approach to the common and rarer issues which confront obstetricians. References have been cited where they are required to underpin and justify the guidance provided but we recommend the reader to consult the national guidelines which are an increasingly common feature of clinical practice and to refer to the *Cochrane Database of Systematic Reviews* in areas where practice is subject to rapid change. That said, we are unapologetic in continuing the tradition, for which this work has been unique, of giving historical context to this endlessly fascinating subject.

TF Baskett

AA Calder

S Arulkumaran

CONTRIBUTORS

Anthony Addei MB ChB FRCA
Consultant Anaesthetist, St George's Hospital, London, UK

Victoria M Allen MD MSc FRCS(C)
Associate Professor, Department of Obstetrics and Gynaecology, Dalhousie University, Halifax, Nova Scotia, Canada

Sir Sabaratnam Arulkumaran PhD DSc FRCS(Ed) FRCOG
Professor Emeritus of Obstetrics & Gynaecology, St George's University of London, UK

Jon FR Barrett MB BCh MD FRCOG FRCS(C)
Chief of Maternal-Fetal Medicine, Sunnybrook Health Sciences Centre; Professor, University of Toronto, Canada

Thomas F Baskett MB FRCS(Ed) FRCS(C) FRCOG
Professor Emeritus, Department of Obstetrics and Gynaecology, Dalhousie University, Halifax, Nova Scotia, Canada

Andrew A Calder MD FRCP(Ed) FRCS(Ed) FRCOG
Professor Emeritus, Department of Obstetrics and Gynaecology, University of Edinburgh, UK

Joanna F Crofts MD MRCOG
NIHR Academic Clinical Lecturer, University of Bristol, UK

Timothy J Draycott MB BS MD FRCOG
Consultant Obstetrician & Health Foundation Improvement Science Fellow, Research into Safety & Quality (RiSQ) Group, University of Bristol, Bristol, UK

Leroy C Edozien LLB PhD FRCOG FWACS
Consultant Obstetrician and Gynaecologist, Manchester Academic Health Science Centre, University of Manchester, St Mary's Hospital, Manchester, UK

John CP Kingdom MD FRCSC(ObGyn & MFM) MRCP(UK) FRCOG
Professor of Obstetrics and Gynaecology, Medical Imaging, Physiology & Pathology, University of Toronto; Gordon C. Letich Chair, Department of Obstetrics & Gynaecology, University of Toronto; Head, Division of Maternal-Fetal Medicine, Department of Obstetrics and Gynaecology, University of Toronto; Rose Torno Chair in Obstetrics & Gynaecology, Staff, Obstetrics & Maternal-Fetal Medicine, Mount Sinai Hospital, Toronto, Canada

Jane E Norman MD FRCOG FMedSci
Professor of Maternal and Fetal Health, Consultant Obstetrician and Director of Tommy's Centre for Maternal and Fetal Health, University of Edinburgh, UK

Robert C Pattinson MD FRCOG FCOG(SA)
Director, MRC Maternal and Infant Health Care Strategies Research Unit, Department of Obstetrics and Gynaecology, University of Pretoria, South Africa

Michael S Robson MB BS MRCOG FRCS(Eng) FRCPI
Consultant Obstetrician and Gynaecologist, The National Maternity Hospital, Dublin, Ireland

Sarah J Stock PhD MRCOG
Clinical Lecturer, MRC Centre for Reproductive Health, University of Edinburgh, UK

Abdul H Sultan MD FRCOG
Consultant Obstetrician and Gynaecologist,
   Croydon University Hospital, UK

Vikram S Talaulikar MD MRCOG
Clinical Research Fellow, St George's Hospital
   and University of London, UK

Ranee Thakar MD MRCOG
Consultant Obstetrician and Gynaecologist,
   Croydon University Hospital, UK

Derek J Tuffnell FRCOG
Consultant Obstetrician and Gynaecologist,
   Bradford Teaching Hospitals NHS
   Foundation Trust, Bradford, UK

Michael J Turner MAO FRCOG FRCPI
Professor of Obstetrics and Gynaecology,
   UCD Centre for Human Reproduction,
   Coombe Women and Infants University
   Hospital, Dublin, Ireland

Andrew D Weeks MD FRCOG
Professor of International Maternal Health and
   Consultant Obstetrician, Sanyu Research
   Unit, University of Liverpool, Liverpool
   Women's Hospital, UK

CHAPTER 1

HUMAN BIRTH

AA Calder

> 'When the child is grown big and the mother cannot continue to provide him with enough nourishment, he becomes agitated, breaks through the membranes, and incontinently passes out into the external world free from any bonds'
> Hippocrates, On Generation, 4th century BC
>
> 'The stimulus for labour may originate in certain states of vital development or physical expansion of the fundus, corpus or cervix uteri and in altered conditions of the fetus, liquor amnii or placenta and the loosening or decadence of the membranes....'
> James Young Simpson
> Lectures on Midwifery, 1860

The safe and effective management of labour and delivery requires a clear understanding on the part of the birth attendant of the anatomy, physiology and biochemistry of human parturition and of its central participants – the mother and infant.

The 20th century, across most of which 'Munro Kerr' has stretched, witnessed the most spectacular growth and advance of medical science and with it a steady improvement in our understanding of the birth process. A hundred years ago the obstetrician's art depended mainly on the insights brought by the giants of 18th century obstetrics, notably William Smellie (1697–1763) and William Hunter (1718–1783), both incidentally born within 20 miles of Munro Kerr's birthplace. Smellie, who became acknowledged as 'The Master of British Midwifery', was the consummate man-midwife and teacher. His monumental *Treatise on the Theory and Practice of Midwifery* (1752), based on his extensive clinical experience, described and defined the birth process as never before and formed the basis for the clinical conduct of labour. His definition of the mechanisms of labour shed light on the convoluted journey through the birth canal which the fetus is required to follow. His *Sett of Anatomical Tables with Explanations and an Abridgement of the Practice of Midwifery* (1754) amplified these fundamental principles. This atlas, for which Smellie employed the Dutch artist Jan van Rymsdyk, was only surpassed 20 years later when

Hunter, employing the same artist, published his spectacular *Anatomy of the Human Gravid Uterus* (1774).

When Munro Kerr was preparing the original *Operative Midwifery* in 1908 there had been little further progress. The relevant anatomy was fairly well understood but the physiology of the myometrium and cervix, and the biochemistry, endocrinology and pharmacology of human labour were almost entirely unknown. At the start of the new millennium the young obstetrician may consider that those mysteries have almost all been solved following a century of discoveries which saw the emergence of oxytocin, oestrogen, progesterone, prostaglandins and many other hitherto unknown substances. But it would be surprising indeed if the close of the 21st century does not reveal an even more complex picture.

CURRENT UNDERSTANDING

As a starting point for the wide range of clinical issues addressed within this textbook, a brief review follows of some of the key elements of basic medical science pertaining to human labour and delivery as currently understood. This, by necessity, will be superficial and selective. For more detailed and comprehensive accounts the reader is referred to current textbooks of reproductive physiology, anatomy, biochemistry and endocrinology.

Myometrial Function

The myometrium is the engine which drives human labour, during which it displays a highly sophisticated and co-ordinated set of forces. The simple objective of these is to efface and dilate the cervix and drive the fetus through the birth canal. In contrast to other smooth muscle systems, the myometrium displays three unique properties which are crucial for its function:

1. It must remain quiescent for the greater part of human pregnancy, suppressing its natural instinct to contract until called upon to do so at the appointed time.

2. During labour it must display a pattern which affords adequate periods of relaxation between contractions without which placental blood flow and fetal oxygenation would be compromised.

3. It possesses the capacity for *retraction*, vital to prevent exsanguination after delivery but also essential during labour. Retraction is a unique property of uterine muscle whereby a shorter length of the muscle fibre is maintained, without the consumption of energy, even after the contraction that produced the decrease in length has passed. As the cervix is effaced and pulled around the fetal presenting part, an inability of the myometrial fibres in the uterine corpus to retract, in essence to steadily reduce their relaxed lengths, would mean that the tension on the cervix could not be maintained.

At its most basic, human labour may be regarded as an interaction between the corpus and the cervix (Fig 1-1). For the maintenance of pregnancy the corpus must be quiescent and the cervix closed and uneffaced. In labour the corpus contracts and the cervix yields. A useful analogy may be to compare this process to the experience of putting on, for the first time, a roll-neck pullover. Just as with the fetus, the head must be flexed to present its smallest diameters to the cervix, or neck of the pullover, which is effaced round the presenting part and ultimately dilated as a result of traction applied by the arms, which are in this connection analogous to the myometrial fibres.

Although it has been conventional to acknowledge a 'lower uterine segment' arising from the uterine isthmus (between the non-pregnant corpus and cervix), in practice it may be more helpful simply to see the boundary between corpus and cervix as the 'fibromuscular junction' which marks the change from a mostly muscular corpus to a predominantly fibrous cervix. Obstetric purists may argue that the concept of a 'lower segment' is helpful in the definition of placenta praevia and in directing the site of contemporary caesarean sections but, those issues apart, it is of little relevance and it is a difficult concept to define either anatomically or physiologically.

At its simplest, contraction of the myometrial cell requires actin and myosin to combine in the contractile filament actomyosin (Fig 1-2). This reaction is catalyzed by the enzyme myosin light-chain kinase, which is heavily calcium dependent. Calcium in turn relies for its availability on oxytocin and prostaglandin F2α, which transport it into the cell and also free it from intracellular stores. On the other hand this

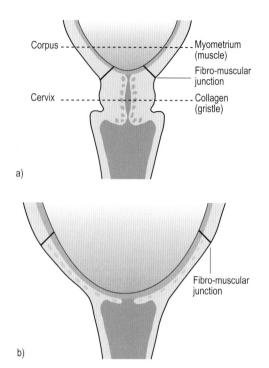

FIGURE 1-1 ■ (a) Diagrammatic representation of the relationship of the uterine corpus and cervix in mid pregnancy. The interface between them is usefully described as the fibro-muscular junction (FMJ). (b) Cervix fully effaced at start of labour, in the primigravida.

reaction is inhibited by progesterone, cyclic AMP and β-adrenergic agents. A particular insight into how the myometrial effort is co-ordinated into a concerted function came from the recognition of the essential requirement for gap junctions (biochemically characterized as Connexin-43) to be formed between individual myometrial cells, allowing cell-to-cell transmission of electrical impulses and ions. Thus, the corpus can display a wave of contractility propagated across its cell population which becomes a functional syncytium rather than a disorganized rabble of individual muscle fibres.

The Cervix

The recognition, little more than 50 years ago, that the cervix possesses a distinct structure based on collagen-rich connective tissue rather than smooth muscle has been fundamental to a better understanding of its function. It is thus not a 'sphincter' of the uterus but rather a tough, rigid obstacle to delivery which has to undergo a profound change in consistency to permit effacement, dilatation, and delivery to take place (Fig 1-3). That change is the process we now describe as 'cervical ripening'. The requisite

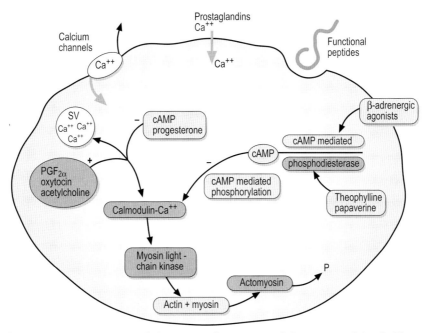

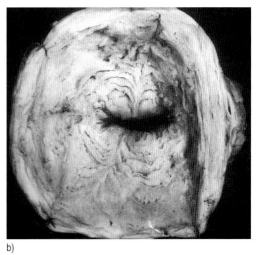

FIGURE 1-2 ■ Schematic representation of the contractile process of the myometrial cell. Those components shown in dark boxes represent contraction, those in light boxes represent relaxation.

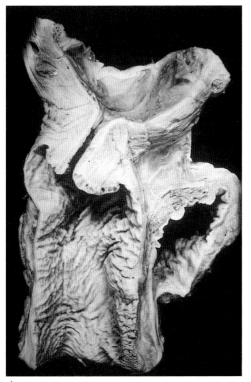

a)

FIGURE 1-3 ■ Original dissections prepared by William Hunter in the 18th century. That on the left (a) shows the lower part of the uterus, cervix, vagina, bladder and urethra in sagittal section in the last few weeks of pregnancy. That on the right (b) shows the cervix from the intrauterine aspect as it undergoes effacement in the last month of pregnancy (the fibro-muscular junction is now at the periphery of this specimen).

loosening and degradation of the collagen bundles is now recognized as having much in common with an inflammatory process, which requires the participation of inflammatory mediators including prostaglandin E2 and cytokines (especially interleukin-8), the recruitment of neutrophils and the synthesis of matrix metalloproteinases including collagenases and elastase (Fig 1-4).

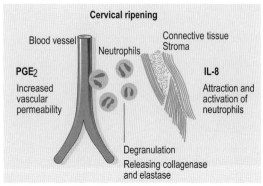

FIGURE 1-4 ■ Schematic representation of the control of cervical ripening. The collagen of the cervical stroma is broken down by matrix metalloproteinases, such as collagenase and elastase derived from neutrophils in an inflammatory-like process which requires them to be drawn into the tissue under the influence of interleukin-8 (IL8) from capillaries which have been dilated and made more permeable by prostaglandin E_2 (PGE$_2$)

BIOLOGICAL CONTROL OF LABOUR – TRIGGERING AND MAINTENANCE

The process by which the labour process is triggered and maintained has been the subject of intensive investigations. The clinical drive to this area of research has been the desire:

- to better understand, prevent or suppress preterm labour with all its complications
- to improve our ability to correct abnormal uterine action and poor progress in labour
- to enhance our capacity to induce effective labour when dictated by clinical circumstances.

The following brief review oversimplifies what is a most complex set of interactions, but it may suffice as a basis for rational clinical intervention. It is now recognized that the trigger for parturition comes from the fetus rather than from the mother. The maturing fetal brain is thought to provoke the release of corticotrophin from the fetal pituitary gland (Fig 1-5). This may be considered analogous to the switching on of pituitary gonadotrophin production at the time of puberty. The fetal adrenal gland responds by releasing two main products, cortisol and dehydro-epiandrosterone sulphate:

- Cortisol stimulates fetal pulmonary surfactant production to mature the lungs for extrauterine function and may also influence other organ systems. This is thought to result in changes in the composition of

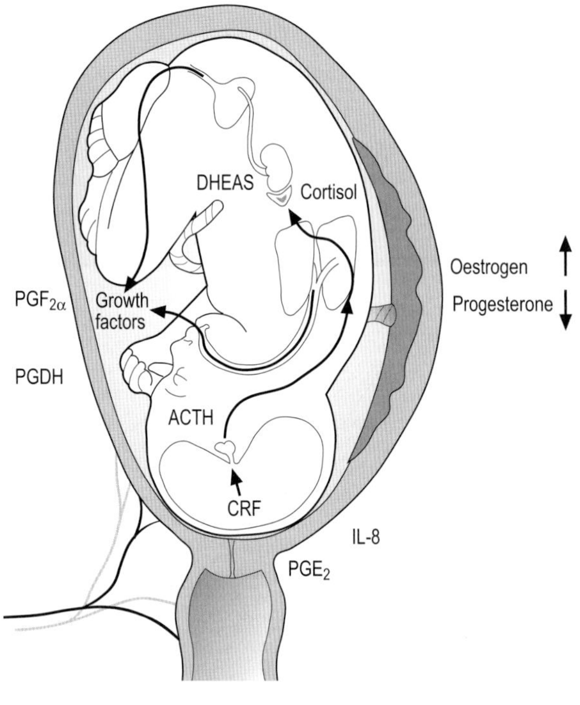

FIGURE 1-5 ■ Fetal control of the onset of labour is thought to result from activation of its hypothalamo–pituitary–adrenal axis, which leads in turn to modification of placental steroid production and activation of prostaglandins in the decidua and cervix.

the amniotic fluid which provoke the release of prostaglandin E2 from the amnion. This may be important for a direct influence on the cervix, especially focused at the internal os as this is the portion of the cervix which lies in intimate contact with the fetal membranes. The internal os needs to ripen first to initiate cervical effacement. To do this the activity of the principal prostaglandin degrading enzyme PG dehydrogenase within the chorion must decline, a phenomenon which has recently been confirmed.

- Dehydro-epiandrosterone sulphate is metabolized in the placenta to enhance oestradiol levels, which may provoke the release of prostaglandin $F_{2\alpha}$ from its richest source, the decidua, thereby exciting myometrial contractions.

Progesterone remains the principal enigma. It is known to inhibit both myometrial contractility and the formation of gap junctions, and is also recognized as supporting the activity of prostaglandin dehydrogenase, but evidence for its withdrawal prior to parturition remains elusive. It seems likely that there is either a process whereby its activity at tissue level declines without a drop in circulating levels, or simply that its influence is overcome by other factors.

We can therefore postulate that a cascade of endocrine changes initiated by the fetal brain results in the activation of a variety of endocrine and inflammatory substances which have the effect of co-ordinating three key events:

- maturing essential fetal organ systems, notably the lungs, for the challenges of extrauterine life
- transforming the rigid cervix into a compliant and readily dilatable structure
- initiating the myometrial contractions which will ultimately drive the fetus through the birth canal.

Figure 1-6 summarizes the key biochemical components which are thought to control the inflammatory-type processes which convert the stroma of the cervix from a rigid structure to a soft and compliant one, and the activation of the myometrial contractility which ultimately brings about its effacement and dilatation.

This brief overview is of necessity simplistic. The control of the birth process requires the participation of a myriad of other factors, such as adhesion molecules and receptors for hormones and prostaglandins, as well as other hormones such as vasopressin and relaxin. Perhaps the most important recent change in thinking has been to see the whole process of parturition as an inflammatory-type event. This has vital consequences for our understanding of those pregnancies which do not follow the normal pattern of labour onset and progress, either because it is delayed or activated prematurely. The role of infection in the latter is gaining increasing importance and it seems likely that some women may be at increased risk of preterm labour on account of an increased susceptibility to infection from deficiency of endogenous antimicrobial substances (Fig 1-7).

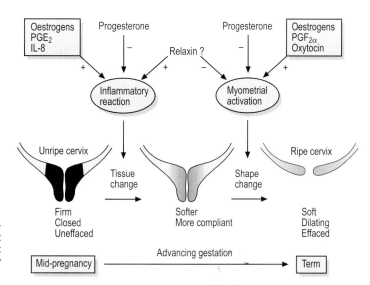

FIGURE 1-6 ■ A schematic representation of the factors which bring about the softening and dilation of the cervix during the transition from pregnancy maintenance to parturition.

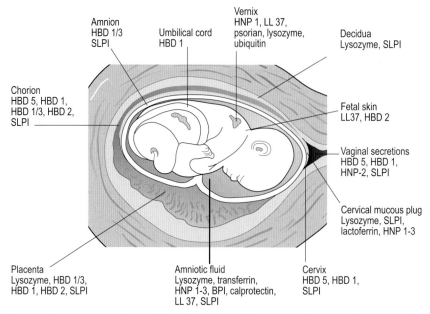

Amnion
HBD 1/3
SLPI

Umbilical cord
HBD 1

Vernix
HNP 1, LL 37,
psorian, lysozyme,
ubiquitin

Decidua
Lysozyme, SLPI

Chorion
HBD 5, HBD 1,
HBD 1/3, HBD 2,
SLPI

Fetal skin
LL37, HBD 2

Vaginal secretions
HBD 5, HBD 1,
HNP-2, SLPI

Cervical mucous plug
Lysozyme, SLPI,
lactoferrin, HNP 1-3

Placenta
Lysozyme, HBD 1/3,
HBD 1, HBD 2, SLPI

Amniotic fluid
Lysozyme, transferrin,
HNP 1-3, BPI, calprotectin,
LL 37, SLPI

Cervix
HBD 5, HBD 1,
SLPI

FIGURE 1-7 ■ Some of the natural antimicrobial substances which may be important in resisting infection during pregnancy. A deficiency of these may predispose to preterm delivery (by permission of Dr Sarah Stock).

BIBLIOGRAPHY

Calder AA, Greer IA. Physiology of labour. In: Phillip E, Setchell M, editors. Scientific foundations of obstetrics and gynaecology. Oxford: Butterworth; 1991.

Calder AA. Normal labour. In: Edmonds DK, editor. Dewhurst's textbook of obstetrics and gynaecology for postgraduates. Oxford: Blackwell; 1999.

Hunter W. Anatomy of the human gravid uterus. Birmingham: Baskerville; 1774.

Kerr JM. Operative midwifery. London: Baillière, Tindall and Cox; 1908.

Olson DM, Mijvoc JE, Sadowsky DW. Control of human parturition. Sem Perinatol 1995;19:52–63.

Smellie W. Treatise on the theory and practice of midwifery. London: D. Wilson; 1752.

Smellie W. Set of anatomical tables with explanations and an abridgement of the practice of midwifery. London: D. Wilson; 1754.

CHAPTER 2

RISK MANAGEMENT IN LABOUR AND DELIVERY

LC Edozien

'While in the later parts of this volume I have described the, at times, complex methods by which obstetric difficulties may be surmounted, I must from the outset make plain to the reader that the foundation of successful and safe obstetrics rests foremost upon prevention rather than upon operative skill. Many of the serious complications of pregnancy and most of the hazards of labour can be prevented, or their dangerous consequences obviated, if they were anticipated'.

PR Myerscough
Munro Kerr's Operative Obstetrics, 10th edition, 1982[1]

INTRODUCTION

The practice of operative obstetrics is underpinned by the Hippocratic exhortation, *primum non nocere* (first, do no harm). Unfortunately, errors do happen and sometimes these result in harm to the patient. Harm may result not only from errors of commission but also from errors of omission (particularly, failure to take preventative action). Intrapartum care is particularly susceptible to patient safety incidents, for a variety of reasons including: there are effectively two patients in one (mother and baby); swift transitions occur from low to high-risk situations; the margins between safety and harm in intrapartum care are thin; high levels of both surgical and medical expertise are often required; and speedy action is frequently essential.

Maternity care providers are obliged to adopt a systematic approach towards reducing the risk of incidents and of harm to patients. Risk management provides this approach. It is the totality of attitudes, structures and processes that are employed in a formal and integrated manner to protect the safety of patients and other service users. It addresses the following basic questions: What could go wrong? What are the chances of it happening and what would be the impact? What can we do to minimize the chance of this happening or to mitigate damage when it has gone wrong? What can we learn from things that have gone wrong, and how can lessons be shared?

The risk of patient safety incidents is likely to be contained more effectively if these questions are addressed proactively and prospectively, rather than by fire-fighting after the event. Often, however, efforts to manage risk during labour and delivery are haphazard rather than tailored, reactive rather than proactive, and diffuse rather than integrated.

One way of facilitating an integrated and proactive approach to risk management is the use of the RADICAL framework, which comprises the following domains in an integrated grid: Raise Awareness, Design for safety, Involve users, Collect and Analyse patient safety data, and Learn from patient safety incidents.[2] RADICAL is both a procedural and cognitive framework; it is a way of conceptualizing risk management, emphasizing the integration of various domains and finding a balance between the individual practitioner's accountability and the responsibilities of the organization.

RAISING AWARENESS

To effectively reduce the occurrence of patient safety incidents on the labour ward, staff need to be aware of the prevalence and underlying causes of these incidents. In this regard, awareness can be raised through local newsletters, clinical and academic meetings, maternity dashboards (a tool to benchmark quality and safety against agreed standards) and multiprofessional education. Local and national statistics concerning legal claims and complaints are also useful and should be widely disseminated.

Are Delivery Units as Safe as They Should Be?

Legal claims for problems occurring in labour are sometimes in excess of £6m per claim. An analysis of maternity claims in the period 2000–2010 published by the UK National Health Service Litigation Authority[3] showed that there were 5087 injury claims out of a total of 5.5m births. Although this amounts to less than one claim for every 1000 births, not every injury results in a claim and claims are the tip of the iceberg; also, not every episode of error in healthcare results in harm. The three most frequent categories of claim were those relating to management of labour (14.05%), caesarean section (13.24%) and cerebral palsy (10.65%). Two of these categories, namely cerebral palsy and management of labour, along with cardiotocograph (CTG) interpretation, were also the most expensive and together accounted for 70% of the total value of all the maternity claims. Other harms which commonly result in claims include perineal trauma and uterine rupture. The key risk management themes that emerged from the project were the need for formal processes to manage risk at all levels; learning and training; supervision and support; protocols and guidance; and learning lessons from patient safety incidents.

Many patient safety incidents are potentially preventable. Previous studies, for example, implicated suboptimal care in half of maternal deaths and three-quarters of intrapartum-related fetal/neonatal deaths.[4,5] High profile investigations and reports indicate that basic safety concerns are not always addressed,[6] and case studies show that a proactive, formal programme to improve safety in childbirth yields measurable improvements.[7,8]

Underlying Causes

Factors that have been implicated in failures of maternity services include systemic deficiencies in the management of high-risk cases; lack of input from consultants (including absence of consultant ward rounds on the labour ward); ineffective teamwork between obstetricians and midwives; workforce deficiencies; failure to recognize severity of a woman's condition; and poor documentation.

Some of these factors (such as workforce issues and the organization of services) are intrinsic characteristics of the department that predispose to the occurrence of incidents ('latent pathogens'), and their control requires an organizational approach. Others relate to individual practitioner knowledge, skills and competencies, and behaviour, which are amenable to correction by individual effort. It is particularly important for doctors and midwives to be aware of the value of non-technical skills in reducing the occurrence of patient safety incidents. These skills include teamwork, leadership and situational awareness.

Situational awareness is being aware of unfolding events and understanding how these affect individual and team goals and objectives; it is the ability to maintain the 'big picture' and think ahead. This is an important attribute on the labour ward. A consistent finding of enquiries into intrapartum-related perinatal deaths was that they were due mainly to clinicians' failure to recognize a problem and take appropriate action. In the National Health Service Litigation Authority (NHSLA) report,[3] only 21% of the claims involved high-risk pregnancies, indicating the need to keep the eye on the ball at all times; the transition from low risk to high risk could be swift. Practices and interventions that help maintain situational awareness include having cardiotocograph readings 'buddied' periodically (a second clinician independently interprets the trace), and the use of checklists.[9] In some obstetric units in the UK, a checklist/sticker is used each time a CTG is interpreted to ensure none of the key elements (baseline rate, accelerations, decelerations, variability, overall classification and plan) is omitted.

Another way of maintaining situational awareness is to continually assess and reassess priorities, ensuring that staff are deployed appropriately and that each woman gets the attention she needs when she needs it.[10] For this purpose, the labour ward whiteboard should be seen and treated as a dynamic rather than static dashboard.

DESIGN FOR SAFETY

Human error cannot be totally eliminated, but the risk of patient safety incidents can be reduced if, at individual and unit levels, we aim to provide care in a way that reflects safety awareness and a commitment to reducing the likelihood of error. Interventions such as clinical practice guidelines, care bundles, communication tools, handover protocols, promotion of hand hygiene, use of a surgical safety checklist and team training fall under this domain.

Clinical Practice Guidance

One safety lesson from 'high-reliability organizations' (such as the aviation industry) is that errors are less likely to happen if processes are standardized and if there is less reliance on memory. Staff should have access to referenced, evidence-based multidisciplinary guidelines for the management of various conditions and scenarios in labour and delivery. Ideally these should be available electronically. Policies and guidelines should be reviewed and updated, following a pre-specified schedule (e.g. every 3 years) and when there are major new research findings that warrant immediate change of practice. The Royal College of Obstetricians and Gynaecologists,[11] Society of Obstetricians and Gynaecologists of Canada,[12] Royal Australia and New Zealand College of Obstetricians and Gynaecologists[13] and the American College of Obstetricians and Gynecologists[14] have produced rich repositories of evidence-based guidelines and clinical standards which are accessible on their websites. The UK National Institute for Health and Clinical Excellence has also produced evidence-based guidelines for intrapartum care.[15] The delivery unit should be proactive in addressing high-risk conditions such as oxytocin induction and augmentation of labour, interpretation of CTG, vaginal birth after caesarean section, operative vaginal delivery, massive obstetric haemorrhage, obesity and management of perineal trauma.

Tools Facilitating Delivery of Safer Care

Teamwork, effective communication, training and avoidance of fatigue are essential for protecting patient safety on the labour ward and in the operating theatre. A variety of tools have been devised to address this.

A care bundle is a group of evidence-based interventions related to a disease or care process that, when executed together, result in better outcomes than when implemented individually. Care bundles have been developed for induction and augmentation of labour and for electronic fetal monitoring, and the care bundle for placenta praevia has been found to be particularly useful and easy to implement.[16]

The use of a surgical safety checklist has been shown to reduce the occurrence of patient safety incidents, and one has been devised specifically for maternity services.[17] Implementation of the checklist is straightforward and facilitates team work.[18]

There should be a personal, recorded handover of care between staff when there is a change of shift and when a patient is transferred from one professional to another. Each delivery unit should have its own structured multidisciplinary intershift handover (SMITH) protocol specifying what should be done before a handover ward round begins, how the handover should be conducted and how action points from the ward round should be documented and followed up.[19]

Interpretation of Cardiotocographs: Beware of Cognitive and Systemic Pitfalls

While it is widely recognized that failure of CTG interpretation is a common antecedent of patient safety incidents, interventions to address the problem are almost always based on the premise that these failures reflect a knowledge deficit. Education on the correct interpretation of CTGs will increase knowledge and promote better interpretation,[20] but it must be complemented by interventions that address other sources of failure to recognize or act on an abnormal CTG. These other sources include team and communication failures, fatigue and loss of situational awareness (discussed above).[21-23]

Oxytocin: Boon or Bane?

The use of oxytocin is one of the most beneficial pharmacological interventions in obstetrics, but its injudicious use is also one of the most common causes of adverse outcomes and litigation. Projects that encourage clinicians to treat oxytocin with respect have been shown to decrease not only the incidence of uterine tachysystole but also the rate of primary caesarean section.[24]

To ensure that this time-honoured drug remains a boon rather than bane, guidelines for its use should be adhered to. The indication for induction or augmentation of labour should be clear, the infusion regime should be followed to the letter, the fetus should be continuously monitored, and uterine contractions and the progress of labour should be carefully assessed. Malpresentation and obstructed labour should be excluded before labour is induced or augmented. Particular care should be taken in multiparous women and those with a uterine scar. In such cases, oxytocin should be used only with the approval of a senior obstetrician. In the event of uterine tachysystole, there should be timely recognition, and the infusion should be reduced or discontinued, depending on the fetal cardiograph. Oxytocin should not be used in labour where there are no facilities for an immediate caesarean section.

The same degree of respect accorded to oxytocin should be extended to other oxytocic drugs such as prostaglandin and misoprostol. In contemporary obstetric practice in the developed world, spontaneous rupture of the multigravid uterus is rare, and the vast majority of ruptures follow the administration of oxytocic drugs (prostaglandin or oxytocin) to induce or augment labour in a scarred uterus. Local guidelines should be categorical about how oxytocics may or may not be used in women scheduled for vaginal birth after caesarean section.

Instrumental Delivery: To Fail to Prepare Is to Prepare to Fail

Approximately 1 in 10 deliveries in the Western world is an instrumental delivery, and morbidity from this operation could be considerable. Obstetricians and midwives should therefore be attuned to patient safety issues in operative vaginal delivery, adequate preparation and pre-application assessment being the key to harm-free care.[25] The path to safety traverses the following:

- The use of non-operative interventions (such as delayed pushing) to reduce the rate of instrumental deliveries
- Making the right decisions as to when instrumental delivery is indicated or contraindicated
- Appropriate management of 'trial of instrumental delivery'
- Ensuring competence and supervision
- Keeping good records of instrumental deliveries
- Maintaining mindfulness and awareness of error-inducing factors

Table 2-1 gives a taxonomy of error in instrumental delivery that could be used to contain risk.

Perineal Trauma: Timely Recognition Is Vital

Interventions such as antenatal perineal massage and perineal guarding or support techniques at delivery could help reduce the incidence of perineal trauma. Often, however, a tear occurs despite the best efforts of the accoucheur. So long as the extent of the tear is correctly recognized and managed, the longer-term outcome is likely to be satisfactory. Problems arise when a third or fourth degree tear has not been recognized or not been managed appropriately. There is clear evidence that structured training of staff improves the outcome of repair,[26] and all units should have processes in place to ensure that staff are competent in repairing perineal tears.

Massive Haemorrhage: Time Is of the Essence

Although a large proportion of cases of massive haemorrhage occur in the absence of risk factors, there is a substantial proportion that are associated with factors such as uterine fibroids, placenta praevia, antepartum haemorrhage, prolonged labour, grandmultiparity and use of oxytocin in labour. The presence of such risk factors should alert the team and pre-emptive measures – such as placement of an intravenous cannula, ready deployment of oxytocic drugs

TABLE 2-1   **Examples of Error in Instrumental Vaginal Delivery. (Reproduced from Edozien, 2007 with permission from Elsevier)**

Type of Error	Description	Possible Consequence	Safe Practice
A: Action			
Operation omitted	Abdominal palpation not done	Level of presenting part misjudged	Use of proforma/ checklist
Operation mistimed	Rotation done during a contraction	Cervical spine injury to the fetus	Rotate only when uterus is relaxed
Operation too long or too short	Prolonged traction	Intracranial injury	Stick to time limits and number of pulls
Operation in wrong	Traction directed forwards and upwards too soon; this causes premature extension of the head, as a result of which a larger diameter of the head emerges at the introitus	Third degree perineal tear	Mind axis of traction
Operation too much	Continuous traction applied	Compression of fetal head	Only apply traction during contraction
B: Information Retrieval			
Information not retrieved	No assessment regarding thromboprophylaxis	Prophylaxis not prescribed	Incorporate this assessment into documentation proforma

TABLE 2-1 Examples of Error in Instrumental Vaginal Delivery. (Reproduced from Edozien, 2007 with permission from Elsevier) (Continued)

Type of Error	Description	Possible Consequence	Safe Practice
	History of diabetes disregarded	Shoulder dystocia not anticipated	Identify background risk factors before offering instrumental delivery
Wrong information retrieved	Mistaken head level or position	Misapplication of instrument; trauma	Double check
	Thinking the cervix is fully dilated when it is not	Cervical tear	
Incomplete information retrieved	Failure to assess moulding	Traumatic delivery; brain injury	Adopt systematic approach to assessment
	Omission of equipment check	Delay in delivery; stress and impairment of cognition	
C: Procedural Checks			
Check omitted or not properly done	Failure to ensure cup does not catch tissue	Vaginal laceration	Training
	Check for proper application of forceps not done	Trauma to baby's face and eye	Understand reason for check
	No check for descent with pull	Undue traction applied	Beware of confirmation bias
	PR not done at end of procedure	Third degree tear missed	Include VE, PR, swab check in documentation
	VE not done at end of procedure. Swabs not counted	Retained swab in vagina	
D: Communication			
Failure to communicate	With woman	Valid consent not obtained	Verbal and eye contact; empathy
	With midwife	Patient given conflicting information	Preoperative briefing
	With senior colleague	Required supervision not provided	
	With anaesthetist	Inadequate analgesia	Team work
	With paediatrician	Neonatal resuscitation delayed	
E: Selection (Choosing from a Number of Options)			
	Wrong ventouse cup type	Avoidable failure of ventouse	
	Ill-advised sequential instrumentation	Neonatal handicap	
F: Cognition			
Failure to anticipate	Failure to anticipate PPH in prolonged labour	Massive haemorrhage	Have Syntocinon infusion ready at delivery
Failure to ask the right questions	No descent despite traction: is position correctly determined? Is pull in the right direction?	Trauma	Situational awareness
	Forceps have less than secure grip of head: is there undiagnosed OP? Is forceps applied over baby's face?	Trauma	Situational awareness

and use of interventional radiology – are taken. When massive haemorrhage occurs, with or without risk factors, the team should be in a position to trigger a 'massive haemorrhage protocol', ensuring a speedy and appropriate response. There is a demonstrable reduction in incidence of postpartum haemorrhage and reduction in associated maternal morbidity in units that have implemented such a protocol and continually rehearsed it.[27]

Shoulder Dystocia: Expect the Unexpected

The possible occurrence of shoulder dystocia may be anticipated when the baby is big, but many cases will occur out of the blue. Labour ward staff must be ready to deal with this emergency at any time. Guidelines for management and documentation are available.[28] Adherence to a shoulder dystocia protocol is enhanced by simulation training (and this does not have to be high-tech simulation).[29] The implementation of a shoulder dystocia protocol and the appropriate training both promote safe practice and improve outcomes.[30,31] Standardized documentation not only helps in cases that are litigated but also in itself promotes safe practice.[32,33]

Obesity: The Little Things Make a Big Difference

Prospective risk assessment will confirm whether or not the unit has the equipment required for safe care of obese (and particularly morbidly obese) women. Approximately one in two morbidly obese women will have a caesarean delivery. There should be a suitable bed and operating table. The table should be capable of providing a left lateral tilt of the obese woman.

Anticipatory care in labour is essential in reducing obesity-related maternal mortality and morbidity.[34] Obese women should have a venous cannula inserted early in labour and the theatre team should be alerted. The abdominal panniculus could make palpation unreliable and it may be difficult to obtain a good quality CTG trace using an abdominal transducer; there should be no hesitation to employ an ultrasound scanner and fetal scalp electrode. Attention should be paid to pressure areas and to hydration. Appropriate thromboprophylaxis should be administered, ensuring the right dose for the woman's body weight.

Training and Supervision: Work in Teams, Train in Teams

Good risk management puts systems in place to ensure the competence and training of all staff. All new staff should have induction and, where appropriate, mentorship and preceptorship arrangements. Robust arrangements should also be in place to ensure that temporary staff have an induction and are competent to perform tasks assigned to them. Training should be multiprofessional and clinical teaching should be combined with teamwork training.[35,36] Adequate arrangements for supervising inexperienced staff should also be in place.

INVOLVE USERS

The involvement of patients, their partners and families, and lay groups should be seen as an index of the quality and safety of care. Often this objective is pursued by having lay representation on labour ward forums, but effective engagement demands more than mere presence at meetings. Service users could be engaged in the *design* or reconfiguration of maternity services to enhance safety and, through patient education, in the protection of their own safety. Clinicians and managers can also involve service users in safety by sharing with them lessons learned from patient safety incidents and keeping them informed of efforts to ensure that harm-free care is provided. Most importantly, there should be open and candid communication with patients and partners when safety incidents happen. The findings of investigations and remedial actions taken should be shared with them.

COLLECT AND ANALYSE PATIENT SAFETY DATA

To ensure that safe care is continually delivered, it is important to collect patient safety data, analyse them and convert the data to information that is intelligible to frontline staff and service users. These data may be collected retrospectively by means of incident reporting. An indicative list of incidents that should be reported is available[37] but this list is indicative rather than exclusive.

Incident reporting is the most common means of collecting safety data on the labour ward, but it must be recognized that valuable data can be obtained by means of a less frequently used modality, prospective risk assessment. Prospective risk assessment is particularly important when new services, devices and working patterns are being introduced. A rise in the number of deliveries as a result of hospital reconfigurations or population movements, for example, will introduce new risks that call for appropriate contingency plans. Quantitative and qualitative data on patient safety can also be derived from 'root cause analyses' of incidents and from analysis of complaints and claims.

Identified risks should be entered into a local risk register. The risk register also contains measures that are in place to control these risks, what further measures are required, the resources for risk control, and time lines for any action points.

Standards of clinical care and of multidisciplinary record keeping should be monitored through periodic criterion-based audits.[38] Each audit should have an action plan and emphasis should be on closing the loop in the audit cycle.[39] Clinical audit should be embedded in an overarching programme of quality and safety improvement, and not for sanctioning individual clinicians.

'*A survey of the health professionals in Malawi showed that they held a favourable opinion about clinical audit. However there are some areas of concerns that should not be overlooked. For instance a third of providers believe that clinical audit will create a feeling of blame among providers who fail to meet standards, and more than a quarter believe that managers will use clinical audit to identify and punish health care providers. Some challenges identified by health care providers that could hinder the implementation of standards include shortage of staff, high workload and inadequate knowledge and skills. Many of the providers surveyed suggested some possible solutions: active involvement of managers in criterion-based audit, and making it crystal clear that information from audit will not be used as a basis of disciplinary sanctions.*'[40]

LEARN FROM EXPERIENCE

A risk management programme is successful only to the extent that it nurtures an environment that facilitates organizational and individual learning from patient safety incidents. A learning organization is one that is able to create new knowledge from patient safety incidents, learn from its experience and that of others, transfer knowledge acquired, and bring about change in its behaviour as a response to the new knowledge.

Safety incidents should be investigated, the level of investigation depending on severity. Major incidents require a Systems Analysis, better known (inappropriately some experts would argue) as 'root cause analysis'. Such investigations should meet defined quality standards and there are protocols for conducting them, such as the London Protocol.[41] Systems Analyses, that potentially could show features within the department that are conducive to the occurrence of harm to patients. These features ('latent pathogens', as they are sometimes called) increase the chance that a clinician at the sharp end will make an error that could result in accidental injury to the patient. They include a lack of explicit protocols, a lack of training, inadequate supervision, communication failures and poor equipment design. The outcome of system analyses should be disseminated within the unit to share lessons and change practice where applicable, without blaming individuals. Lessons learned should inform the design of services and can be used to raise awareness of the causes, consequences and prevention of patient safety incidents.

When things go wrong, it is important to provide support for staff. A learning environment cannot be nurtured unless this support is provided.

CONCLUSION

Patient safety is at the core of medical professionalism. The approach to risk management outlined in this chapter combines individual clinician accountability for safe practice with organizational responsibility for ensuring that appropriate defences are in place to protect patient safety and to learn from safety incidents. This combination is critical to the safe conduct of labour and delivery.

REFERENCES

1. Myerscough PR. Munro Kerr's Operative Obstetrics. 10th ed. London: Baillière Tindall; 1982. p. 3.
2. Edozien LC. The RADICAL framework for implementing and monitoring healthcare risk management. Clinical Governance: An International Journal 2013;18: 165–75.
3. National Health Service Litigation Authority. Ten years of maternity claims: an analysis of NHS Litigation Authority data. London: NHSLA; 2012.
4. Department of Health. Why Mothers Die 1997–1999. Report of the Confidential Enquiries into Maternal Deaths in the United Kingdom. London: RCOG Press; 2001.
5. Maternal and Child Health Research Consortium. Confidential enquiry into stillbirths and deaths in infancy. 8th Annual Report. London: Maternal and Child Health Research Consortium; 2001.

6. Healthcare Commission. Review of maternity services provided by North West London Hospitals NHS Trust. London: Healthcare Commission; 2005.

7. Pettker CM, Thung SF, Norwitz ER, Buhimschi CS, Raab CA, Copel JA, et al. Impact of a comprehensive patient safety strategy on obstetric adverse events. Am J Obstet Gynecol 2009;200:492.e1–8.

8. Grunebaum A, Chervenak F, Skupski D. Effect of a comprehensive obstetric patient safety program on compensation payments and sentinel events. Am J Obstet Gynecol 2011;204:97–105.

9. Fausett MB, Propst A, Van Doren K, Clark BT. How to develop an effective obstetric checklist. Am J Obstet Gynecol 2011;205:165–70.

10. Sen R, Paterson-Brown S. Prioritisation on the delivery suite. Curr Obstet Gynaecol 2005;15:228–36.

11. Royal College of Obstetricians and Gynaecologists. RCOG guidelines. Available at http://www.rcog.org.uk/guidelines (accessed 7 Nov 2012).

12. Society of Obstetricians and Gynaecologists of Canada. Clinical guidelines. Available at http://www.sogc.org/guidelines/index_e.asp (accessed 7 Nov 2012).

13. Royal Australian and New Zealand College of Obstetricians and Gynaecologists. College statements & guidelines. Available at http://www.ranzcog.edu.au/womenshealth/statements-a-guidelines/college-statements-and-guidelines.html (accessed 7 Nov 2012).

14. American Congress of Obstetricians and Gynecologists. http://www.acog.org/.

15. National Institute for Health and Clinical Excellence. Intrapartum care: management and delivery of care to women in labour. Clinical guidelines, CG55 London; September 2007.

16. Royal College of Obstetricians and Gynaecologists, Royal College of Midwives, National Patient Safety Agency. Safer Intrapartum Care Project. Care bundles. London: Royal College of Obstetricians and Gynaecologists; 2010.

17. Available at http://www.nrls.npsa.nhs.uk/resources/?EntryId45=83972.

18. Kearns RJ, Uppal V, Bonner J, Robertson J, Daniel M, McGrady EM. The introduction of a surgical safety checklist in a tertiary referral obstetric centre. BMJ Qual Saf 2011;20:818–22. doi: 10.1136/bmjqs.2010.050179.

19. Edozien LC. Structured multidisciplinary intershift handover (SMITH): a tool for promoting safer intrapartum care. J Obstet Gynaecol 2011;31:683–6.

20. Pehrson C, Sorensen JL, Amer-Wåhlin I. Evaluation and impact of cardiotocography training programmes: a systematic review. BJOG 2011;118:926–35. doi: 10.1111/j.1471-0528.2011.03021.x.

21. Santo S, Ayres-de-Campos D. Human factors affecting the interpretation of fetal heart rate tracings: an update. Curr Opin Obstet Gynecol 2012;24:84–8.

22. MacEachin SR, Lopez CM, Powell KJ, Corbett NL. The fetal heart rate collaborative practice project: situational awareness in electronic fetal monitoring – a Kaiser Permanente Perinatal Patient Safety Program Initiative. J Perinat Neonatal Nurs 2009;23:314–23.

23. Miller LA. System errors in intrapartum electronic fetal monitoring: a case review. J Midwifery Womens Health 2005;50:507–16.

24. Krening CF, Rehling-Anthony K, Garko C. Oxytocin administration: the transition to a safer model of care. J Perinat Neonatal Nurs 2012;26:15–24.

25. Edozien LC. Towards safe practice in instrumental vaginal delivery. Best Pract Res Clin Obstet Gynaecol 2007;21:639–55.

26. Andrews V, Thakar R, Sultan AH. Outcome of obstetric anal sphincter injuries (OASIS) – role of structured management. Int Urogynecol J Pelvic Floor Dysfunct 2009;20:973–8.

27. Rizvi F, Mackey R, Barrett T, McKenna P, Geary M. Successful reduction of massive postpartum haemorrhage by use of guidelines and staff education. BJOG 2004;111:495–8.

28. Royal College of Obstetricians and Gynaecologists. Shoulder dystocia. Green-top guideline No. 42. 2nd ed. London: RCOG; 2012.

29. Grobman WA, Hornbogen A, Burke C, Costello R. Development and implementation of a team-centered shoulder dystocia protocol. Simul Health 2010;5: 199–203.

30. Grobman WA, Miller D, Burke C, Hornbogen A, Tam K, Costello R. Outcomes associated with introduction of a shoulder dystocia protocol. Am J Obstet Gynecol 2011;205:513–7.

31. Draycott TJ, Crofts JF, Ash JP, Wilson LV, Yard E, Sibanda T, et al. Improving neonatal outcome through practical shoulder dystocia training. Obstet Gynecol 2008;112:14–20.

32. Clark SL, Belfort MA, Dildy GA, Meyers JA. Reducing obstetric litigation through alterations in practice patterns. Obstet Gynecol 2008;112:1279–83.

33. Moragianni VA, Hacker MR, Craparo FJ. Improved overall delivery documentation following implementation of a standardized shoulder dystocia delivery form. J Perinat Med 2011;40:97–100. doi: 10.1515/JPM.2011.112.

34. Edozien LC. Multimodal framework for reducing obesity-related maternal morbidity and mortality. In: Mahmood T, Arulkumaran S, editors. Obesity: a ticking time bomb for reproductive health. London: Elsevier; 2013.

35. Siassakos D, Crofts JF, Winter C, Weiner CP, Draycott TJ. The active components of effective training in obstetric emergencies. BJOG 2009;116:1028–32.

36. Merién AE, van de Ven J, Mol BW, Houterman S, Oei SG. Multidisciplinary team training in a simulation setting for acute obstetric emergencies: a systematic review. Obstet Gynecol 2010;115:1021–31.

37. Royal College of Obstetricians and Gynaecologists. Improving patient safety: risk management for maternity and gynaecology. Clinical Governance Advice No. 2. London: RCOG; September 2009.

38. Panigrahy R, Welsh J, MacKenzie F, Owen P, Perinatal Effectiveness Committee in Glasgow (PEC). A complete audit cycle of management of third/fourth degree perineal tears. J Obstet Gynaecol 2008;28:305–9.

39. Dupont C, Deneux-Tharaux C, Touzet S, Colin C, Bouvier-Colle MH, Lansac J, et al, Pithagore group. Clinical audit: a useful tool for reducing severe postpartum haemorrhages? Int J Qual Health Care 2011;23: 583–9.

40. Kongnyuy EJ, van den Broek N. Criteria for clinical audit of women friendly care and providers' perception in Malawi. BMC Pregnancy Childbirth 2008;8:28.

41. Vincent C. Understanding and responding to adverse events. N Engl J Med 2003;348:1051–6.

CHAPTER 3

AUDIT AND STANDARDS OF INTRAPARTUM CARE

MS Robson

> 'You only know what you measure and what you cannot measure must be made measurable'.
> *Gallileo*

INTRODUCTION

From the available literature it is clear that intrapartum care is provided in many different ways and with variable outcomes, for which there will be many reasons. The intention of this chapter is not to suggest one way of providing care but rather persuade professionals that we should standardize the way we examine the quality of care that we provide so we can improve it. We need to encourage midwives and obstetricians to know more about events and outcomes in their own unit. Clinically relevant information is needed on a continuous and timely basis in order to rationalize decision-making. To do this we need to introduce the concept of a Multidisciplinary Quality Assurance Programme (MDQAP)[1] for labour and delivery.

MULTIDISCIPLINARY QUALITY ASSURANCE PROGRAMME

Figure 3-1 describes this concept in the context of labour and delivery. Similar programmes have been suggested elsewhere.[2] Quality Assurance should be applied to the subject as a whole. Audit, classification of information, assessing management and modifying management, when applicable, should be applied to the processes involved in achieving it. All these components are crucial to achieving quality, but accurate and complete information collection is paramount. At the present time, setting standards and benchmarking interventions and outcomes are used as assessment of quality in a healthcare organization. Good information collection itself must be the first quality standard. Information must be easily available, quality controlled and validated.

AUDIT

Audit is defined as the formal examination and recording of the results and is divided into structure (representing resources), process (the way that resources are applied) and outcome (the result of intervention). Recently more emphasis has been placed on auditing processes rather than outcomes, but patients are primarily interested in outcome. Quality is related to outcome and this will guide processes. A more practical definition of audit is continuously looking at your outcomes in a standardized way at the most senior level on a regular basis, resulting in a formal written annual report documenting the quantity and quality of care.[3]

High-quality audit has long been undervalued as a guide for the development and support of clinical practice, as opposed to other forms of evidence-based medicine. The reason is that audit requires time, resources, discipline and leadership. The challenge from a practical point of view is to combine routine documentation of notes with audit and the ability to use them for teaching, education and research without duplication of effort. The information needs to be relevant, carefully defined, accurately collected, timely and available. Information collection needs adequate resources and meticulous organization.

INFORMATION COLLECTION

No judgement or assessment of management, indeed no knowledge of what is actually taking place in a delivery unit is possible unless a reliable system to collect information is in place.

The information collection system must not depend on individuals but must be part of a general organizational approach to the labour ward. A senior midwife and obstetrician should be responsible for organization of information collection.

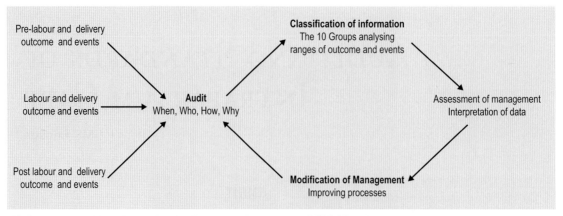

FIGURE 3-1 ■ Multidisciplinary Quality Assurance Programme (MDQAP) – Labour and Delivery. (Reproduced from Robson M, Hartigan L, Murphy M. Methods of achieving and maintaining an appropriate caesarean section rate. Best Pract Research Clin Obstet Gynaecol 2013; 27:297–308 with permission.)

Information collection must be carefully planned and certain principles must be remembered. To ensure quality information the amount of information collected needs to be continually reviewed so that the quantity does not exceed the resources required to collect it. The information must be collected by people who understand the relevance and importance of the information. A team approach is essential and the collection shared between staff.

Information collection still depends upon manual collection in many cases and the partogram is commonly used for that purpose. The partogram can be reproducible so that one copy can be kept on the labour ward for inspection and the other kept in the medical record. Collection of information is usually contemporaneous and is only transferred to an electronic register after delivery.

Computer software programmes have been designed to collect information contemporaneously but the programmes still need to be designed to satisfy the principles of information collection previously described. Otherwise there will be no benefit. The advantages of being able to review cases with partograms, fetal and maternal monitoring simultaneously, as well as all the events and outcomes recorded will be significant if used appropriately. However, a standard way of recording, retrieving and analysing is needed so that a large number of cases can be quickly and easily reviewed. The software programmes need to be '*user tempting*' to ensure that they are embraced by users. There should also be simple ways of checking complete information collection and accuracy. Analysis of the information collected using classification systems will help achieve this.

Finally, apart from collection of physical outcome of mothers and babies there needs to be some method of integrating the mother's satisfaction about the care provided into the software programme.

INFORMATION RETRIEVAL, PRESENTATION AND DISSEMINATION

Most clinicians require standard clinical information to assess the quality of care, resolve clinical problems and identify any changes in outcome as a result of modifications of guidelines or methods of care.

The information therefore needs to be presented in a standard way on a regular basis with flexibility for more detailed investigation. An annual clinical report including detailed information on labour and delivery as well as neonatal outcome is essential. International standardization will enable learning from each other but only when a common language has been developed.

LABOUR EVENTS AND OUTCOME

In collecting information about labour and delivery there are two main types of information and Table 3-1 summarizes some basic information that is useful to collect: firstly, epidemiological data such as age, height, body mass index, medical conditions, ethnicity and other case-mix variables; secondly, there is what is commonly known as *interventions*, which refer to events (or outcomes) carried out by professionals involved in the mothers' care. Although these are performed with the intention of improving care, many interpret them as interference with a normal physiological process. The difficulty with a generic term like *interventions* is that there

---

TABLE 3-1   Maternal and Fetal Information

Maternal	Fetal
Age of women	Birth weight
Ethnicity	Gestation
Booking weight and height (BMI)	Apgar score (<7 at 5 min)
Total number of women (to construct the 10 groups)	Cord pH (pH<7.0)
Spontaneous labour	Erb's palsy
Inductions (fetal, maternal, no medical reasons)	Encephalopathy
Prelabour CS indications (fetal, maternal, no medical reason)	Admissons to ICU
Number of CS (to analyse distribution of CS)	Admissons to ICU >24 h
Number of CS in 1st stage of labour (fetal, dystocia)	Days at facility for the newborn
Number of CS in 2nd stage of labour (fetal, dystocia)	Stillbirths (<37 and ≥37weeks)
Artificial rupture of membranes	Intrapartum deaths
Oxytocin (1st stage)	Neonatal deaths (≤7 and ≤28 days)
Oxytocin (2nd stage)	Cerebral palsy
Epidural	
Vaginal operative delivery (ventouse or forceps)	
Duration of labour	
Episiotomy	
3rd or 4th degree tears	
Postpartum haemorrhage	
Blood transfusion	
Peripartum infectious morbidity	
Peripartum hysterectomy	
Days at facility for the mother	
Maternal deaths	

CS, caesarean section.

is no distinction in how the mother, midwife or medical staff perceive the particular event or outcome in question. Even more confusing is the fact that what may be an intervention to one woman may not be an intervention to another; indeed it may be a desired event or outcome. In order to clarify matters the term intervention should be avoided. Instead, all events that take place should be recorded whether they are processes carried out by professionals or occur as a result of the care provided. Some labour events are also labour outcomes, in that the mother, midwife or medical staff consider them to affect the health or satisfaction of either the mother or baby. All events and outcomes need to be defined in a standard way.[3]

Caesarean section is a case in point; an event that may take place in the process of labour and delivery. It may also be an outcome either negative or positive or indeed neither, depending on the circumstances of the delivery. Induction of labour, artificial rupture of membranes, use of oxytocin and length of labour are other examples of events that may also be outcomes or may affect the incidence of other outcomes.

The third type of information that is collected in labour and delivery is information used to classify the epidemiological data and the events and outcomes.

INDICATIONS

While recording numbers of events and outcomes should be straightforward, recording why we carry out certain procedures has been less successful. This needs to be clarified if we are to improve care. The most common examples in labour and delivery are induction of labour and caesarean section; their indications have been difficult to define and implement consistently. A further problem is the increase in numbers of indications used. This presents a problem for classification and obtaining an overview of care; in particular why the procedures are being carried out and whether they can be justified in terms of other outcomes.

If an appropriate caesarean section rate is to be described, then indications for caesarean section have to be standardized. Pre-labour caesarean sections should ideally be classified into fetal, maternal or no medical indication. If more than one indication exists then one main indication should be chosen, with the other indications added in a hierarchical manner.

A definition for no medical indication or maternal request is required.[4] Practically it might be best defined as 'at the time of the request by the woman, in the opinion of the obstetrician there is a greater relative risk of a significant adverse outcome to mother or baby by carrying out a caesarean section than awaiting spontaneous labour and delivery or inducing labour'.

A medical indication for a caesarean section must be one that is used consistently in similar circumstances. Otherwise the indication should be recorded as maternal request. This does not mean to say it is inappropriate care to carry out a caesarean section after counselling the woman,[5] but only that it should be classified as maternal request and also include the reason for that request. Variances in the application of indications can be studied by analysing them in different groups of women. Importantly though, it is not inconceivable that an indication for caesarean section recorded as maternal request today may well, with change in practice and outcomes from labour and delivery, become a medical indication in the future and also vice-versa.

The terms elective and emergency caesarean section are difficult to define and are rarely applied in a standard way. An elective caesarean section might best be defined as a planned procedure (greater than 24 hours), carried out during routine working hours, at greater than 39 weeks, in a woman who is neither in labour nor has had labour induced. All other caesarean sections would be audited as emergency or possibly more appropriately as non-elective caesarean sections. The reasons why they were recorded as non-elective could be recorded using the rationale described above. This adds an organizational element as well as clinical to the definition of elective and emergency and would be helpful in assessing an appropriate caesarean section rate.

Indications for caesarean sections in labour need to be simple, replicable and allow for improvement of care. Management of labour depends on ensuring fetal wellbeing and achieving efficient uterine action and they are also the reasons why caesarean sections are carried out in labour. It is therefore logical that indications for caesarean sections in labour might be classified into fetal or dystocia so that management can be assessed. A fetal indication would be defined by convention when a caesarean section is carried out for suspected fetal distress (for whatever reason), but without the use of oxytocin. All other caesarean sections performed in labour are classified as a form of dystocia. No formal definition of dystocia is suggested as each delivery unit will have their own interpretation but this will not preclude them from using the following classification. Rather, the subclassification of dystocia will depend upon whether the progress in labour had been less than 1 cm/hour (inefficient uterine action) or more than 1 cm/hour (efficient uterine action). Inefficient uterine action is then subdivided into poor response (despite maximum treatment with oxytocin), inability to treat adequately (for fetal reasons), inability to treat adequately (because of the uterus overcontracting) or lastly no treatment (oxytocin not given because thought to be inappropriate: for example in labour with a malpresentation, in a woman with a previous caesarean section, when a woman declines oxytocin or indeed declines labour itself).

This classification, shown in Table 3-2, differentiates between suspected fetal distress without oxytocin as opposed to suspected fetal

TABLE 3-2	**Classification for Caesarean Sections in Labour**	
Fetal Distress (No Oxytocin)		
Dystocia	IUA (inefficient uterine action <1 cm/hr)	Poor response. Maximum dose[1] reached
		Inability to reach maximum dose[1] because of fetal intolerance
		Inability to reach maximum dose[1] because of over-contractions or not following unit protocol
		No oxytocin given
	EUA (efficient uterine action >1 cm/hr)	Cephalopelvic disproportion
		Malposition (occipito posterior or occipito transverse)

[1]Maximum dose refers to individual unit's protocol.

TABLE 3-3	Indications for Induction of Labour

Fetal reasons
Preclampsia/hypertension
Post dates (≥42 weeks)
Pre-Labour Spontaneous Rupture of Membranes
Maternal reasons/pains
Non-medical reasons or dates <42 weeks

distress after oxytocin was started, but when the primary problem was dystocia.

The distribution of the results with oxytocin use reflects the way that dystocia is diagnosed and how oxytocin is used in labour in the delivery unit.[6] In particular the incidence, timing, dose and regimen of oxytocin. Applying this classification to different groups of women[6] gives different results that can be used to analyse caesarean section rates and their implications more rationally.

Indications for induction of labour are also difficult to define. A possible solution, initially at least, is shown in Table 3-3 which has proven useful in order to get an overview.[6] More detail about each induction can be included in a hierarchical manner within these six groups.

CLASSIFICATION OF INFORMATION

For the MDQAP to be successful there is clearly a need for quality information, but as important is the need to classify, structure and organize information so that it can be easily used by clinicians on a daily basis to assess and improve care.

Classification systems are used in medicine to transform crude data and information into useful information so that clinical care can be improved. They are based on the identification of different concepts that may each have several parameters. The purpose of a classification system usually determines its structure, but the ideal classification will satisfy different purposes. The main groups of the classification must be robust enough to be unlikely to need changes. The groups or categories of the classification need to be prospectively identifiable so that outcomes can be improved in those same patients in the future. The groups or categories must be mutually exclusive, totally inclusive and clinically relevant. The classification system must be simple to understand and easy to implement.

10-GROUP CLASSIFICATION

The philosophy of the 10-group classification system in assessing maternity care is based on the premise that all epidemiological information, as well as maternal and fetal events and outcomes will be more clinically relevant if initially analyzed within the 10 groups.

The 10-group classification system (TGCS) shown in Table 3-4 with the number of caesarean sections in each group, complies with the principles of a classification system described above.[7] If implemented on a continuous basis, it would allow the critical assessment of perinatal care leading to change if thought necessary. The obstetric concepts, with their parameters, used to classify the women in the TGCS are the category of the pregnancy, the previous obstetric record of the woman, the course of labour and delivery and the gestational age of the pregnancy. The concepts and their parameters are all prospective, mutually exclusive, totally inclusive, simple and easy to understand and organize.[7]

Importantly, they are clinically relevant to midwives and obstetricians because the information they depend on is required whenever an assessment is made of a pregnant woman who is either in labour or about to deliver. It therefore makes sense that all maternal and fetal information is viewed within these concepts and parameters or combinations of them and thus the 10-group classification was formed. The groups were chosen on the basis that they provide the best clinical and organizational overview relative to the number of groups. They allow a comparison between delivery units, permitting more specific analysis of the labour events and outcomes including their indications and epidemiological variables. Each of the 10 groups can and should be further subdivided when required. Groups 1 and 2 should be analysed separately and also together, as should Groups 3 and 4.

The philosophy of the 10-group classification in assessing maternity care is based on the premise that all epidemiological information as well as maternal and fetal events and outcomes will be more clinically relevant if initially analysed within the 10 groups, their obstetric concepts or parameters. This is particularly important in assessing caesarean section rates, but also other outcomes.[8] The system can also be used to classify any group of women defined by other fetal and maternal information. For example, all women over the age of 35 or different ethnic groups can be classified into the 10 groups and analysed and compared with a standard population.

TABLE 3-4   **10-group Classification System**

Groups	Overall Caesarean Section (CS) Rate (%) 1977/9250 (21.4%) National Maternity Hospital 2011			
	NUMBER OF CS OVER TOTAL NUMBER OF WOMEN IN EACH GROUP	RELATIVE SIZE OF GROUPS (%)	CS RATE IN EACH GROUP (%)	CONTRIBUTION MADE BY EACH GROUP TO THE OVERALL CS RATE (%)
1. Nulliparous, single cephalic, ≥37 weeks, in spontaneous labour	179/2389	25.8 2389/9250	7.5 179/2389	1.9 179/9250
2. Nulliparous, single cephalic, ≥37 weeks, induced or CS before labour*	475/1368	14.8 1368/9250	34.7 475/1368	5.1 475/9250
3. Multiparous (excluding prev. CS), single cephalic, ≥37 weeks, in spontaneous labour	30/2751	29.7 2751/9250	1.1 30/2751	0.3 30/9250
4. Multiparous (excluding prev. CS), single cephalic, ≥37 weeks, induced or CS before* labour	109/871	9.4 871/9250	12.5 109/871	1.2 109/9250
5. Previous CS, single cephalic, ≥37 weeks	571/936	10.1 936/9250	61.0 571/936	6.2 571/9250
6. All nulliparous breeches	204/219	2.4 219/9250	93.2 204/219	2.2 204/9250
7. All multiparous breeches (including prev. CS)	113/133	1.4 133/9250	85.0 113/133	1.2 113/9250
8. All multiple pregnancies (including prev. CS)	134/212	2.3 212/9250	63.2 134/212	1.5 134/9250
9. All abnormal lies (including prev. CS)	35/35	0.4 35/9250	100 35/35	0.4 35/9250
10. All single cephalic, ≤36 weeks (including prev. CS)	127/336	3.6 336/9250	37.8 127/336	1.4 127/9250

*Groups 2 and 4 are commonly divided into a (inductions) and b (prelabour caesarean sections).

CLASSIFICATION OF CAESAREAN SECTION AND INDUCTION OF LABOUR

At the present time there is no accepted classification system for caesarean sections. The biggest single step to try and achieve and maintain appropriate caesarean section rates would be to agree a classification for caesarean sections and to use that classification in reporting for all deliveries. The 10-group classification system has been recommended as appropriate for this purpose.[9]

The indications for caesarean section should be analysed within each group of women because the definition and the management will vary in each group and will have different risk–benefit ratios. The 10-group classification can be used to assess any caesarean section rate in absolute terms, but also to compare with other lower or higher caesarean section rates either within the same delivery unit from previous years, or with other delivery units elsewhere. It would be possible to see how the sizes of the different groups vary and also in which groups of women there is a difference in caesarean section rates. It will not immediately explain the reasons, and further analysis would be required, but it will allow a useful overview from which to start. From this it will be possible to identify different groups of women and change the management according to available evidence.[10]

In general, groups 1, 2 and 5 contribute two-thirds of the overall caesarean section rate, with group 5 being the largest individual contributor.[11–13] Group 5 contains women with at least one previous caesarean section and a single cephalic pregnancy at term and needs to be subdivided into prelabour caesarean section, spontaneous and induced labour.

Induction of labour and the contribution it makes to caesarean section rates remains a controversial issue. The 10-group classification allows a unique analysis of that contribution. The two groups of women that are relevant in the study of induction are single cephalic nulliparous women (Group 2a) and single cephalic multiparous (without a previous scar) women (Group 4a) (see Table 3-4). The denominator that is used to study the incidence and indications for the inductions is the total number of women in Groups 1 and 2, and Groups 3 and 4 respectively.

ASSESSMENT OF MANAGEMENT – INTERPRETATION OF INFORMATION

Standardized Classification of Continuous Audit of Labour and Delivery Is Required to Assess Care

What is needed now is more detailed standard analysis on specific groups of women by maternity units who manage labour and delivery in different ways but use the 10-group classification as a standard basis for analysis. Information collection should be complete and interpretation can only be carried out if all the information is available. The use of amniotomy, oxytocin, indications and methods of induction of labour, and management of women with previous caesarean section should all be examined within the 10-group classification, but at the same time looking at other relevant fetal and maternal outcomes. Further detailed analysis of different groups may be required.

Modification of Management

Modification of management is the most challenging part of any quality assurance programme. With quality information most women and professionals will arrive at the same conclusion. Regular meetings are required with one person taking responsibility for leadership. There must be multidisciplinary agreement to ignore previous biases and use both audit and current literature to stimulate a common approach. Guidelines need to be carefully thought out and remain flexible. Modification of management can only take place if there is a mechanism in place for changing management. Good communication is necessary so that everyone is aware of the changes, especially those most closely involved. Modification is only safe if there is a continual audit present in the labour ward to spot quickly problems that may occur as a result of change. All modifications must be assessed after a stipulated time period.

The 10-group classification allows more focussed analysis of management and allows specific changes in processes, if necessary, in certain groups of women.[10] Its success depends on the integrity of the MDQAP and in particular continuous audit and classification of information.

REFERENCES

1. Robson M, Hartigan L, Murphy M. Methods of achieving and maintaining an appropriate caesarean section rate. Best Pract Res Clin Obstet Gynaecol 2013;27: 297–308.
2. Main EK, Morton CH, Hopkins D, Giuliani G, Melsop K and Gould J. Cesarean deliveries, outcomes, and opportunities for change in California: toward a public agenda for maternity care safety and quality. Palo Alto, CA: CMQCC; 2011. Available at http://www.cmqcc.org (accessed 12 Sept 2012).
3. Robson M. In: Creasy R, editor. Labour ward audit. Management of labor and delivery. US: Blackwell Science; 1997. p.559–70, 1–12.
4. Visco AG, Viswanathan M, Lohr KN, Wechter M, Gartlehner G, Wu JM, et al. Cesarean delivery on maternal request: maternal and neonatal outcomes. Obstet Gynecol 2006;108:1517–29.
5. National Institute of Health and Clinical Excellence. Caesarean section. NICE Guideline 2011:1–282.
6. Robson M. National Maternity Hospital Clinical Report 2010:105–29.
7. Robson M. Classification of caesarean sections. Fetal Matern Med Rev 2001;12:23–39.
8. Homer CSE, Kurinczuk JJ, Spark P. A novel use of a classification system to audit severe maternal morbidity. Midwifery 2010;26:532–6.
9. Torloni MR, Betran AP, Souza JP, Widmer M, Allen T, Gulmezoglu M, et al. Classifications of cesarean section: a systematic review. PLoS One 2011;6(1):e14566.
10. Robson MS, Scudamore IW, Walsh SM. Using the medical audit cycle to reduce cesarean section rates. Am J Obstet Gynecol 1996;174:199–205.
11. Brennan DJ, Robson MS, Murphy M, O'Herlihy C, et al. Comparative analysis of international cesarean delivery rates using 10-group classification identifies significant variation in spontaneous labor. Am J Obstet Gynecol 2009;201:308.e1–8.
12. Brennan DJ, Murphy M, Robson MS, O'Herlihy C, et al. The singleton, cephalic, nulliparous woman after 36 weeks of gestation: contribution to overall cesarean delivery rates. Obstet Gynecol 2011;117:273–9.
13. Stivanello E, Rucci P, Carretta E, Pieri G, Seghieri C, Nuti S, et al. Risk adjustment for inter-hospital comparison of caesarean delivery rates in low-risk deliveries. PLoS One 2011;6:e28060.

CHAPTER 4

COMPETENCE AND SKILLS TRAINING

TJ Draycott

> 'I look forward to the great advances in knowledge that lie around the corner, but I do sometimes wonder whether the vast sums of money now being spent on research might not produce more rapid and spectacular improvement in health if devoted to the application of what is already known'.
> Max Rosenheim
> President, Royal College of Physicians, 1968

Improving maternal and perinatal care, and reducing preventable intrapartum harm in particular, is a global priority. Improved training for intrapartum care is at least part of the solution, but this must be both effective and sustainable.

As early as 1760 a French midwife, Madame du Coudray, recognized that training deficiencies for accoucheurs could directly cause harm[1] and moreover that training on an 'obstetric machine' (mannequin) could reduce these preventable harms:

> 'But when difficulties arise they are absolutely unskilled, and until long experience instructs them they are the witness or the cause of many misfortunes, of which the least terrible is the death of the mother or the child and even both. These subjects could have been useful to the state, and mothers would not have to lose their fertility in the flower of youth; one learns on the machine in little time how to prevent such accidents'.

Over 250 years after Madame du Coudray was commissioned to start a national training programme across France, at first glance we appear to have made little progress; a systematic review of obstetric emergencies training published in 2003 concluded that few methods of obstetric skills training had been evaluated, and there was minimal evidence of their effectiveness.[2]

However, since 2003, a nascent evidence base for intrapartum skills training has emerged and I will present a review of the current evidence for effective and sustainable intrapartum skills training to improve care and perinatal outcomes.

PREVENTABLE HARM

Women,[3] their families and insurers[4] value safety in labour highest. However, in 2008 the UK-based Kings Fund report 'Safe Births: everybody's business'[5] observed that while the overwhelming majority of births in England are safe, some births are less safe than they could and should be. This observation accurately summarizes almost the last century of obstetric care in the UK.

In 1917 the UK Medical Research Committee reported that '52% of infant deaths were avoidable' and in 1924 the author of a national UK Maternal Mortality Report described maternal deaths as a 'burden of avoidable suffering'.

Although perinatal outcomes have improved over the last century, the proportion of 'avoidable suffering' has remained depressingly static since these early reports: >50% of intrapartum stillbirths were deemed avoidable with better care in the 4th CESDI (Confidential Enquiry into Stillbirths and Deaths in Infancy) report, published in 1997[6] and the most recent CMACE (Centre for Maternal and Child Enquiries) report 'Saving Mothers' Lives', published in 2011, still identified substandard care in 70% of Direct deaths and 55% of Indirect deaths.[7]

The investigation of the root cause of these maternal and perinatal deaths reveals a consistent set of themes related to substandard care, including failure to recognize problems; failure to seek senior input;[4,8] poor or non-existent team working;[8] and the requirement to improve skills, with emphasis on teams and not individuals.[9]

Improving maternal and perinatal care is also a global priority; the World Health Organization (WHO) has estimated that 1500 women die every day from preventable complications of pregnancy and childbirth.[10] Worldwide, there are approximately four million neonatal deaths each year, with a similar number of stillbirths[11] and these have become the focus for two of the Millennium Development Goals.

Finally, this preventable harm is extraordinarily expensive. Substandard care and its sequelae cost the NHS £3.1 billion in the decade 2000–2010;[4] individual, family and societal costs notwithstanding.

SKILLS TRAINING

Improved multiprofessional training appears to be one of the most promising strategies to improve perinatal outcomes across the world, localized for best fit, with a parallel evaluation of outcomes to ensure a positive effect.

Training has been recommended almost annually since the 1990s; as early as 1996, the 5th Confidential Enquiry into Stillbirths and Deaths in Infancy recommended a 'high level of awareness and training for all birth attendants'.[8] Annual 'Skill Drills' have been recommended by both the Royal College of Midwives (RCM)[12] and the Royal College of Obstetricians and Gynaecologists (RCOG),[13] as well as national bodies on both sides of the Atlantic; the Joint Commission on Accreditation of Healthcare Organizations (JCAHO) in the USA[9] and the maternity Clinical Negligence Scheme for Trusts (CNST) whose Risk Management standards have mandated training in the UK since 2000.[14] Moreover, teamwork training has also been recommended.[8,9]

Training is not magic, nor is it automatically effective; therefore we must ensure that training improves outcomes. There are now numerous studies evaluating the effectiveness of skills training for obstetric emergencies, with increasing evidence that practical training is associated with improvements in clinical outcomes.[15–18] However, not all training has been associated with such positive effects and there are a number of studies where training either did not improve clinical outcome[19,20] or was associated with an increase in perinatal morbidity.[21] Where training has been demonstrated to be effective it should be widely implemented and can be included in national guidance.[22]

Intrapartum care demands sensitivity, clinical skill and acumen from a multiprofessional team of carers. Training should address all of these elements, and this is likely to require a broad range of training techniques and tools. The Kings Fund recognized that: "maternity units could easily provide their own simulation-based training … Any such training should include clinical skills, communication, team working, and awareness of roles within the team".[5]

I will review some different elements of intrapartum training, particularly training for electronic fetal heart rate monitoring (EFM), the use of simulation for technical skills training and also some new evidence for teamwork training.

ELECTRONIC FETAL HEART RATE MONITORING

'Make the right way the easiest way'.

All practitioners involved in intrapartum care should ensure that they have the knowledge and skills to interpret the cardiotocograph (CTG) and act appropriately, with the aim of providing high-quality, defensible care. However, this does not appear to be the case for some carers at least.

The evidence linking brain injury to intrapartum care is inconsistent but it is a major source of litigation.[4] The recent NHS Litigation Authority (NHSLA) report concluded that the most effective way to reduce the financial and human cost of maternity claims is to continue to improve the management of risks associated with maternity care, focusing on preventing incidents involving the management of women in labour, including the interpretation of CTG traces.

A Swedish study reviewed the outcomes of infants (>33 weeks) born in Stockholm County between 2004 and 2006 and found that there was substandard care during labour in two-thirds of infants with a 5-minute Apgar score of <7. The main reasons for the substandard care were related to misinterpretation of the CTG and not acting on a pathological CTG in a timely fashion.[23] These findings were almost exactly replicated in Norway over a similar time period.[24]

A recent systematic review concluded that training can improve CTG competence and clinical practice, but further research is needed to evaluate the type and content of training that is most effective.[25]

One of the problems with CTG interpretation is that it is difficult and requires a holistic assessment of the woman, her labour and appropriate action as well as the fetal heart rate pattern itself. Improving outcomes in labour when EFM is used is dependent on more than just CTG interpretation alone. The National Institute of Clinical Excellence (NICE) in the UK have produced two guidelines that helpfully standardize the interpretation of intrapartum CTGs; however, they are each >100 pages long,[26,27] which makes them difficult to implement at the coalface of care.

Intrapartum CTG Proforma	Reassuring (Acceptable)		Non-Reassuring	Abnormal	North Bristol NHS Trust
Baseline rate (bpm)	110 - 160 Rate:		100 - 109 Rate: 161 - 180 Rate:	Less than 100 Rate: More than 180 Rate: Sinusoidal pattern for 10 minutes or more	Comments:
N.B. Rising baseline rate even within normal range may be of concern if other non-reassuring/abnormal features present.					
Variability (bpm)	5 bpm or more		Less than 5 bpm for 40 - 90 minutes	Less than 5 bpm for 90 minutes	Comments:
Accelerations	Present		None for 40 minutes	Comments:	
Decelerations	None		Typical variable decelerations with more than **50%** of contractions for more than **90** minutes	Atypical variable decelerations with more than **50%** of contractions for more than **30** minutes	Comments:
	Typical variable decelerations with more than **50%** of contractions but for less than **90** minutes		Atypical variable decelerations with more than **50%** of contractions for less than **30** minutes	Late decelerations for more than **30** minutes	
	Typical or atypical variable decelerations with less than **50%** of contractions		Late decelerations for less than **30** minutes		
	True early decelerations		Single prolonged deceleration up to than **3** minutes	Single prolonged deceleration for more than **3** minutes	
N.B. If CTG has any non-reassuring or abnormal features from commencement of monitoring, it may not be appropriate to wait 30 or 90 minutes before requesting review					
Opinion	*Normal CTG* (All 4 features reassuring)		*Suspicious CTG* (1 non-reassuring feature)	*Pathological CTG* (2 or more non-reassuring or 1 or more abnormal features)	
Cont's: :10	Maternal pulse:		Liquor color:	Dilatation (cm):	Gestation (wks):
Action:					RVJ0191 (1GD)
Date:	Time:	Signature: .... Print: .... Designation:			

FIGURE 4-1 ■ CTG sticker consistent with NICE 2007 Intrapartum Guideline.

CTG stickers that summarize the guidelines into a simple stick-on format (Fig 4-1) have been successfully introduced into practice with an associated 50% reduction in 5-minute Apgar scores of <7 minutes and hypoxic ischaemic encephalopathy in a UK unit.[17] However, the sticker itself does not magically improve outcomes; all staff in the unit should be trained annually to use the sticker, its use should be mandated for all staff whenever a CTG is reviewed and other contrary tools and systems should be stopped. Finally, the use of stickers should be 'policed' using notes audits and the effect on outcomes such as low Apgar scores.

Stickers have been recommended in Sweden[23] and, where they have been introduced as part of a multiprofessional training programme there have been significant improvements in infants born in poor condition in both the USA[28] and Australia.[29]

Multiprofessional training for CTG interpretation, using standardized tools can be effective and both the tools and the training should be implemented more widely.

SIMULATION AND OBSTETRIC SKILLS TRAINING

Obstetric emergencies are rare and it is axiomatic that they should be managed by experienced staff; indeed, this is almost ubiquitously recommended. However, experience is difficult to acquire because of their rarity, but may be gained in part through simulation.

Simulation permits individual health professionals and teams to inculcate skills and cultures in preparation for safe, effective clinical care, whilst gaining confidence and becoming more efficient. Simulation is an educational device, not a place or a technology: it can be as simple as trousers with red material to reproduce some of the visual clues for postpartum haemorrhage (PPH) or as complex as a high-technology simulation centre.

We should not overestimate the effect of simulation; a recent review of simulation-based medical education (SMBE) recognized that some but not all SMBE was associated with improvements in clinical outcome.[30] There is an important need to test whether obstetric simulation training programmes are effective, sustainable and cost-effective.

ECLAMPSIA

One of the first published descriptions of obstetric simulation was an eclampsia drill.[31] Simulating eclampsia enabled departmental staff to develop and 'road test' an eclampsia box containing the equipment, drugs and guidelines required to manage the clinical condition.

Subsequently a randomized-controlled trial comparing effectiveness of different methods and sites for multiprofessional training for eclampsia across a whole region demonstrated marked improvement in care after training.[32] Following training, there were significant improvements in completion of basic tasks (87% pre vs. 100% post) and the administration of magnesium sulphate (61% pre vs. 92% post) in simulated eclampsia. Time taken to commence administration of magnesium sulphate was on average nearly 2 minutes quicker following training.[32]

Simulation training for eclampsia is gaining in importance as the rate of eclampsia is falling in the UK, whereas substandard care appears to be increasing, particularly for pre-eclampsia and eclampsia, where >90% of deaths were associated with substandard care[7] in the last triennial enquiry. The introduction of simple tools like the eclampsia box described above and regular rehearsal using local drills appears to be the most effective and sustainable method of training for eclampsia.

SHOULDER DYSTOCIA

Shoulder dystocia, including training, is covered in Chapter 12.

VAGINAL BREECH DELIVERY

Planned vaginal breech birth has become increasingly uncommon since the publication of the Term Breech Trial,[33] but competence in assisted vaginal breech delivery remains an important skill for accoucheurs to care for women who choose vaginal breech birth, and also for those women who present very late in labour (see Chapter 16).

As with shoulder dystocia, practical simulation using high-fidelity models provides an opportunity for staff to practise management. There is a report of significant improvement in residents' ability to perform simulated breech deliveries following training on a birth simulator including a patient-actor.[34]

INSTRUMENTAL DELIVERY

There is good evidence that when delivery needs to be expedited, a single instrument application is the safest method of delivery, followed by caesarean section and then two instrument applications (ventouse and forceps), with failed instrumental delivery and caesarean as the most dangerous.[35]

Therefore, appropriate and safe use of forceps and vacuum remains an essential obstetric skill,[36] but UK obstetric trainees have identified that training for operative birth, particularly rotational deliveries, can be difficult to acquire.[37] Simulation and virtual reality models may offer more training opportunities.

Dupius and colleagues developed a high-fidelity model that allows the trajectory of the application of forceps blades to be tracked using spatial sensors.[38] Senior obstetricians demonstrated a superior technique, but after training the abilities of junior staff improved.[38] Other models have been developed to simulate appropriate traction. After practical training both the correct forces and successful delivery were achieved more often in simulated instrumental births.[39,40]

MATERNAL COLLAPSE

Maternal cardiac arrest is rare, complicating approximately 1 in 30000 pregnancies in the UK[41] and it is therefore imperative that all healthcare professionals can provide basic resuscitation. In the 2007 CEMACH Report[41] resuscitation skills were considered poor in an unacceptably high number of maternal deaths. This and the most recent report[7] both recommend that all clinical staff should undertake regular training to improve basic, intermediate and advanced life support skills.

Perimortem caesarean section is an essential part of Advanced Cardiac Life Support for cardiac arrest/collapse in pregnancy. Simulation provides an opportunity to practise skills for this very rare problem and improved care after cardiac arrest has been described after simulation training in a general hospital setting.[42] A small US study also found improved outcome in an obstetric setting.[43]

However, results of training in an obstetric setting across a whole health system have been disappointing: a recent retrospective cohort study investigated the use of perimortem caesarean section in the Netherlands between 1993 and 2008 following the introduction of obstetric training in 2004. The rate of perimortem caesarean increased from 12% to 35% after the introduction of training.[44] However, maternal outcomes remained poor, most likely due to delay in performing the caesarean as none were carried out within 5 minutes of the cardiac arrest.[44]

NEONATAL RESUSCITATION

A systematic review concluded that perinatal mortality might be reduced if birth attendants receive practical neonatal resuscitation training, but the evidence of effect is weak.[45] More recent studies have evaluated the effect of the World Health Organization Essential Newborn Care course, a neonatal rather than obstetric training course. One study using a before-and-after implementation design was associated with improvements in midwives' skills and knowledge.[46] There was also a reduction in early neonatal deaths among low-risk women who delivered in first-level clinics in Zambia.[47] A cluster randomized-controlled trial to assess this neonatal resuscitation intervention could not replicate the original results.[48]

Following the introduction of the 3-day Essential Newborn Care course in six countries there was neither a significant reduction in the rate of early neonatal deaths, nor in the rate of perinatal death. Interestingly, there was an unexpected reduction in the rate of stillbirth. It is plausible that the observed reduction in stillbirths might have been the result of training because before training infants born without obvious signs of life may have been misclassified as stillbirths. After training, resuscitation was more likely to be attempted, with a possible reduction in those births previously misclassified as stillbirths.

Promising preliminary observations of the effect of the Helping Babies Breathe programme have recently been published.[49] This is an educational training programme for low-resource countries that aims to improve neonatal resuscitation using basic simulation scenarios.

TRAINING IN LOW-RESOURCE SETTINGS

A recent WHO review of intrapartum training in low- and middle-income countries concluded:

'Where in-service training can be provided at a low cost, it may be worthwhile to do so, given that some improvements in care process can be expected. However, in general, such training may be associated with high cost and therefore for most settings it is difficult to justify the conduct of routine in-service neonatal and paediatric training courses primarily based on models developed in high-income countries'.[50]

The authors propose that the success of in-service training of healthcare professionals depends on a number of factors, but two are especially important: appropriately skilled instructors in sufficient numbers; with suitable, locally adapted training materials. Many courses have been developed that include simulations of obstetric emergencies to train staff in low-resource settings.

Challenges, in addition to those outlined above, include the wide variation in local settings, practices and staffing, as well as under-resourced health services that are often overwhelmed. Care must be taken to avoid inappropriate 'square peg in a round hole' introduction of non-localized courses from high-income settings.

For example, staff identified poor training as a contributor to substandard care and poor outcomes during a confidential enquiry into maternal deaths at a regional hospital in Tanzania[51] but the introduction of ALSO (Advanced Life Support in Obstetrics) training from the USA did not improve outcomes.[52]

More work is required to understand the specific requirements for, and local adaptation of, training in developing world settings.

TEAMWORKING AND TEAMWORK TRAINING

Conventional healthcare training has typically focused on specific, technically skilled tasks in professional silos, whereas intrapartum care is team based and multiprofessional. Therefore, it is self evident that training should be similarly so and this has been recognized by a number of national bodies.[9,41]

Teamwork training recognizes that people make fewer errors when they work in effective teams. Each member of the team can understand their responsibilities when processes are planned and standardized and team members can 'look out' for one another, trapping errors before they cause an accident.[53]

The aviation model of training is often proposed, but the comparison is even more often overstated: flying a plane is not like caring for a woman in labour, and there is at least one very appealing suggestion that medical care is more like handling baggage at an airport than taking off and landing the plane. Baggage comes in different sizes and shapes, involves complex transfers, and is often in poor condition. Baggage handling is a task that shares with managing patients a staggering amount of co-ordination, time-pressured decision-making, frustrating delays, and tracking systems for non-standardized raw material that needs to be handled safely.[54]

At least in an intensive care setting it has been recognized that teamwork interventions must be tailored to the highly specific demands of the medical setting[55] and this definitely applies to an intrapartum setting.

EFFECTIVE TEAMWORK TRAINING FOR INTRAPARTUM CARE

There is evidence to support training for obstetric emergencies in multiprofessional teams; most notably improved obstetric and perinatal outcomes after the introduction of multiprofessional clinical groups with integrated team training.[56] However, isolated teamwork training does not appear to be effective in intrapartum care.[19,57]

Those training programmes associated with improvements in perinatal outcome were all conducted 'in-house', training 100% of staff, reported the introduction of system changes, often suggested by their staff after participating in the training and trained all staff together incorporating teamwork principles into clinical training scenarios.[56,57]

In-house training appears to be the most efficient and cost-effective means of training all staff in an institution. It can also address specific local issues and can be used as a driver for system changes.[56,58,59] Moreover, training within the local environment may be the most effective way of improving outcomes.[60]

Some clinical teams possess characteristics that make them more efficient than others, and so are better able to achieve good outcomes by performing key actions in a timely manner. However, these characteristics are not explained by differences in knowledge or skill;[61] training needs to emphasize teamworking.

Finally, in one obstetric study, more efficient teams that administered magnesium sulphate within the allocated time (10 minutes) were likely to have:[62]

- Stated (recognized and verbally declared) the emergency earlier
- Managed the critical task using closed-loop communication (task clearly and loudly delegated, accepted, executed and completion acknowledged)
- Had significantly fewer exits from the labour room compared with teams who did not and used a structured form of communication.

These skills should be taught during training and where they have been integrated into training there have been associated improvements in decision-delivery intervals and neonatal outcomes after category 1 births.[15]

LEADERSHIP – ROLES AND RESPONSIBILITIES

Team leadership involves providing direction, structure and support for other team members. The team leader is often the most senior obstetrician present but may be the midwifery co-ordinator or anaesthetist, and whoever knows the team members' roles and responsibilities and has adequate experience to anticipate the possible end to an emergency.[63] It is essential that the team leader is nominated, declared verbally and accepted by the rest of the team as early as possible.[63]

COMMUNICATION

Obstetric emergency situations occur in the presence of a conscious patient with close relatives, where the safety of a much loved and anticipated baby is at stake. These events are often remembered forever.

Poor maternal experience is another significant complication of pregnancy and birth. UK based research showed that over 25% of new mothers were not satisfied with communication by the medical staff and there was a significant association between satisfaction with communication by medical staff and overall satisfaction with care.[64]

Training in communication both to the patient and amongst team members is important to ensure that the needs of the mother and birth partner are also considered.

Communication can be improved after training using patient actors[65,66] and it is noteworthy that the patient actors reported that their perception of their safety during the drill could be improved by information provided about the:

- Cause of emergency
- Condition of the baby
- Aims of treatment

Once again these simple elements could usefully be included in training programmes to improve communication with patients.

COMMON THEMES OF EFFECTIVENESS

A review of training programmes associated with improvement in clinical outcomes was published in 2009.[56]

Common features of clinically effective training programmes were:

- Multiprofessional training
- Training of all staff in an institution
- Training staff locally within the unit in which they work
- Integrating teamwork training with clinical teaching
- Use of high-fidelity simulation models
- Institution-level incentives for training (e.g. reduced hospital insurance premiums)
- Use of self-assessment to directed infra-structural changes.

CONCLUSION

Reducing preventable harm is a priority for accoucheurs, women and insurers across the globe. Intrapartum skills training appears to offer a direct route to improvement; however, the effect of intrapartum training programmes has been at least inconsistent, if not conflicting. The questions that remain are to whom the training is best given and in which environment.

Expense of research, the need for collaboration and standardized guidance for training as well as the technical costs of developing new and more advanced simulators and training programmes are reasons for caution. More and better research should be undertaken to investigate training and in particular the effect of training at scale. The reduced morbidity and mortality burden from better care means that financial benefits from investment in intrapartum training will follow proof of its effectiveness.

There is an accruing evidence base for intrapartum skills training and also the characteristics of effective training. Therefore, with the current evidence intrapartum training should be local, multiprofessional, mandatory for all staff and ideally supported by institution incentives (most often insurance based) to train.

REFERENCES

1. Gelbart NR. The king's midwife :a history and mystery of Madame Du Coudray. Berkeley, CA: University of California Press; 1999.
2. Black RS, Brocklehurst P. A systematic review of training in acute obstetric emergencies. BJOG 2003;110:837–41. PubMed PMID: 14511966.
3. Kingdon JN, Singleton V, Gytte G, Hart A, Gabbay M, Lavender T. Choice and birth method: mixed-method study of caesarean delivery for maternal request. BJOG 2009;116:886–95.
4. NHS Litigation Authority. Ten Years of maternity claims: an analysis of NHS Litigation Authority data. London: NHS Litigation Authority; 2012.
5. Kings Fund. Safe births: Everybody's business. An independent inquiry into the safety of maternity services in England. London: Kings Fund; 2008.
6. Maternal and Child Health Research Consortium. CESDI 4th Annual Report. Care during labour and delivery. London, 1997.
7. Draycott T, Lewis G, Stephens I. Executive summary, Eighth Report of the Confidential Enquiries into Maternal Deaths in the UK. BJOG 2011;118(Suppl. 1): e12–21.
8. Confidential Enquiry into Stillbirths and Deaths in Infancy. 7th Annual Report. London: CESDI; 2000.
9. Joint Commission on Accreditation of Healthcare Organizations. Sentinel Event Alert 2004.
10. World Health Organisation. Making pregnancy safer 2011. Available at http://www.who.int/making_pregnancy_safer/topics/maternal_mortality/en/index.html (cited 25 April 2011).
11. Lawn JE, Cousens S, Zupan J. 4 million neonatal deaths: When? Where? Why? Lancet 2005;365:891–900.
12. Royal College of Midwives. Clinical risk management Paper 2: shoulder dystocia. London: RCM; 2002.
13. Report RCoOaGRCoMJWP. Towards Safer Childbirth: minimum standards for the organisation of labour wards. London: RCOG Press; 1999.
14. NHS Litigation Authority. CNST standards – maternity manual. London: NHSLA; 2000.
15. Siassakos D, Hasafa Z, Sibanda T, Fox R, Donald F, Winter C, et al. Retrospective cohort study of diagnosis-delivery interval with umbilical cord prolapse: the effect of team training. BJOG 2009;116:1089–95.
16. Draycott TJ, Crofts JF, Ash JP, Wilson LV, Yard E, Sibanda T, et al. Improving neonatal outcome through practical shoulder dystocia training. Obstet Gynecol 2008;112:14–20.
17. Draycott T, Sibanda T, Owen L, Akande V, Winter C, Reading S, et al. Does training in obstetric emergencies improve neonatal outcome? BJOG 2006;113:177.182.
18. Scholefield H. Embedding quality improvement and patient safety at Liverpool Women's NHS Foundation Trust. Best Prac Res Clin Obstet Gynaecol 2007;21: 593–607.
19. Nielsen PE, Goldman MB, Mann S, Shapiro DE, Marcus RG, Pratt SD, et al. Effects of teamwork training on adverse outcomes and process of care in labor and delivery: a randomized controlled trial. Obstet Gynecol 2007;109:48–55.
20. Markova V, Sorensen JL, Holm C, Norgaard A, Langhoff-Roos J. Evaluation of multi-professional obstetric skills training for postpartum hemorrhage. Acta Obstet Gynecol Scand 2012;91:346–52.
21. MacKenzie IZ, Shah M, Lean K, Dutton S, Newdick H, Tucker DE. Management of shoulder dystocia: trends in incidence and maternal and neonatal morbidity. Obstet Gynecol 2007;110:1059–68.
22. Crofts J, Fox R, Montague I, Draycott T. Royal College of Obstetricians and Gynaecologists. Greentop guideline 42: Shoulder dystocia. London: RCOG; 2012.
23. Berglund S, Petterson H, Cnattigius S, Grunewald C. How often is a low Apgar score the result of substandard care during labour? BJOG 2010;117:968–78.
24. Andreasen S, Backe B, Jorstad RG, Oian P. A nationwide descriptive study of obstetric claims for compensation in Norway. Acta Obstet Gynecol Scand 2012;91:1191–5.

25. Pehrson JS, Amer-Wåhlin I. Evaluation and impact of cardiotocography training programmes: a systematic review. BJOG 2010;118:926–35.
26. National Institute for Clinical Excellence. NICE Clinical Guideline 55 – intrapartum care. London: National Institute for Clinical Excellence; 2007.
27. Royal College of Obstetricians and Gynaecologists Clinical Effectiveness Unit. The use of electronic fetal monitoring. The use and interpretation of cardiotocography in intrapartum fetal surveillance. Evidence-based Clinical Guideline Number 8. London: RCOG; 2001.
28. Weiner C. The implementation of PROMPT at the Kansas University Medical Centre. In: Draycott T, editor. Personal Communication. Kansas, 2012.
29. Victorian Managed Insurance Authority. VicPROMPT Pilot Project Evaluation Report: An evaluation of the VicPROMPT pilot project: a multi-professional obstetric emergencies training program 2010–2011. Melbourne: VMIA; 2012.
30. McGaghie WC, Draycott TJ, Dunn WF, Lopez CM, Stefanidis D. Evaluating the impact of simulation on translational patient outcomes. Simul Healthc 2011; 6(Suppl):S42–7.
31. Draycott T, Broad G, Chidley K. The development of an eclampsia box and fire drill. Br J Midwifery 2000;8: 26–30.
32. Ellis D, Crofts JF, Hunt LP, Read M, Fox R, James M. Hospital, simulation center, and teamwork training for eclampsia management: a randomized controlled trial. Obstet Gynecol 2008;111:723–31.
33. Hannah ME, Hannah WJ, Hewson SA, Hodnett ED, Saigal S, Willan AR. Planned caesarean section versus planned vaginal birth for breech presentation at term: a randomised multicentre trial. Term Breech Trial Collaborative Group. Lancet 2000;356:1375–83.
34. Deering S, Brown J, Hodor J, Satin AJ. Simulation training and resident performance of singleton vaginal breech delivery. Obstet Gynecol 2006;107:86–9.
35. Murphy DJ, Liebling RE, Verity L, Swingler R, Patel R. Early maternal and neonatal morbidity associated with operative delivery in second stage of labour: a cohort study. Lancet 2001;358:1203–7.
36. Patel RR, Murphy DJ. Forceps delivery in modern obstetric practice. BMJ 2004;328(7451):1302–5.
37. Royal College of Obstetricians and Gynaecologists. RCOG trainees survey. London: RCOG; 2009.
38. Dupuis O, Moreau R, Silveira R, Pham MT, Zentner A, Cucherat M, et al. A new obstetric forceps for the training of junior doctors: a comparison of the spatial dispersion of forceps blade trajectories between junior and senior obstetricians. Am J Obstet Gynecol 2006;194: 1524–31.
39. Moreau R, Pham MT, Brun X, Redarce T, Dupuis O. Assessment of forceps use in obstetrics during a simulated childbirth. Int J Med Robot 2008;4:373–80.
40. Leslie KK, Dipasquale-Lehnerz P, Smith M. Obstetric forceps training using visual feedback and the isometric strength testing unit. Obstet Gynecol 2005;105: 377–82.
41. Lewis G. Saving Mothers' Lives: reviewing maternal deaths to make motherhood safer 2003–5. The Seventh Report of the Confidential Enquiries into Maternal Deaths in the United Kingdom. London: CEMACH; 2007.
42. Wayne DB, Didwania A, Feinglass J, Fudala MJ, Barsuk JH, McGaghie WC. Simulation-based education improves quality of care during cardiac arrest team responses at an academic teaching hospital: a case-control study. Chest 2008;133:56–61.
43. Fisher N, Eisen LA, Bayya JV, Dulu A, Bernstein PS, Merkatz IR, et al. Improved performance of maternal-fetal medicine staff after maternal cardiac arrest simulation-based training. Am J Obstet Gynecol 2011;205:239 e1–5.
44. Dijkman A, Huisman CM, Smit M, Schutte JM, Zwart JJ, van Roosmalen JJ, et al. Cardiac arrest in pregnancy: increasing use of perimortem caesarean section due to emergency skills training? BJOG 2010; 117:282–7.
45. Bhutta ZA, Darmstadt GL, Hasan BS, Haws RA. Community-based interventions for improving perinatal and neonatal health outcomes in developing countries: a review of the evidence. Pediatrics 2002;115(Suppl. 2): 519–617.
46. McClure EM, Carlo WA, Wright LL, Chomba E, Uxa F, Lincetto O, et al. Evaluation of the educational impact of the WHO Essential Newborn Care course in Zambia. Acta Pædiatrica 2007;96:1135–8.
47. Carlo WA, McClure EM, Chomba E, editors. Impact of World Health Organization (WHO) Essential Newborn Care Course (ENC) training: a multicenter study. Baltimore: Annual Meeting of the Pediatric Academic Societies; 2009.
48. Carlo WA, Goudar SS, Jehan I, Chomba E, Tshefu A, Garces A, et al. Newborn-care training and perinatal mortality in developing countries. N Engl J Med 2010;363:614–23.
49. Musafili A, Essen B, Baribwira C, Rukundo A, Persson LA. Evaluating Helping Babies Breathe: training for healthcare workers at hospitals in Rwanda. Acta Paediatr 2013;102:e34–8.
50. Kawaguchi A, Mori R. The In-service training for health professionals to improve care of the seriously ill newborn or child in low- and middle-income countries. Geneva: World Health Organization; 2010.
51. Sorensen BL, Elsass P, Nielsen BB, Massawe S, Nyakina J, Rasch V. Substandard emergency obstetric care – a confidential enquiry into maternal deaths at a regional hospital in Tanzania. Trop Med Int Health 2010;15: 894–900.
52. Sorensen BL, Rasch V, Massawe S, Nyakina J, Elsass P, Nielsen BB. Impact of ALSO training on the management of prolonged labor and neonatal care at Kagera Regional Hospital, Tanzania. Int J Gynaecol Obstet 2010;111:8–12.
53. Helmreich RL. On error management: lessons from aviation. BMJ 2000;320:781–5.
54. Bosk CL, Dixon-Woods M, Goeschel CA, Pronovost PJ. Reality check for checklists. Lancet 2009;374:444–5.
55. Reader TW, Cuthbertson BH. Teamwork and team training in the ICU: where do the similarities with aviation end? Crit Care 2011;15:313.
56. Siassakos D, Crofts JF, Winter C, Weiner CP, Draycott TJ. The active components of effective training in obstetric emergencies. BJOG 2009;116:1028–32.
57. Riley W, Davis S, Miller K, Hansen H, Sainfort F, Sweet R. Didactic and simulation nontechnical skills team training to improve perinatal patient outcomes in a community hospital. Jt Comm J Qual Patient Saf 2011;37: 357–64.
58. Siassakos D, Fox R, Hunt L, Farey J, Laxton C, Winter C, et al. Attitudes toward safety and teamwork in a maternity unit with embedded team training. Am J Med Qual 2011;26:132–7.
59. Thompson S, Neal S, Clark V. Clinical risk management in obstetrics: eclampsia drills. Qual Saf Health Care 2004;13:127–9.
60. Siassakos D, Crofts J, Winter C, Draycott T, on behalf of the SaFE Study Group. Multiprofessional 'fire-drill' training in the labour ward. J SOGC 2009;11:55–60.
61. Siassakos D, Draycott TJ, Crofts JF, Hunt LP, Winter C, Fox R. More to teamwork than knowledge, skill and attitude. BJOG 2010;117:1262–9.

62. Siassakos D, Bristowe K, Draycott TJ, Angouri J, Hambly H, Winter C, et al. Clinical efficiency in a simulated emergency and relationship to team behaviours: a multisite cross-sectional study. BJOG 2011;118: 596–607.

63. Bristowe K, Siassakos D, Hambly H, Angouri J, Yelland A, Draycott T, et al. Teamwork for clinical emergencies: interprofessional focus group analysis and triangulation with simulation. Qual Health Res 2012;10:1383–94.

64. Kirke P. Mothers' views of care in labour. BJOG 1980;87:1034–8.

65. Siassakos D, Bristowe K, Hambly H, Angouri J, Crofts JF, Winter C, et al. Team communication with patient actors: findings from a multisite simulation study. Simul Healthc 2011;6:143–9.

66. Crofts JF, Bartlett C, Ellis D, Winter C, Donald F, Hunt LP, et al. Patient-actor perception of care: a comparison of obstetric emergency training using manikins and patient-actors. Qual Saf Health Care 2008;17:20–4.

CHAPTER 5

ASSESSMENT AND MANAGEMENT OF LABOUR

MS Robson

ON THE QUALIFICATIONS OF AN ACCOUCHEUR

'Those who intend to practice midwifery, ought first of all to make themselves masters of anatomy, and acquire competent knowledge in surgery and physic ... and of practising under a master, before he attempts to deliver by himself. He should also embrace every occasion of being present at real labours ... Over and above the advantages of education, he ought to be endued with a natural sagacity, resolution, and prudence; together with that humanity which adorns the owner, and never fails of being agreeable to the distressed patient'.

William Smellie
A Treatise on the Theory and Practice of Midwifery, London: D. Wilson, 1752, pp446–447

INTRODUCTION

The aim of care in labour is a healthy mother and baby and an emotionally fulfilling experience. Childbirth is a sentinel event in the life of a woman and her family. Failure to look after women and their babies adequately, especially in their first labour, may leave permanent physical and emotional scars and result in women rejecting the care offered. In their next pregnancy they may request delivery by caesarean section or alternatively have no further children.

Labour is a dynamic process depending on physiological and anatomical factors. A normal labour is considered by most as an unassisted vaginal delivery, following spontaneous labour at term resulting in a healthy mother and baby within a reasonable length of time. This is a retrospective definition and has recently been the focus of attention.[1,2] Every delivery unit should have a clear vision of what they are trying to achieve and ensure the statement is prominently positioned in the delivery ward.

GENERAL PRINCIPLES OF LABOUR

Overview

In understanding labour it is important to talk about women who are actually in labour. This means a correct diagnosis. Efficient uterine action is the key to normality in labour and the correct diagnosis of labour is the most important single decision. Quality care in labour is achieving efficient uterine action and simultaneously ensuring fetal and maternal wellbeing.

Nulliparous labour is completely different to multiparous labour and spontaneous labour must be differentiated from induced labour. Single cephalic pregnancies must be distinguished from breech and multiple pregnancies and preterm labour from term labour.

The singleton cephalic nulliparous woman at term in spontaneous labour represents the key challenge and the most significant experience to the woman and her family. The singleton cephalic multiparous woman (without a previous scar) at term in spontaneous labour is the other main group of women and the contrast between the two must never be forgotten.

With these principles in mind a rational approach to the care of women in labour can be developed.

Antenatal Preparation for Labour

The better prepared and more confident a woman and her partner are before labour and delivery the better the effect on every aspect of her outcome both physically and emotionally. Reassurances should be given that continuous, sympathetic and informed support will be forthcoming and that labour will not be allowed to last for too long. Preparation should be specific about how the diagnosis of labour is made and the importance of the part the mother has to play in the second phase of the second stage of labour (pushing phase). The graphic representation of labour on the partogram should be explained so that the woman is aware of the progress of her labour. The common events that take place in labour and the reasons for them should be explained. The difference between spontaneous and induced labour should also be emphasized and the methods used to ensure fetal wellbeing should be demonstrated. The relief of pain is discussed, with the emphasis on convincing the expectant mother she has nothing to fear on the basis that the duration of labour will be limited and she will never be left alone. The organization and planning of antenatal preparation is crucial and must be credible. Nulliparous and multiparous women should have separate preparation for their labours.

Management of the Labour Ward

When discussing labour, emphasis is always placed on the management of labour. Less emphasis, if any, is put on the management of the labour ward. A well-organized labour ward is essential to provide the best care and achieve the most out of available personnel and equipment. The adequacy and use of resources has to be continually challenged.

The predominant professional carer for the woman and fetus in labour should be the midwife but they together with obstetricians, paediatricians and anaesthetists must integrate their expertise to provide the best outcome for each woman. Each professional must have their own clinical responsibilities, but lines of communication must be clear between professional groups and between junior and senior staff.

Assessment of the Woman Before Labour

Much is written about defining high- and low-risk women before labour. This is important, but the purist view on labour would be that most women are healthy and have well grown babies before going into labour. Once in labour the principles of labour remain the same and abnormalities of labour relate most commonly to poor progress.

Diagnosis of Labour

'If the os uteri remains close shut, it may be taken for granted, that the woman is not yet in labour, not withstanding the pains she may suffer'
  William Smellie
    A Treatise on the Theory and Practice of Midwifery. London. D Wilson, 1752, p180

The most single important aspect about labour is the diagnosis. In most labours there is usually little doubt.

The diagnosis of labour is made by history and examination. The woman will present with a history of regular, painful intermittent contractions. The frequency, length and strength of the contractions may vary and be subjective. A history of ruptured membranes and loss of the mucous plug is strongly supportive. Cervical effacement and dilatation on vaginal examination confirms the diagnosis.

The cervix in nulliparous and multiparous women is different. The nulliparous cervix is tubular shaped. The multiparous cervix is of comparable size but is cone shaped. The length of the cervix should be recorded in centimetres and the cervix in nulliparous women should not be considered to be 'dilated' until effacement (thinning) of the cervix has taken place (Fig 5-1).

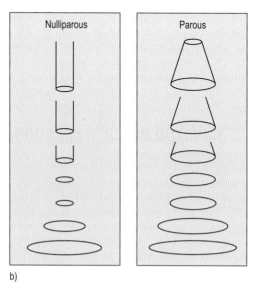

| The nulliparous cervix is tubular in shape and, although constricted somewhat at either end, both internal os and external os usually allow a fingertip to pass | |
| The parous cervix is pyramidal in shape with an internal os of comparable size but an external os that hangs loose to the extent that it may allow two fingers or more to pass | |

a)

Nulliparous Parous

b)

FIGURE 5-1 ■ Diagramatic representation of cervical effacement (a) and dilatation of the nulliparous and the parous cervix (b). (Reproduced with permission from O'Driscoll K, Meagher D, Robson M. Active Management of Labour. 4th ed. London: Mosby, 2003.)

There is no exact formula for the confirmation of the diagnosis of labour. In practice it represents a decision to commit a woman to delivery. Parity and gestation should be taken into consideration but a fixed cervical dilatation as a prerequisite for the diagnosis of labour may be clinically inappropriate. Error in diagnosis can occur when women were either wrongly diagnosed in labour when they were evidently not, or a missed diagnosis of labour when the woman returns fully dilated within a few hours. The difficulty arises more commonly in nulliparous women and has greater implications than in multipara. Occasionally the woman may return completely demoralised and with an exhausted uterus; so that a labour that may have benefited from early assistance instead results in a prolonged labour with subsequent short-term and long-term consequences.

The diagnosis of labour is therefore crucial and also ensures that, right or wrong, a prospective decision is always made, either accepting the diagnosis of labour or rejecting it. Otherwise it is impossible to audit results, and standards cannot be set. Occasionally, deferring a decision for an hour is appropriate but encouraging indecision on a labour ward may be counterproductive.

'The most important single issue of care in labour is diagnosis. When the initial diagnosis is wrong, all subsequent care is likely to be also wrong'.

KIERAN O'DRISCOLL[3]

The quality of decision-making can only be assessed by continuous audit looking at length of labour, oxytocin and caesarean section rates within the 10 groups.[4]

Care of the Mother and Fetus

The woman's general condition should always be checked at the beginning of labour, including general observations and urinalysis. Confirmation of the frequency, length and strength of the uterine contractions, the lie of the fetus, the presentation and descent of the head into the pelvis is carried out by abdominal examination.

Fetal wellbeing is confirmed by assessing the size of the baby; the colour, quantity and consistency of the liquor gives information regarding the fetus's condition prior to labour and how it may respond to labour. The liquor may become meconium stained during labour, signifying possible fetal compromise. The fetal heart rate may be monitored either by Pinard stethoscope, hand held Doppler or continuous electronic monitoring.

Stages of Labour

Labour is divided into three stages. The first and second stages rely on anatomical criteria and this may be disadvantageous as labour is essentially a dynamic process. In normal labour the transition from the first to the second stages is of little clinical significance and the important events are the diagnosis of labour and the maternal urge to push. The importance of defining the first and second stages of labour becomes more relevant if the labour does not progress normally. Because normal labour can only be confirmed retrospectively, there is difficulty in defining exactly when a normal labour becomes abnormal and requires treatment. Indeed, this definition will be different depending on the gestation, the parity, and whether the pregnancy is singleton cephalic. It will also depend on what the initial dilatation of the cervix was at the diagnosis of labour.

The Partogram

The partogram for recording the progress of labour was introduced after the classical studies of Emmanuel Friedman[5] in the USA and subsequently the pragmatic innovations of Hugh Philpott in Africa.[6,7] Elements of Philpott's partogram were incorporated into the current World Health Organization's partogram (Fig 5-2). Partograms vary but the important component is a graphical plot of the progress in labour to assist decision-making. This is emphasized in the partogram used in Active Management of Labour[3] where no allowance for the latent phase is made (Fig 5-3). The graphical plot is measured in *centimetres dilated* on the *x* axis against *hours in labour* on the *y* axis. The partogram records other information about labour events and labour outcomes contributing to the audit of labour and may exist in different colours for easy distinction between nulliparous and multiparous women. Carbon copies may be used so that copies of the partogram can be kept separately on the labour ward for inspection after the woman has delivered.

Spontaneous Onset of Labour and Favourable Predictive Factors

The most important aspect about the management of normal labour is the fact that there has been spontaneous onset. The risk of *intervention* is much less in spontaneous labour, and much less again in multiparous women (without a

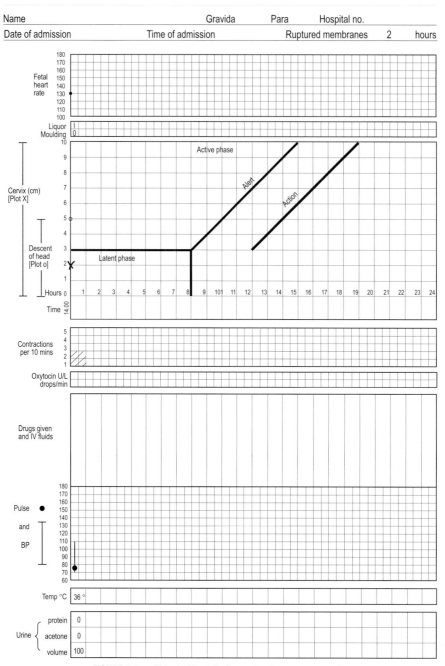

FIGURE 5-2 ■ World Health Organization partograph.

previous scar) than in other groups of women. A greater dilatation of the cervix at the time of diagnosis of labour and presentation to the delivery ward does not necessarily reflect the length of time in labour, but is more likely to reflect efficient uterine action especially when the history of contractions has not been long. This and engagement of the presenting part are good predictors of normal labour. On the contrary, a long history of contractions without onset of labour or only 1 cm dilated on admission are less favourable predictive factors as is labour at later gestations.[8] This is especially true in nulliparous women where the requirement for artificial rupture of the membranes, oxytocin acceleration (augmentation), caesarean delivery and other interventions increase steadily from 37 weeks to 42 weeks.

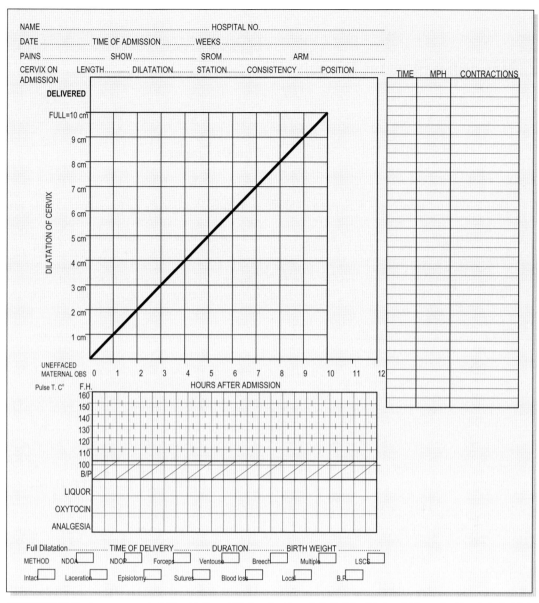

FIGURE 5-3 ■ Partogram used at The National Maternity Hospital, Dublin (National Maternity Hospital, Dublin).

Personal Attention

Personal attention in labour cannot be overemphasized and is undervalued in most delivery units. The fear of being left alone is common. It is important that a woman's morale is maintained from the beginning of her labour. The longer her labour, the more difficult it is to achieve this; and the greater her loss of composure, the more difficult it becomes for her to recover it. The final result can be panic, from which the individual may never fully recover.

The solution is a commitment in each delivery unit to every expectant mother of continuous personal attention through labour. This can only be carried out effectively if there is a limitation on the duration of labour. The ability to provide continual personal attention is the best indicator of the quality of care afforded in any delivery unit and mothers regard it as the most important contribution to their care.

Although childbirth has long ceased to present a serious physical challenge to healthy women in western society, the emotional impact of labour remains a matter of common concern.[3]

NORMAL AND ABNORMAL LABOUR

Efficient uterine action is the key to normality.

Agreement of what is normal and abnormal labour is not universal between either women or professionals. It is time to replace natural and normal with an open concept of the good. Furthermore, what makes the professional healthcare practitioner professional is his or her knowledge of means and consequences, not his or her opinion about what is good or bad.[9]

All professionals should have similar aims in labour. The controversy in the management of labour arises when does *normal* becomes *abnormal* and whether early *intervention* can prevent more *major intervention* later. Labour should not be thought of as either normal or abnormal but a gradation in terms of events and outcomes and the term *intervention* should be replaced by events and outcomes as they have different implications for individual women and professionals.

In discussing abnormal labour a distinction needs to be made between the abnormalities of labour (inefficient uterine action, malposition and cephalopelvic disproportion) which take place in the woman with a singleton, cephalic pregnancy at term in spontaneous labour, and other women with obstetrical abnormalities who happen to be in labour, such as induction of labour, women with a previous uterine scar, malpresentations and multiple pregnancies.

Dystocia

Dystocia is defined as difficult or prolonged labour (poor progress) and is common in nulliparous women but rare in multiparous women who have delivered vaginally previously. Progress in labour depends on the powers (uterine efficiency), the passenger (size, position and attitude of the fetus) and the passage (pelvic bony and soft tissues both inside and outside the uterus).

Inefficient Uterine Action

Inefficient uterine action (dysfunctional labour, inco-ordinate uterine action) is the most common cause of poor progress in spontaneous labour in nulliparous women, but it is rare in multiparous women. The most common causes of inefficient uterine action leading to a dystocic labour in nulliparous women are an error in the diagnosis of labour, delay in diagnosis of inefficient uterine action, delay in treatment of inefficient uterine action, inappropriate treatment or appropriate treatment of inefficient uterine action but with no response. In addition there may be labours in which the diagnosis has been made and treatment initiated, but there is an inability to treat at the appropriate dose of oxytocin because of either fetal intolerance or uterine tachysystole.

The Passenger

The fetus will vary in size and the larger the fetus, the higher all intervention rates are, including the length of labour. The fetal head may also vary in terms of its position and attitude. This may be a primary phenomenon, or more rarely associated with variants or abnormalities in pelvic bony or muscular architecture. The most common abnormal cephalic malposition is the occipito-posterior position. This may be persistent or transient in labour. It is associated with dystocic labours, most commonly secondary to inefficient uterine action. Persistent occipito-posterior position is associated with extension of the fetal head resulting in a larger unfavourable diameter presenting in the pelvis. The occipito-transverse position occurs when normal rotation has been incomplete, and is abnormal if persistent late in the second stage. Transverse arrest should not be thought of as the result of a physical obstruction, as the term may imply, but rather the expression of an inadequate driving force. It is not the cause of delay, it is the result. In the presence of efficient uterine action or in multiparous labour these problems are rare.

Cephalic malpresentations, such as face or brow presentation, should always be considered and excluded (see Chapter 11).

The Pelvis

Pelvimetry is not useful in deciding whether a pelvis is adequate, unless there is a history of bony disease or trauma. It is important to remember that the pelvic passage includes the passage within the uterus as well as the passage outside the uterus in the pelvis. Rarely there may be other reasons in the pelvis contributing to poor progress, including pelvic soft tissue masses, fibroids, or congenital or iatrogenic abnormalities of the uterus or vagina.

The cervix, whose purpose is to keep the fetus safely in the uterus during the pregnancy, should also be included under this heading. During normal labour the cervix dilates secondary to uterine contractions, but dilatation of the cervix also depends on complex physiological changes within the cervix, which alter its structure. Previous operations on the cervix such as cone biopsy may result in cervical incompetence and preterm labour; alternatively it may result in fibrosis preventing normal physiological changes and cervical dilatation from taking place.

Cephalopelvic Disproportion and Obstructed Labour

Cephalopelvic disproportion is used to describe an anatomical disproportion between the size of the fetal head and the size of the pelvis. Its use should be restricted to the nulliparous woman with a vertex presentation. It is wrongly thought to be a common cause of dystocic labours. Unfortunately, it is very difficult to be certain of the diagnosis and should only be considered in the presence of efficient uterine action, which means full cervical dilatation with a short labour progressing at more than 1 cm/hour, a single cephalic vertex presentation with an occipito-anterior position. The diagnosis should only be made in labour. In practice true cephalopelvic disproportion is rare and most women with a previous diagnosis of cephalopelvic disproportion will deliver vaginally in their next pregnancy if they are allowed to go into spontaneous labour.

The term obstructed labour rather than cephalopelvic disproportion should be used in multiparous women, although they both imply that for anatomical reasons the fetus is unable to be delivered safely vaginally. They share the assumption that in both situations there is efficient uterine action. This is almost certainly true in obstructed labours in multiparous women, but not necessarily certain in most cases of suspected cephalopelvic disproportion in nulliparous women. Obstructed labour in multipara, like true cephalopelvic disproportion in nulliparous women, is very rare, but in the multipara is a dangerous condition which, if unrecognized, can lead to uterine rupture. The nulliparous uterus is virtually immune to rupture; the sole exception is manipulation with instruments and rare connective tissue disorders.

The multiparous uterus is rupture prone, particularly if there is a previous scar and is often associated with prostaglandins and oxytocin (see Chapter 15).

DIAGNOSIS AND MANAGEMENT OF POOR PROGRESS IN LABOUR

Prolonged Latent Phase, Primary Dysfunctional Labour and Secondary Arrest

These terms relate to poor progress in labour. They have been classically described in relation to the partogram but their use is best restricted to nulliparous women where they are all most commonly due to inefficient uterine action. Their application in multiparous women in whom inefficient uterine action is rare is misleading. They all are difficult to define and their usefulness in labour is open to question, in particular the term *latent phase* and its relationship to the diagnosis of labour in nulliparous women.

What is important to remember is that the diagnosis and subsequent treatment of poor progress generally occurs in nulliparous women and typically at three points in the labour. Firstly, early on in labour (0–4 cm dilatation representing prolonged latent phase or primary dysfunctional labour), then in the middle of labour (5–9 cm representing primary dysfunctional labour or secondary arrest) and finally at full dilatation (10 cm usually representing secondary arrest but if progress has been less than 1 cm/hour possibly still primary dysfunctional labour). Therefore inefficient uterine action, should always be considered the cause of poor progress in nulliparous women especially when progress has been less than 1 cm/hour.

In multiparous women poor progress when labour is correctly diagnosed is rare. After 5 cm it is even more unusual and should never be assumed to be inefficient uterine action unless obstructed labour has been excluded and uterine contractions documented as poor.

Assessing Progress in Labour

Abdominal and vaginal examinations are performed to assess progress in labour (Table 5-1). Progress in the first stage of labour is assessed by cervical dilatation. Cervical dilatation less than 1 cm/hour is generally considered poor progress but different rates of progress in spontaneous labour are used to define normal progress. Other clinical indices that sometimes are used to assess progress in the first stage are the consistency and thickness of the cervix and descent of the head both on abdominal and vaginal examination. Position of the fetal head to assess progress in the first stage of labour is not useful. In the second stage of labour, progress is assessed by the descent and rotation of the fetal head. Vaginal assessments carried out during a contraction give the most information about dilatation and descent.

Physiologically the important vaginal assessments in labour are within one of three divisions: confirmation of labour (0–4 cm), half way along (5–9 cm) and full dilatation with the head on the perineum (10 cm).

TABLE 5-1	**Factors to be Assessed at Vaginal Examination in Labour**	
Presentation	cephalic	
	breech/foot	
	shoulder/arm	
	umbilical cord	
Cervix	effacement	
	dilatation	
	oedema	
	application to presenting part	
Fetal head	station	
	position	
	flexion/deflexion	
	caput	
	asynclitism	
	moulding	
Membranes	intact/ruptured	
Amniotic fluid	volume:	
	– absent/scant/normal/abundant	
	content:	
	– clear	
	– meconium (thin/thick)	
	– blood	

Nulliparous Women

Poor progress or dystocia in labour is the most common abnormality in spontaneous labour in nulliparous women and inefficient uterine action is the most common cause of this dystocia.

In nulliparous women, the treatment of poor progress in the absence of fetal problems is early artificial rupture of the membranes. If there continues to be poor progress an oxytocin infusion to accelerate (augment) labour is started. Having excluded inefficient uterine action as a possible cause, if there continues to be poor progress then operative intervention is required, either by vaginal delivery if possible, or by caesarean section. There is no agreement on the timing of these interventions. Only continuous audit of outcome will help to confirm whether they are appropriate.

The management of poor progress in the second stage of labour in nulliparous women has become more important with the increasing use of epidural analgesia. The first phase of the second stage of labour (full dilatation but the head high and the sagittal suture in the transverse position) should be managed as a physiological continuation of the first stage.

In women in whom the progress in labour in the first stage of labour has been adequate and not required acceleration (augmentation) with oxytocin, but the head is high, in the transverse position and the woman has no urge to push, the vaginal examination is repeated after 1 hour. If the head is still high at that time, in the transverse position and the woman has no urge to push then an oxytocin infusion is started. Organized pushing is then started 1 hour later.

However, if 1 hour after full dilatation the head has descended, is in the occipito-anterior position and the woman has the urge to push (second phase of the second stage) then pushing is commenced and only if there is no progress after 10 minutes is oxytocin started.

If at the time of diagnosis of full dilatation the head is low, is in the occipito-anterior position and the woman has the urge to push then pushing is also commenced and if there is no progress after 10 minutes oxytocin is also started.

If at the time of diagnosis of full dilatation the woman's labour is already being accelerated (augmented) with oxytocin then pushing is commenced if the head is low, is in the occipito-anterior position and the woman has the urge to push. If not, then pushing is commenced after 1 hour.

Vaginal operative delivery for poor progress in the second stage of labour usually takes place after an hour of pushing (see Chapter 10).

Multiparous Women

In multiparous women inefficient uterine action is very unlikely as a cause of poor progress, especially if the cervix has reached 5 cm dilatation. The reasons for poor progress in multiparous women that need to be excluded are a malpresentation or an abnormal position or attitude of the fetus. However, a large fetus with the vertex presenting in an occipito-anterior position may also cause obstructed labour. If there is initial efficient uterine action in a multiparous woman followed by no cervical dilatation, the diagnosis of obstructed labour should be considered.

In multiparous women the treatment of poor progress in the absence of any fetal problems is early artificial rupture of the membranes. If there continues to be poor progress, obstructed labour should be excluded. If this is diagnosed in the first stage of labour then the treatment is caesarean section. Management of poor progress in the second stage of labour can be difficult in multiparous women, but should be rare. Operative delivery will be necessary and occasionally by caesarean section. Oxytocin to accelerate labour at full dilatation in multiparous labour is not recommended.

The main cause of inefficient uterine action in a multiparous woman in labour is an error in diagnosis of labour or possibly secondary to epidural analgesia. Both usually present with poor progress at a much earlier cervical dilatation. The decision to accelerate (augment) labour in the multiparous woman should only be made by a senior obstetrician and only carried out after vaginal examination to exclude obstructed labour.

Risks of Treatment with Oxytocin and Assessment of Contractions

It is the effect on the uterus and baby that is important, not the dose of oxytocin.

Treatment of poor progress in labour with oxytocin should never be carried out if there is any suspicion of fetal distress. The nulliparous uterus should be considered immune to rupture, but the multiparous uterus prone to rupture. Oxytocin should therefore only be given to accelerate (augment) the multiparous uterus with caution. Rupture of the multiparous uterus can take place in the absence of oxytocin if prolonged, obstructed labour is not treated appropriately by caesarean section.

The assessment of uterine contractions is best carried out by clinical examination. In nulliparous women the number of contractions should not exceed seven in 15 minutes. However, oxytocin should always be started if there is poor progress, providing there is no evidence of fetal distress, as inefficient uterine action is common. Starting oxytocin may not always make the contractions more frequent, but instead more efficient. Fifteen minutes for assessment rather than 10 minutes is recommended because there is a longer time to assess the contractions. (The following definitions of excessive uterine contractions have been proposed by the American College of Obstetricians and Gynecologists: tachysystole, more than five contractions in 10 minutes averaged over 30 minutes and hypertonus, a contraction lasting ≥ 2 minutes.)[10,11]

In multiparous women the assessment of contractions is more critical as the likelihood of inefficient uterine action is rare and therefore the requirement for oxytocin is much less. In addition the risks of oxytocin in multiparous women are much greater. In multiparous women the number of contractions should not exceed five in 15 minutes. This is chosen because of the potential risk of oxytocin in multiparous labour.

The dose of oxytocin has been much debated in the literature, and can range from a starting dose of 1–5 mU/minute, increasing every 15–30 minutes to a maximum of 30 mU/minute. Each unit should decide on the dose and timing of incremental increase, but there are advantages to using a standard oxytocin dose for all women on each labour ward. The safeguards in monitoring contractions, described above, must be strictly observed and the essential factor is not the dose of oxytocin, but the effect that takes place on the uterus and the fetus. In this context the terms tachysystole, hypertonus and hyperstimulation should be clearly understood. Tachysystole refers to overcontracting of the uterus and hypertonus refers to a prolonged contraction (≥ 2 minutes). When either of them results in an adverse effect on the fetus then the term hyperstimulation should be used. The critical endpoint is the potential effect on the fetus, manifest by a non-reassuring fetal heart rate pattern. Thus, any oxytocin-induced contraction pattern that leads to a non-reassuring fetal heart rate pattern constitutes hyperstimulation for that particular uterus and fetus.

The Duration of Labour

The implications of prolonged labour were aptly summarized by Kieran O'Driscoll as follows:[12]

'Prolonged labour presents a picture of mental anguish and physical morbidity which often leads to surgical intervention and may produce a permanent revulsion to childbirth, expressed by the mother as voluntary infertility; it constitutes a danger to the survival and subsequent neurological development in the infant. The harrowing experience is shared by relatives and by doctors and nurses to the extent that few complications so tarnish the image of obstetrics'.

Measuring the duration of labour makes a significant contribution to the audit of everyday clinical practice. It should be considered as one of the basic parameters of labour. The failure to define it in the past has prevented the proper clinical assessment of the impact that duration of labour has on every aspect of the delivery suite and the provision of maternity care.

The length of labour should be defined from the time of diagnosis to delivery of the baby. The reasons why duration of labour is so defined are that professional responsibility begins when the diagnosis is made, and duration can be recorded accurately for purposes of comparison. Mothers will often themselves tend to recall duration of labour in this way.

More than any other objective measurement, duration of labour determines the impact of childbirth particularly on mothers, but also on babies, and also on those who care for both of them. It also has an effect on the efficient organization of the delivery ward and therefore indirectly affects every aspect of a woman's care.

Most women's morale starts to deteriorate after 6 hours in labour, and after 12 hours the rate of deterioration increases dramatically. The incidence of fetal hypoxia and operative deliveries increases. Shorter labours will also mean that personal attention for each woman in labour is a realistic possibility.

Contentious Issues

The current contentious issues are the timing of amniotomy in labour, the incidence, dose and regimen of oxytocin to accelerate (augment) labour and the optimal length of labour. Taking the National Maternity Hospital philosophy of Active Management of Labour as an example, amniotomy is performed at the diagnosis of labour, there is no allowance made for a latent phase and vaginal examinations are performed earlier in nulliparous women as compared to multiparous women to assess progress and the requirement for oxytocin. The maximum dose of oxytocin used is 30 mU/minute.[3]

Other approaches to labour and delivery will be different, but all these issues are interrelated and they will only be solved by continuous audit within standard groups of women and subsequent comparison between units. Audit must include unit policies on amniotomy, frequency of vaginal examination, oxytocin administration, operative delivery rates and their indications, neonatal outcome, methods of fetal surveillance and maternal satisfaction. These issues are discussed further in Chapter 3.

REFERENCES

1. Society of Obstetricians and Gynaecologists of Canada. Joint Policy Statement on Normal Childbirth. J Obstet Gynaecol Can 2009;31:602–3.
2. NCT/RCM/RCOG. Making normal birth a reality. Consensus Statement 2007;8(Nov):1–8.
3. O'Driscoll K, Meagher D, Robson M. Active management of labour. 4th ed. London: Mosby; 2003.
4. Robson MS. Classification of caesarean sections. Fetal Maternal Med Rev 2001;12:23–9.
5. Friedman EA. Primigravid labor. A graphicostatistical analysis. Obstet Gynecol 1955;6:567–89.
6. Philpott RH, Castle WM. Cervicographs in the management of labour in primigravidae. I: The alert line for detecting abnormal labour. J Obstet Gynaecol Br Cwlth 1972;79:592–8.
7. Philpott RH, Castle WM. Cervicographs in the management of labour in primigravidae.II: The action line and treatment of abnormal labour. J Obstet Gynaecol Br Cwlth 1972;79:599–602.
8. Saunders N, Paterson C. Effect of gestational age on obstetric performance: when is 'term' over? Lancet 1991;338:1190–2.
9. Wackerhausen S. What is natural? Deciding what to do and not to do in medicine and health care. Br J Obstet Gynaecol 1999;106:1109–12.
10. American College of Obstetricians and Gynecologists. Technical Bulletin No.218. Dystocia and the augmentation of labor. Washington DC: ACOG; 1995.
11. American College of Obstetricians and Gynecologists. Practice Bulletin No. 107. Induction of labor. Obstet Gynecol 2009;114:386–97.
12. O'Driscoll K, Jackson RJA, Gallagher JT. Prevention of prolonged labour. BMJ 1969;2:447–50.

CHAPTER 6

FETAL SURVEILLANCE IN LABOUR

S Arulkumaran

> 'By applying the ear to the mother's belly; if the child is alive you hear quite clearly the beats of its heart and easily distinguish them from the mother's pulse'.
> François Mayor
> Biblioth Universelle des Sciences et Arts. Geneva: 1818; 9:249

The fetus is exposed to maximal hypoxic stress during labour as the uterine contractions reduce perfusion to the placenta and may compress the umbilical cord, thus reducing blood flow into the placenta. Such reduced flow is greater in cases of fetal intrauterine growth restriction as the placenta is small. Some cotyledons may be infarcted and cord compression is more likely if there is oligohydramnios. Depending on the risk identified, appropriate surveillance would help to reduce perinatal morbidity or mortality. Emergencies can arise in labour that may cause acute fetal compromise as in cases of placental abruption, cord prolapse or uterine rupture. Clinical vigilance and prompt action are needed in such cases. Assessment of the fetal condition by auscultation or advanced methods should be related to the clinical situation for the best outcome for the mother and the new-born.

INTERMITTENT AUSCULTATION

Available evidence suggests that intermittent auscultation (IA) is adequate in low-risk pregnancies. Electronic fetal monitoring (EFM) reduces neonatal convulsions and increases operative interventions, but has not been shown to reduce cerebral palsy.[1,2] Most national organizations accept IA to be adequate and appropriate for low-risk pregnancies and recommend continuous EFM for high-risk pregnancies.[3-5] Auscultation of the fetal heart rate (FHR) should be for 1 full minute soon after a contraction, every 15 minutes in the first stage and every 5 minutes in the second stage of labour. If IA cannot be provided as recommended or the mother wishes to have EFM, it should be provided. Low risk before labour may become high risk during labour and this should prompt conversion to EFM.

Intermittent auscultation is practised with a fetal stethoscope (Pinard or De Lee) or by using a Doppler device. Increasingly the mother prefers the latter as the family enjoy listening to the FHR. The practice of listening for 15 seconds and multiplying by four to calculate the rate per minute gives rise to erroneous FHR/min because of the possibility of multiplying the error by four. Doppler devices electronically calculate and provide digital display of the FHR and are accurate.

Prior to IA, recording the latest time the woman felt fetal movements reassures that the fetus is healthy. The baseline FHR should be auscultated and recorded on admission. Further reassurance is derived by the attendant and mother palpating for fetal movements (FM) and recording that event and the auscultated acceleration of the FHR >15 beats above the baseline at the time of FM. As a next step auscultation should be performed immediately after contraction that should identify any FHR deceleration. Such 'intelligent auscultation' may reveal the presence of accelerations with FHR and no decelerations and is equivalent to a reactive cardiotocograph (CTG) trace. It is likely that the baseline variability will be normal in a reactive CTG with FHR accelerations and FMs.

> 'One day whilst examining a patient near term and trying to follow the movements of the fetus with the stethoscope I was suddenly aware of a sound that I had not noticed before; it was like the ticking of a watch. At first I thought I was mistaken, but I was able to repeat the observation over and over again. On counting the beats I found that these occurred 143–148 times per minute and the patient's pulse was only 72 per minute'.
> Jacques Alexandre Kergaradec
> Memoire sur l'auscultation, appliqué a l'etude de la grossesse. Paris: Mequignon-Marvis, 1822

The deceleration that returns to the baseline rate before the contraction abates is unlikely to be harmful to the fetus provided the duration of decelerations is less than the duration of the

FHR at the baseline rate so as to generate adequate perfusion. Auscultation with a fetal stethoscope during a contraction is uncomfortable for the mother and there is attenuation of the fetal heart sound with thickening of the contracting myometrium. A Doppler device can be used during and just after a contraction. Most of the 'harmful' FHR decelerations are late, atypical variable and prolonged decelerations and should be identified by auscultation immediately after a contraction. Subsequent to the initial 'intelligent auscultation' the attendant can listen every 15 minutes in the first stage and every 5 minutes in the second stage of labour for 1 minute just after a contraction. Should there be audible abnormality of the FHR (rise in baseline rate, decelerations), or difficulty in auscultation, or should a high-risk factor become evident in labour (e.g. meconium, bleeding or blood-stained liquor, need for oxytocin augmentation), the process of IA should be converted to continuous EFM.

HIGH-RISK PREGNANCY AND CONTINUOUS EFM

EFM provides a continuous recording of the FHR with the use of a trans-abdominal ultrasound transducer or a fetal scalp electrode after the membranes have ruptured. Those identified as high risk (Table 6-1) during the antenatal period or in labour should be offered continuous EFM. The FHR is recorded on the upper 'cardio' channel and the contractions are recorded on the lower 'toco' channel of the recording graph paper and this CTG displays the FHR in relation to the contractions.

TABLE 6-1 **High-Risk Factors that Would Suggest the Need for EFM**

Maternal	Fetal
Pre-eclampsia	Intrauterine growth restriction (IUGR)
Diabetes	Prematurity
Prelabour rupture of membranes (>24 hours)	Prolonged pregnancy (>42 weeks)
Previous caesarean section	Breech presentation
Antepartum haemorrhage	Abnormal fetal function tests
Maternal medical disorders	Oligohydramnios/ meconium-stained liquor
Induced labour	Multiple pregnancy

There are four features in the FHR trace recorded by electronic FHR monitors: baseline rate, baseline variability, accelerations and decelerations. These are described below and are based on the NICE guidelines (National Institute of Clinical Excellence, UK).[3]

Baseline Fetal Heart Rate

Each fetus will exhibit its own baseline rate. It is deduced by drawing a line where the FHR is steady for a period of 2 minutes without the transient changes of accelerations and/or decelerations. The normal baseline rate at term is 110–160 beats per minute (bpm).

Baseline Variability

Baseline variability is the 'wiggliness' of the baseline and is a reflection of the integrity of the autonomic nervous system and its influence on the heart rate. The ascending limb is due to the sympathetic and the descending limb is due to the parasympathetic activity of the fetal autonomic nervous system. The baseline variability is assessed by measuring the bandwidth of the 'wiggliness' seen at the baseline rate during a 1-minute segment of the FHR trace. The normal baseline variability is 5–25 bpm. When it is <5 bpm the baseline variability is reduced – which may be due to fetal sleep, drugs that act on the central nervous system, hypoxia, brain haemorrhage, infection, chromosomal or congenital malformation of the brain or heart.

Accelerations

Accelerations are a sudden rise of the FHR from the baseline by >15 beats for a duration of >15 seconds. These are usually associated with activity in the brain associated with FM ('somatic nervous system'). Two such accelerations in a 15-minute CTG trace are termed *reactive* and this usually indicates a non-hypoxic fetus.[6] It is very unusual for the neonate to be acidotic at birth if the FHR trace was reactive just before delivery.[7]

Decelerations

Decelerations are a sudden fall of the baseline rate of >15 bpm for >15 seconds. The shapes of the decelerations and relationship to contractions vary. Decelerations indicate a transient stress to the fetus. Based on the shape and timing of decelerations to the contractions, one can identify the cause of the stress.

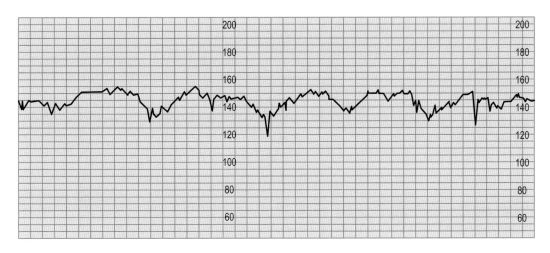

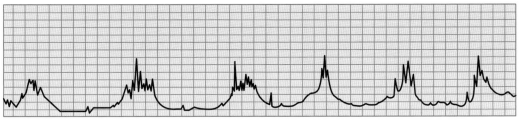

FIGURE 6-1 ■ Early decelerations.

Early decelerations are 'mirror images' of contractions and are associated with head compression in the late first and second stages of labour (Fig 6-1). There is a slow reduction in FHR as the intensity of contraction increases – the lowest FHR or nadir of the deceleration is at the peak or acme of the contraction. There is slow recovery of the FHR to the baseline rate as the contraction abates and returns to the baseline. Since they are 'uniform' decelerations and are reflective of head compression causing vagal stimulation they should be seen only in the late first stage or second stage of labour. Early decelerations are not due to hypoxia and generally they do not decelerate >40 bpm below the baseline rate.

Variable decelerations are 'non-uniform' and have a precipitous fall from the baseline rate and a quick recovery back to the baseline FHR. They vary in shape, size and timing in relation to contractions. They are due to cord compression. They can also be due to head compression, being common with malpresentations and malpositions and when this is the case they do not have the slight increase in the FHR just prior to and at recovery of the FHR known as 'shouldering'. Those due to cord compression have a transient slight increase in the baseline FHR just before and after the deceleration ('shouldering') due to baroreceptor-mediated responses. These pre and post humps that are described as 'shouldering' are shown in Fig 6-2. Variable decelerations due to cord compression may be relieved by change of position of the mother or by amnioinfusion.[8]

Atypical variable decelerations (Fig 6-3). In a pregnancy, more than one mechanism of stress may operate on the fetus. There may be cord compression due to oligohydramnios causing variable decelerations and the same pregnancy may be associated with placental insufficiency, and with contractions the fetus may also exhibit late decelerations. When both mechanisms operate (cord compression and uteroplacental insufficiency at the same time) there may be a variable followed by late deceleration and these are known as 'combined' or 'biphasic' decelerations. The merger of the two of these can present as variable deceleration with late recovery of the FHR to the baseline rate, i.e. after the contraction has reached the baseline pressure. Variable decelerations with duration >60 seconds and depth >60 beats, and those with absence of baseline variability during the deceleration and between variable decelerations at the baseline rate, or an overshoot of the returning heart rate, or the absence of shouldering after being initially present, are classified as atypical variable decelerations. Atypical variable decelerations are considered an abnormal feature in a CTG trace, whilst simple variable decelerations are considered a non-reassuring feature.[3]

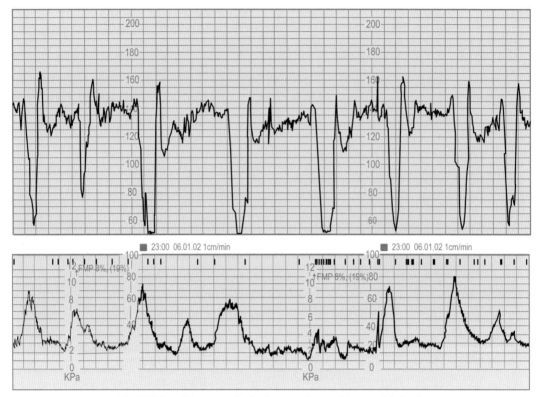

FIGURE 6-2 ■ Simple variable decelerations with 'shouldering'.

Late decelerations start towards the end or soon after the contraction peaks and the rate does not recover until well after the contraction has ceased. There is a lag of greater than 20 seconds before the onset of the contraction and that of the deceleration. When blood flow and oxygen supply to the intervillous space are critically reduced the FHR slows – an effect mediated via chemoreceptors. Typical late decelerations are shown in Figure 6-4. The combination of late decelerations (however subtle) with persistent tachycardia and reduced baseline variability is the most pathological FHR pattern and is almost invariably associated with fetal hypoxia (Fig 6-5).

FETAL BEHAVIOURAL STATE IN THE CTG – 'CYCLING'

Non-hypoxic fetuses have alternate '*active*' and '*quiet*' sleep epochs on the CTG and this is referred to as 'cycling'. During the active sleep epoch there are several accelerations and good baseline variability. During the quiet epoch there are no or occasional accelerations and the baseline variability may be reduced to <5 bpm. The quiet period can be 15–40 minutes and rarely more than 90 minutes unless influenced by medication.[9] In the late first stage of labour the CTG may show a long quiet epoch when the head is deeply in the pelvis or after a narcotic is given for pain relief. Occasionally, a healthy fetus that has accelerations and good baseline variability may show segments of reduced variability and shallow decelerations during the quiet epoch but this period does not usually last for >40 minutes, and rarely >90 minutes, and seems to be associated with fetal breathing episodes.[10]

The absence of cycling indicates the possibility of an insult or injury that may have already happened or it may be that the fetus is hypoxic or has sustained some injury such as infection or prior hypoxic insult. If the trace was reactive and cycling and then becomes pathological one may be able to identify the time of the insult. If the trace is pathological from the time of admission then the insult/injury may have already taken place and the timing of injury may be difficult to ascertain. A reactive heart rate pattern of a fetus that exhibits cycling from early labour to near full dilatation is shown in Figure 6-6.

Cycling with an 'active' followed by a 'quiet' sleep pattern suggests that the baby is well oxygenated and likely to be non-hypoxic and

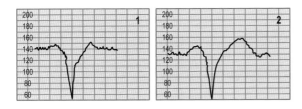

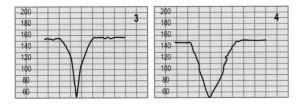

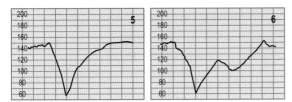

FIGURE 6-3 ■ (1) Typical variable deceleration with shouldering; (2) atypical variable deceleration with overshoot; (3) atypical variable deceleration with loss of shouldering; (4) atypical variable deceleration showing loss of variability, and a depth of deceleration of 60 beats for >60 seconds; (5) atypical variable deceleration with late recovery; (6) atypical variable deceleration with a variable and late component.

'neurologically normal'. Absence of cycling may be due to drugs, infection, cerebral haemorrhage, chromosomal or congenital malformation, or previous brain damage. A previously brain damaged fetus may or may not show cycling but the cord pH is likely to be normal if there are accelerations. Such infants may exhibit signs of neurological damage later on in life.

> 'The foetal pulsation is much more frequent than the maternal pulse ... being about 130 or 140 in the minute; however, it is not necessarily observed to beat always at this rate ... This variation may depend upon a variety of inherent vital causes in the foetus ... An obvious explanation, however, is muscular action on the part of the foetus; and we shall very generally observe the pulsation of the foetal heart increased in frequency after such. The external cause which we shall find most frequently to operate on the fetal circulation, is uterine action, particularly when long continued, as in labour'.
> Evory Kennedy
> Observations on Obstetric Auscultation. Dublin: Longman, 1833

IDENTIFICATION OF INDIVIDUAL FEATURES OF CTG TRACE AND THEIR CLASSIFICATION

The NICE guidelines have provided a framework to categorize the CTG as normal, suspicious or pathological.[3] Once the trace is categorized as suspicious or pathological by the attendant he/she has to seek the possible cause and take action. Action may be one or more of the following: observation and continue with labour, hydration, stopping oxytocin, repositioning the mother, tocolysis, fetal scalp blood sampling, or delivery by the most appropriate route. This decision will depend on the parity, cervical dilatation, rate of progress of labour, and risk factors based on the past and current obstetric history. The mother should be told of the issues involved and the possible actions needed, which should be based on informed choice and with her consent.

Classification of the Individual Features of the FHR Trace[3]

See Table 6-2.

Classification of the Cardiotocograph[3]

- *Normal* – all four features are reassuring.
- *Suspicious* – one of the features is non-reassuring.
- *Pathological* – ≥2 non-reassuring features; ≥1 abnormal feature.

The course of action necessary may vary even within the pathological category. If there is one feature that is abnormal (e.g. only atypical variable decelerations), simple remedial action/s (stopping oxytocin, hydration, repositioning the woman, tocolytics) and observation may be adequate. On the other hand if three features are abnormal (tachycardia, reduced baseline variability and atypical variable or late decelerations) the remedial actions may be those indicated earlier and in addition may include fetal scalp blood sampling (FBS) for pH or delivery, as thought to be most appropriate depending on the clinical situation.

Sinusoidal Pattern

Sinusoidal pattern is a description of the trace where the FHR appears like a sine wave form (Fig 6-7) but has none of the other features of baseline variability, accelerations or decelerations. Sinusoidal pattern was first described in

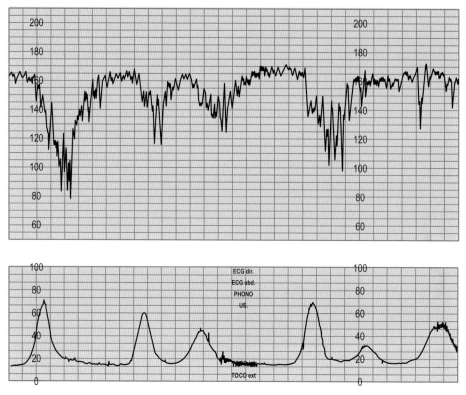

FIGURE 6-4 ■ Late decelerations. The deceleration starts at or beyond the acme of the uterine contraction (lag >20 seconds), is uniform in shape and does not recover until well after the contraction is over.

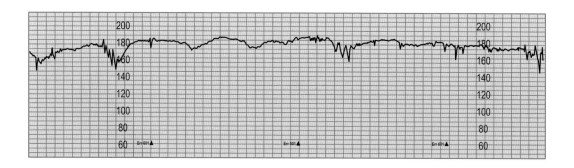

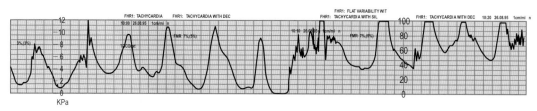

FIGURE 6-5 ■ Combination of late decelerations, persistent tachycardia and reduced baseline variability – the FHR pattern most consistently associated with fetal hypoxaemia/hypoxia.

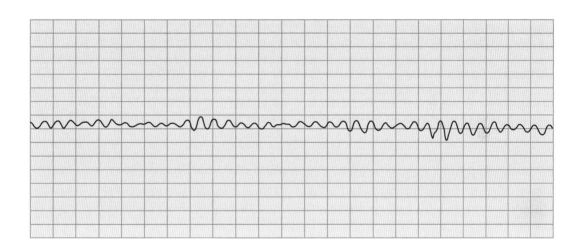

FIGURE 6-6 ■ Active epochs with accelerations and good baseline variability, alternating with quiet epochs with hardly any acceleration and reduced baseline variability, can be seen in a CTG trace from the beginning to the end of labour.

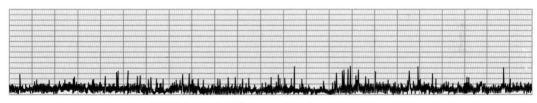

FIGURE 6-7 ■ A CTG trace with sinusoidal pattern.

TABLE 6-2   Features of the FHR Trace – Adapted from NICE Guidelines[3]

	Baseline Rate (bpm)	Variability (bpm)	Decelerations	Accelerations*
Reassuring	110–160	≥5	None Early	Present
Non-reassuring	100–109	<5 for ≥40 min but <90 min	Variable for >50% over 90 mins	
	161–180		Single prolonged <3 min	
Abnormal	<100	<5 for >90 min	Atypical variable &/or late for >50% of contractions over a 30 min period	
	>180	Sinusoidal pattern for >10 min	Single prolonged deceleration >3 min	

*The absence of accelerations with an otherwise normal CTG is of uncertain significance.

fetuses with severe anaemia – pathological sinusoidal pattern.[11] Fetuses that are healthy and thumb sucking, as observed in an ultrasound examination, can also exhibit a physiological sinusoidal pattern.[12] Doppler velocimetry of the middle cerebral artery shows increased velocity and is currently used to detect fetal anaemia.[13] The following are the known reasons for fetal anaemia that could give rise to a sinusoidal pattern.

Blood Group Antibodies that Cross the Placenta

In Rhesus iso-immunization higher concentration of antibodies can give rise to in utero anaemia. Maternal blood tests will reveal the presence of Rhesus antibodies and the concentration of antibodies can be measured. Presence of anti-Kell and anti-Duff antibodies can cause fetal anaemia. ABO blood group antibodies usually cause neonatal jaundice rather than fetal anaemia. Lewis a and b and M and N blood group antibodies are less likely to cause fetal anaemia.

Haemoglobinopathy

Alpha-thalassaemia in the fetus results in anaemia that may be associated with a sinusoidal pattern.

Usually the mother presents in early third trimester with oedema and signs of pre-eclampsia. Ultrasound examination may reveal polyhydramnios, hyperplacentosis and hydrops fetalis ('Bart's hydrops' due to four gene deletions). In these cases the mother may be a known thalassaemia carrier. Termination of pregnancy should be offered, as the fetus with Bart's hydrops does not survive. Currently, in utero stem cell therapy is being studied to salvage these fetuses.

Fetal Infection

Parvo virus infection is known to cause fetal anaemia. If a mother comes with a history of reduced or no FM after a flu-like infection, an ultrasound examination would be useful in the presence of a sinusoidal pattern. A fetus appropriate for gestational age with reduced movement and with poor tone (open palm), or a hydropic fetus with ascites is suggestive of fetal anaemia. Referral to a fetal medicine unit would be necessary to make a definitive diagnosis and possible therapy by intrauterine blood transfusion.

Feto-Maternal Transfusion

This is a well-known cause of fetal anaemia and may show a pseudo-sinusoidal pattern (Fig 6-8).

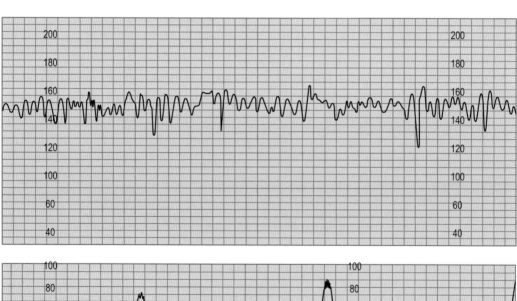
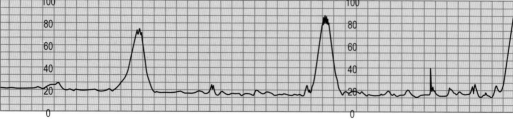

FIGURE 6-8 ■ A CTG trace with pseudo-sinusoidal pattern.

The Kleihauer–Betke test should identify fetal cells in maternal blood to confirm that the cause of anaemia is feto-maternal haemorrhage.

MONITORING UTERINE CONTRACTIONS

Interpretation of the FHR pattern in labour is not possible without relating it to uterine contractions. Contractions are monitored by palpating the uterus between the uterine fundus and the umbilicus. By counting the number of contractions over a 10-minute period the frequency of uterine contractions can be accurately assessed. The duration of contractions can be assessed to some degree of accuracy by palpation. The baseline pressure and the amplitude or strength of contraction cannot be deduced by palpation. The observed uterine activity is usually charted in specific boxes provided on the partogram. There are five boxes and depending on the number of contractions over 10 minutes the boxes are shaded. If the contractions last for <20 seconds, dots are used; if the duration is 20–40 seconds oblique lines are drawn; and if it is >40 seconds the boxes are completely shaded (Fig 6-9).

External tocography is performed by placing a transducer firmly across the abdomen over the uterus, midway between the uterine fundus and the umbilicus. With uterine contraction the upper part of the uterus expands anteriorly pushing the diaphragm or button on the toco transducer to produce the contraction curves. The baseline pressure can be set to 20 mmHg by using an automatic adjustment switch or by turning the toco knob on the machine. The contraction curves recorded will help to calculate the frequency and the duration accurately but not the baseline pressure or the amplitude of the uterine contractions.

Fluid-filled intrauterine catheters can show inaccurate readings associated with blockage by vernix and blood clots. Disposable transducer tipped catheters that are easy to insert are used to record the baseline pressure, frequency, duration and amplitude of contractions accurately. The area under each contraction above the baseline pressure can be quantified as the uterine activity in kilopascals every 15 minutes and annotated on the CTG trace[14] (Fig 6-10). The uterine activity in normal nulliparous and multiparous labour was studied[15,16] with a view to utilizing these values for induction and augmentation of labour. However, randomized-controlled trials did not show any benefit using

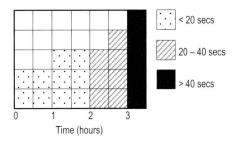

FIGURE 6-9 ■ Quantification of uterine contractions by clinical palpation. Frequency per 10 minutes is recorded by shading the equivalent number of boxes. The type of shading indicates the duration of each contraction.

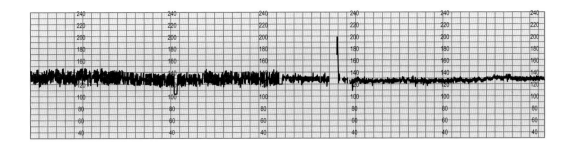

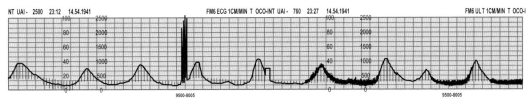

FIGURE 6-10 ■ Quantification of uterine activity by using electronic technology.

intrauterine catheters for induced or augmented labour when compared with external tocography,[17,18] and hence is not recommended for routine use. Palpation of uterine contractions is the norm in low-risk labour and external tocography in high-risk labour.

> 'The discharge of meconium pending labour, in cases where the head presents, is dwelt upon by some as proving the death of the child. But its palpable insufficiency in this respect has been so well pointed out by Dr. Denman and indeed must be so obvious to every practical man, that it is deemed unnecessary to dwell upon it here, further than to state that it merits no confidence whatsoever, as a proof of the death of the fetus'.
> Evory Kennedy
> Observations on Obstetric Auscultation.
> Dublin: Longman, 1833

MECONIUM-STAINED AMNIOTIC FLUID

Meconium is the passage of bowel contents that usually occurs after birth but can happen in utero. The appearance of meconium in the amniotic fluid usually starts at term and the incidence increases with the period of gestation and is considered a function of maturing peristalsis.[19] An alternative explanation is that the meconium is passed due to hypoxia causing relaxation of the fetal anal sphincter. It is rare to find meconium-stained fluid in the preterm period. When it is found preterm it is usually due to infection and can be associated with listeriosis.[20]

It is not common to find meconium in cases of acute hypoxia, like cord prolapse or placental abruption. The chance of developing acidosis is greater in the presence of thick compared with light meconium-stained fluid in the presence of a pathological FHR pattern.[21] It is also known that when the FHR is pathological in the presence of meconium, acidosis develops faster compared with clear fluid.[22] Hence, the presence of meconium is an indication for continuous EFM. If the FHR is reactive and normal the chance of acidosis is minimal and there is no need to do FBS to establish the fetal condition. On the other hand, if the CTG becomes pathological in the presence of meconium, FBS should be considered at an earlier stage. In clinical practice the presence of thick meconium with scanty fluid is of concern, as oligohydramnios may be due to reduced placental function.

An additional concern is the possibility of meconium aspiration during labour or at the time of birth. Meconium aspiration has no correlation to fetal acidaemia. No clear mechanism as to why the fetus aspirates meconium is known.[23] It is postulated that it may be associated with hypoxic episodes in utero. Suctioning the oropharynx and nasopharynx at birth was the routine, but current evidence does not support the practice in order to prevent stimulation that may cause the fetus to aspirate.[24] If the baby does not cry, suction followed by laryngoscopy for signs of meconium below the vocal cords should be carried out and, if present, gastric and bronchial lavage is performed to minimize the chances of meconium aspiration syndrome. The chemical pneumonitis caused by meconium can be fatal. Amnioinfusion is practised in some centres to dilute the meconium in the amniotic fluid and reduce in utero meconium aspiration.[25] In 2010, Cochrane reviewed 13 trials consisting of 4143 women where the intervention group had saline amnio-infusion. This was found to benefit babies in settings where there were inadequate facilities for continuous monitoring. Additional research is needed to fully evaluate the benefits to the mother and baby.[26]

FETAL SCALP BLOOD SAMPLING

Prolonged bradycardia (deceleration), or a trace with markedly reduced baseline variability and late or atypical variable decelerations that are preterminal patterns, warrant immediate delivery without FBS. Placental abruption, scar rupture or cord prolapse also necessitate immediate delivery. Excluding the above, other changes in the CTG may be of concern but do not always reflect fetal hypoxia and acidosis. The parity, cervical dilatation, progress of labour and obstetric risk factors (e.g. the presence of meconium, intrauterine growth restriction, etc.) may dictate the need for FBS, close observation in anticipation of vaginal delivery, or delivery. With pathological CTG a policy of awaiting spontaneous delivery or instrumental delivery in a short time may be acceptable in a multipara in the late first stage of labour who shows good progress of labour, whilst a caesarean section may be more appropriate if there is thick meconium in a primigravid who is 3–4 cm dilated. FBS may be considered if the woman is 5–6 cm dilated without any risk factors with a pathological CTG. Good analysis of the clinical situation and the CTG should reduce the incidence of FBS without compromising the fetus.

Cochrane reviews suggest that the relative risk of having a caesarean section with EFM without the use of FBS is 1.72 (1.38–2.15) and with FBS it is 1.24 (1.05–1.48).[27] The cut-off

TABLE 6-3	Actions Based on FBS Levels	
pH	Condition	Action
<7.20	Acidosis	Immediate delivery
7.20–7.25	Pre-acidosis	Consider another FBS in 30 minutes
>7.25	Normal	Observe the CTG and if it does not improve consider another FBS based on the clinical situation and the evolving CTG pattern

values in Table 6-3 are considered for action based on FBS.

If the result of the last FBS was closer to but above 7.25, or the CTG is getting worse (rise in baseline FHR, increase in the depth and duration of decelerations, reduction in variability), or there are additional risk factors like meconium, perform the FBS within an hour. Considering the rate of decline of the pH and the progress in labour between the FBS time intervals, one may be able to make the clinical decision whether to allow more time for labour to progress or to deliver the fetus.

FBS is contraindicated where it is likely to lead to permanent fetal compromise such as in cases of HIV; herpes; hepatitis B carriers; suspected or confirmed cases of intrauterine infection; and in those with bleeding disorders. The intermittent nature of FBS may need several samples to make a clear decision and is a cause of discomfort to the mother. The difficulty in obtaining fetal scalp blood samples has made adjunctive methods of ascertaining the fetal condition more attractive. The methods that are used in place of FBS or as an adjunct are described below.

ALTERNATE OR ADJUNCTIVE METHODS OF ASSESSING FETAL HEALTH

Fetal Stimulation Tests

Stimulation of an adult brought unconscious to an emergency department is a standard procedure and the level of arousal is considered a marker of the level of insult to the central nervous system. Extending the same principle, investigators have shown that FHR acceleration in response to an external stimulus is likely to be associated with a fetus that is not acidotic. Clarke

et al showed that the fetal scalp pH was greater than 7.20 when it responded with a FHR acceleration to the stimulation of FBS.[28] The type of stimulation was extended to the use of Allis tissue forceps applied to the scalp[29,30] and then to a vibroacoustic stimulus through the maternal abdomen.[31,32] When the fetus responded with an acceleration the fetal pH was >7.20, but when there was no response about 50% of the fetuses were acidotic. Concern was raised about stress to the fetus by the vibroacoustic stimulus because of prolonged periods of tachycardia following such stimulus in some fetuses.[33] Measurement of catecholamines in the umbilical cord blood during indicated cordocentesis has not shown any such increase after vibroacoustic stimulation.[34] Fear of auditory damage has been alleviated by follow-up testing at 4 years of age.[35,36]

Despite such reassurance the method has not found favour in many countries except North America. A meta-analysis reviewed the likelihood ratios and 95% confidence intervals (CI) for some of the available observational studies on vibroacoustic stimulation tests.[37] The Cochrane review points to the difficulty in recommending this method due to the absence of randomized-controlled trials.[38] More studies are needed to establish this as an acceptable method in clinical practice.

Fetal Pulse Oximetry

Pulse oximetry is used in intensive care and anaesthesia to monitor oxygen saturation in the adult. The same principle has been adapted for use to monitor the fetus in labour. Oxygen saturation is very variable in the fetus and the normal range fluctuates between 30% and 80%.[39] The sensors are placed apposed to the fetal cheek and held in position by the design which exerts counter pressure on the lower uterine segment to press the sensing surface against the fetal skin. Fetal scalp oximetry sensors that can be secured to the scalp have become available. Based on animal experiments and observational studies in the human fetus, the threshold value for action has been identified as 30% over a period of 10 minutes.[40] A number of prospective studies have assessed the feasibility and usefulness of this methodology in busy labour ward settings.[41]

The latest Cochrane review (2012) considered six trials involving 7654 women. Although there was a reduction in CS (Caesarean Section) rate for fetal concerns, there was no difference in overall CS rate between the CTG only and CTG and pulse oximetry arm.[42] Further randomized trials are needed before recommending pulse oximetry into routine clinical practice.

Fetal ECG Waveform Analysis

Animal experimental work consistently showed an elevation of the ST segment or rise in the T wave with increasing hypoxia.[43,44] It has been observed that the degree of hypoxia prior to such changes depends on the myocardial glycogen in each species. Myocardial glycogen is mobilized to glucose in response to catecholamine release associated with hypoxic stress and the ST changes are due to entry of glucose into the cells with potassium (K^+). The fetal ECG signal is obtained with the help of a spiral electrode applied to the scalp of the fetus.[45,46] A maternal skin electrode is needed and computer software in the ST waveform analyser (STAN 21 or 31- Neoventa, Goteborg, Sweden) formulates a sample ECG from 30 received complexes and analyses the T/QRS ratio.

The computer analysis of ECG to identify the baseline rise or episodic rise of T/QRS ratio is based on identifying the lowest T/QRS ratio for that fetus. This is done by the computer calculating the lowest T/QRS for 20 minutes by a moving window method (e.g. 4.20–4.40 hours, 4.21–4.41 hours and so on). The lowest T/QRS ratio for the previous 3 hours is considered for calculating the rise in T/QRS ratio. Therefore, the event log requires 20 minutes before automatic ST analysis can begin. During the first 20 minutes of use and when there is a decrease in signal quality with discontinuous T/QRS ratios (there should be at least 10 signals in a 10-minute window for computer analysis), manual data analysis is required. If the machine is disconnected from the woman, and then reconnected within 3 hours, the computer retains the lowest 20-minute T/QRS ratio in memory from the previous 3 hours for that fetus. This enables it to provide the analysis with change in T/QRS ratio once the equipment is reconnected.

In addition to rise in the T/QRS ratio (Fig 6-11) there may be changes in the ST segment – these are known as biphasic ST waveform (Fig 6-12). If the ST waveform changes are above the isoelectric line it is called biphasic grade I, if it cuts the isoelectric line, it is biphasic grade II and if the changes are below the isoelectric line it is grade III. The change is due to repolarization of the ventricle and is a function of the flow of current from endocardium to epicardium. These changes are seen often in a preterm fetus and may be due to the thickness of the myocardium; hence, ST analysis is not used in fetuses less than 36 completed weeks. In addition to chronic hypoxia it may be seen in the initial phases of acute hypoxia, in cases of

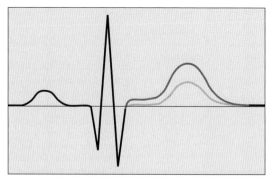

FIGURE 6-11 ■ Fetal ECG waveform analysis. The rise in ST segment and increase in T wave height with hypoxia, epinephrine (adrenaline) surge and anaerobic metabolism.

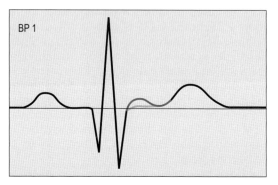

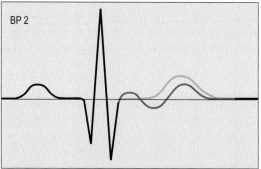

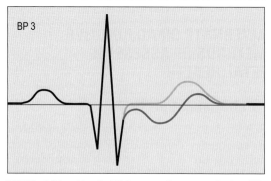

FIGURE 6-12 ■ Fetal ECG waveform analysis. BP1 biphasic grade 1 (ST change is above the isoelectric line). BP2 biphasic grade 2 (ST change cuts the isoelectric line). BP3 biphasic grade 3 (ST change is below the isoelectric line).

myocardial dystrophy and with maternal fever and infection.

If the biphasic events occur in a continuous manner the computer will flag it as an ST event and will indicate whether the biphasic ST changes were continuous for >5 minutes or >2 minutes. If the biphasic events are more than a couple it will be flagged as an ST event. More than two episodes with a suspicious CTG trace and more than one episode with a pathological trace is an indication for intervention.

Significant ST events identified by the ST analyser are flagged and described according to the type (e.g. baseline T/QRS rise, episodic rise in T/QRS, continuous biphasic patterns >2 or 5 minutes, or episodes of biphasic patterns) and *magnitude* of change. These STAN events need to be correlated with the CTG, which needs to be visually interpreted. If one is unable to categorize the CTG as suspicious or pathological then FBS may be required to resolve the situation. The STAN guidelines for taking action are given in Table 6-4. Actions does not mean operative delivery; if there are reversible features like stopping oxytocin, change of posture of the mother and hydration, those should be undertaken whilst observing the improvement of the CTG. If there is no improvement then operative delivery may be indicated.

The results of six randomized-controlled trials consisting of 16 295 women were evaluated by Cochrane to assess the benefits of ECG plus CTG in labour.[47] Those who had ECG waveform analysis as an adjunct to CTG had fewer blood samples and less total operative deliveries. However, there was no reduction in CS rates. The earlier trials showed significant reduction in metabolic acidosis and neonatal encephalopathy[48,49] but the recent Cochrane analysis of a larger cohort did not show the same benefit.

Fetal Scalp Lactate Measurements

Metabolic acidosis is reflected by a measure of pH and BE (Base Excess) or by lactate. The build-up of lactate is related to hypoxia >10 minutes. The duration of hypoxia will determine the lactate levels and it takes hours to clear even after the hypoxia is corrected.

A prospective randomized study compared lactate with pH analysis at FBS and found no significant differences in caesarean section rates, or cord artery pH.[50] Lactate analysis needs only 5 µL of blood and a bedside hand-held monitor, compared with 35 µL needed for most automatic pH and blood gas analyses. Hence, FBS for lactate is more successful than for pH and BE.

Scalp blood lactate correlates well with umbilical arterial and venous lactate, indicating that it could be used for clinical decision-making.[51] The surrogate measures considered for subsequent neurological outcome of the new-born such as Apgar scores, cord arterial pH and base deficit have good correlation with cord blood lactate levels.[52,53] The use of lactate or pH and base deficit has similar sensitivity, specificity and predictive values for perinatal complications.[54] Cochrane reviewed two studies consisting of 3348 mother–baby pairs to evaluate the use of lactate in labour and concluded that the perinatal outcome was the same in the lactate arm as in the the pH and base excess calculation arm.[55] The chance of getting a result was better with lactate because of the small volume needed for analysis. The numbers were too small to show any reduction in CS rates.

TABLE 6-4 **STAN Guidelines – The Use of CTG and STAN Event (The Type and the Magnitude) for Decision-Making**

ST Events	Normal CTG	Intermediary CTG	Abnormal CTG	Preterminal CTG
Episodic T/QRS rise	• Expectant management	• > 0.15	• > 0.10	• Immediate delivery
Baseline T/QRS rise	• Continued observation	• > 0.10	• > 0.05	
Biphasic ST		• 3 Biphasic log messages[†]	• 2 Biphasic log messages[†]	

These guidelines may indicate situations in which obstetric intervention* is required.

*Intervention may include delivery or maternal–fetal resuscitation by alleviation of contributing problems such as overstimulation or maternal hypotension and hypoxia.

[†]The time span between the Biphasic messages should be related to the CTG pattern and the clinical situation.

INTRAPARTUM MATERNAL PYREXIA AND NEONATAL ENCEPHALOPATHY

There are several risk factors for neonatal encephalopathy and maternal pyrexia is being increasingly identified as a major determinant. A study from Western Australia reported an odds ratio for neonatal encephalopathy of 3.82 for maternal pyrexia, compared with 4.29 for persistent occipito-posterior position and 4.44 for an acute intrapartum event.[56] Intrapartum fever is also associated with epidural use.[57] In a series of 4915 low-risk term labours, after controlling for epidural use the odds ratio for neonatal encephalopathy with intrapartum pyrexia was 4.7 (1.3–17.4).[58] There was also a higher incidence of metabolic acidosis (odds ratio 2.91; 1.14–7.39), and admission to neonatal intensive care (odds ratio 1.78; 1.1–2.89).

Not only the incidence of neonatal encephalopathy but the incidence of cerebral palsy is increased in women who have pyrexia exceeding 38°C in labour, with an odds ratio as high as 9.3 (CI 2.7–31.0).[59]

CONCLUSIONS

Labour poses a threat to the fetus because the contractions needed to cause cervical dilatation and descent of the head can also reduce the blood supply to the utero-placental area and may cause cord compression. Appropriate fetal surveillance based on the perceived risk should be offered. The woman and her partner's wishes need to be considered. In the UK low-risk mothers are offered IA. Those with increased risk are offered EFM. Historical studies on EFM showed reduction in intrapartum stillbirths, but the subsequent randomized studies have not shown reduction in perinatal mortality and morbidity. One reason may be that most studies were in low-risk labours and were underpowered to show a significant difference in the rare events of hypoxic ischaemic encephalopathy, cerebral palsy or intrapartum deaths. Several studies, including the recent analysis by the National Health Service Litigation authority, have shown that there was significant incidence of substandard care.[60] Inability to interpret the CTG, failure to incorporate the clinical picture, delay in intervention and poor communication are the main factors.[61] Studies based on neuroimaging suggest that 27% of cases of cerebral palsy in term infants may be due to intrapartum asphyxia – few may be pure intrapartum and the majority may

be due to a combination of antepartum and intrapartum risk factors.[62]

In order to overcome the difficulties in interpretation of CTGs the RCOG and RCM have combined with e-learning for Health Care in the UK to produce an electronic learning package on intrapartum surveillance that is free of charge for all NHS staff.[63] Trials are ongoing to look at computer analysis of CTG (INFANT Trial) and computerized ECG and CTG interpretation in high-risk women in labour. The NHS Litigation Authority (NHSLA) report also has shown reduction of mistakes in CTG interpretation, which suggests continuing education may have been effective.[60] (These issues are discussed further in Chapter 7.)

In concluding we recommend the following basic principles be followed when interpreting a CTG in labour:[64]

- Accelerations and baseline variability are hallmarks of fetal health
- Accelerations without baseline variability should be considered suspicious
- Periods of decreased variability without decelerations may represent quiet sleep
- Hypoxic fetuses may have a normal baseline FHR of 110–160 bpm with no accelerations and baseline variability of <5 for >40 minutes
- In the presence of baseline variability <5 bpm even shallow late decelerations <15 bpm are ominous in a non-reactive trace
- Abruption, cord prolapse and scar rupture can cause acute hypoxia and should be suspected and managed clinically (may give rise to prolonged decelerations/bradycardia)
- Fetal hypoxia and acidosis may develop faster with an abnormal trace when there is scanty fluid with thick meconium, intrauterine growth restriction, intrauterine infection with pyrexia, bleeding and/or pre- or post-term labour
- In preterm fetuses (especially <34 weeks), hypoxia and acidosis can increase the likelihood of respiratory distress syndrome and may contribute to intraventricular haemorrhage, warranting early intervention in the presence of an abnormal trace
- Hypoxia can be made worse by oxytocin, epidural analgesia and difficult operative deliveries
- During labour, if decelerations are absent, asphyxia is unlikely although it cannot be completely excluded
- Abnormal patterns may represent the effects of drugs, fetal anomaly, fetal injury or infection and not only hypoxia.

Acknowledgements

The authors acknowledge Mr Donald Gibb and Elsevier for permission to reproduce in Chapters 6 and 7 some of the figures from *Fetal Monitoring in Practice*, 2nd edn. Oxford: Butterworth 1997.

REFERENCES

1. Thacker SB, Stroup DF, Chang M. Continuous electronic heart rate monitoring for fetal assessment during labor (Cochrane review). Chichester: John Wiley; 2004. The Cochrane Library p. 1.
2. Alfirevic Z, Devane D, Gyte GML. Comparing continuous electronic monitoring of the baby's heartbeat in labour using cardiotocography (CTG, sometimes known as EFM) with intermittent monitoring (intermittent auscultation, IA). Published Online: 8 Oct 2008. Available at http://summaries.cochrane.org/CD006066/comparing-continuous-electronic-monitoring-of-the-babys-heartbeat-in-labour-using-cardiotocography-ctg-sometimes-known-as-efm-with-intermittent-monitoring-intermittent-auscultation-ia
3. National Institute of Clinical Excellence. Intrapartum care: care of healthy women and their babies during childbirth. This guideline is an update of 'Electronic fetal monitoring: the use and interpretation of cardiotocography in intrapartum fetal surveillance' (Guideline C) issued in May 2001. Clinical guideline 55 – 2007. Available at http://publications.nice.org.uk/intrapartum-care-cg55
4. Society of Obstetricians and Gynaecologists of Canada. Fetal health surveillance: antepartum and intrapartum – consensus guideline. J Obstet Gynaecol Can 2007;29(Suppl. 4):S1–56. http://www.sogc.org/guidelines/documents/gui197CPG0709.pdf
5. American College of Obstetricians and Gynecologists. ACOG Practice Bulletin No. 106: Intrapartum fetal heart rate monitoring: nomenclature, interpretation, and general management principles. Obstet Gynecol 2009;114:192–202. doi: 10.1097/AOG.0b013e3181aef106.
6. Kubli FW, Hon EH, Khazin AF, Takemura H. Observations on heart rate and pH in the human fetus during labour. Am J Obstet Gynecol 1969;109:1190–206.
7. Beard RW, Filshie GM, Knight CA, Roberts GM. The significance of the changes in the continuous fetal heart rate in the first stage of labour. J Obstet Gynaecol Br Commw 1971;78:865–81.
8. Miyazaki FS, Nevarez F. Saline amniotic infusion for relief of repetitive variable decelerations: a prospective randomized study. Am J Obstet Gynecol 1985;153:301–3.
9. Spencer JAD, Johnson P. Fetal heart rate variability changes and fetal behavioural cycles during labour. Br J Obstet Gynaecol 1986;93:314–21.
10. Schifrin B, Artenos J, Lyseight N. Late-onset fetal cardiac decelerations associated with fetal breathing movements. J Matern Fetal Neonat Med 2002;12:253–9.
11. Modanlou HD, Freeman RH. Sinusoidal fetal heart rate patterns; its definition and clinical significance. Am J Obstet Gynecol 1982;142:1033–8.
12. Nijhuis JG, Staisch KJ, Martin C, Prechtel HFR. A sinusoidal like fetal heart rate pattern in association with fetal sucking. Report of 2 cases. Eur J Obstet Gynecol Reprod Biol 1984;16:353–8.
13. Mari G, Deter RL, Carpenter RL, Rahman F, Zimmerman R, Moise KJ Jr, et al. Noninvasive diagnosis by Doppler ultrasonography of fetal anemia due to maternal red-cell alloimmunization. Collaborative Group for Doppler Assessment of the Blood Velocity in Anemic Fetuses. N Engl J Med 2000;342:9–14.
14. Steer PJ. The measurement and control of uterine contractions. In: Beard RW, editor. The current status of fetal heart rate monitoring and ultrasound in obstetrics. London: RCOG Press; 1977.
15. Gibb DMF, Arulkumaran S, Lun KC, Ratnam SS. Characteristics of uterine activity in nulliparous labour. Br J Obstet Gynaecol 1984;91:220–7.
16. Arulkumaran S, Gibb DMF, Lun KC, Ratnam SS. The effect of parity on uterine activity in labour. Br J Obstet Gynaecol 1984;91:843–8.
17. Chua S, Kurup A, Arulkumaran S, Ratnam SS. Augmentation of labor: does internal tocography produce better obstetric outcome than external tocography? Obstet Gynecol 1990;76:164–7.
18. Arulkumaran S, Ingemarsson I, Ratnam SS. Oxytocin titration to achieve preset active contraction area values does not improve the outcome of induced labour. Br J Obstet Gynaecol 1987;94:242–8.
19. Miller FC. Meconium staining of the amniotic fluid. Clin Obstet Gynecol 1979;6:359–61.
20. Buchdahl R, Hird M, Gibb DMF. Listeriosis revisited: the role of the obstetrician. Br J Obstet Gynaecol 1990;97:186–9.
21. Arulkumaran S, Yeoh SC, Gibb DMF. Obstetric outcome of meconium stained liquor in labour. Singapore Med J 1985;26:523–6.
22. Steer PJ. Fetal distress. In: Crawford J, editor. Risks of labour. Chichester: John Wiley; 1985. p. 11–31.
23. Wiswell TE, Bent RC. Meconium staining and meconium aspiration syndrome. Unresolved issues. Pediatr Clin North Am 1993;40:955–81.
24. Vain NE, Szyld EG, Prudent LM, Wiswell TE, Aguilar AM, Vivas NI. Oropharyngeal and nasopharyngeal suctioning of meconium stained neonates before delivery of their shoulders: multicentre, randomised controlled trial. Lancet 2004;364:597–602.
25. Fraser WD, Hofmeyr J, Lede R, Faron G, Alexander S, Goffinet F, et al. Amnioinfusion for the prevention of the meconium aspiration syndrome. N Engl J Med 2005;353:909–17.
26. Hofmeyr GJ, Xu H. Amnioinfusion for meconium-stained liquor in labour. Published online: 8 Aug 2010. Available at http://summaries.cochrane.org/CD000014/amnioinfusion-for-meconium-stained-liquor-in-labour
27. Neilson JP. Fetal scalp blood sampling as adjunct to heart rate monitoring. In: Enkin MW, Keirse MJ, Renfew MJ, Neilson JP, editors. Pregnancy and childbirth module of the Cochrane database of systematic reviews. Cochrane Collaboration, Issue 2. Oxford: Update software UK; 1995.
28. Clarke SL, Gimovsky ML, Miller FC. Fetal heart rate response to scalp blood sampling. Am J Obstet Gynecol 1983;144:706–8.
29. Clarke SL, Gimovsky ML, Miller FC. The scalp stimulation test: a clinical alternative to fetal scalp blood sampling. Am J Obstet Gynecol 1984;148:274–7.
30. Arulkumaran S, Ingemarsson I, Ratnam SS. Fetal heart rate response to scalp stimulation as a test for fetal well-being in labour. Asia Oceania J Obstet Gynecol 1987;13:131–5.
31. Edersheim TG, Hutson JM, Druzin ML, Kogut EA. Fetal heart rate response to vibratory acoustic stimulation predicts fetal pH in labor. Am J Obstet Gynecol 1987;157:1557–60.
32. Ingemarsson I, Arulkumaran S. Reactive FHR response to sound stimulation in fetuses with low scalp blood pH. Br J Obstet Gynaecol 1989;96:562–5.

33. Spencer JAD, Deans A, Nicolaidis P, Arulkumaran S. Fetal response to vibroacoustic stimulation during low and high fetal heart rate variability episodes in late pregnancy. Am J Obstet Gynecol 1991;165:86–90.

34. Fisk NM, Nicolaidis P, Arulkumaran S. Vibroacoustic stimulation is not associated with sudden fetal catecholamine release. Early Hum Dev 1991;25:11–17.

35. Arulkumaran S, Skurr B, Tong H. No evidence of hearing loss due to fetal acoustic stimulation test. Obstet Gynecol 1991;78:283–5.

36. Nyman M, Barr M, Westgren M. A four year follow up of hearing and development in children exposed to in utero vibro-acoustic stimulation. Br J Obstet Gynaecol 1992;99:685–8.

37. Skupski DW, Rosenberg CR, Eglinton GS. Intrapartum fetal stimulation tests: a meta-analysis. Obstet Gynecol 2002;99:129–34.

38. East CE, Smyth RMD, Leader LR, Henshall NE, Colditz PB, Lau R, Tan KH. Vibroacoustic stimulation for fetal assessment in labour in the presence of a non-reassuring fetal heart rate trace. Cochrane Database Syst Rev. 2013;1:CD004664.

39. Chua S, Yeong SM, Razvi K, Arulkumaran S. Fetal oxygen saturation during labour. Br J Obstet Gynaecol 1997;104:1080–3.

40. Kuhnert M, Seelbach-Goebel B, Di Renzo GC, Howarth E, Butterwegge M, Murray JM. Guidelines for the use of fetal pulse oximetry during labour and delivery. Prenatal Neonatal Med 1998;3:423–33.

41. Chua S, Rhazvi K, Yeong SM, Arulkumaran S. Intrapartum fetal oxygen saturation monitoring in a busy labour ward. Eur J Obstet Gynecol Reprod Biol 1999;82:185–9.

42. East CE, Begg L, Colditz PB. Fetal pulse oximetry for fetal assessment in labour. Published online: 17 Oct 2012. Available at http://summaries.cochrane.org/CD004075/fetal-pulse-oximetry-for-fetal-assessment-in-labour

43. Rosen KG, Dagbjartsson A, Henriksson BA, Lagercrantz H, Kjellmer I. The relationship between circulating catecholamines and ST waveform in fetal lamb electrocardiogram during hypoxia. Am J Obstet Gynecol 1984;149:190–5.

44. Greene KR, Dawes GS, Lilja H, Rosen KG. Changes in the ST waveform of the lamb electrocardiogram with hypoxia. Am J Obstet Gynecol 1982;144:950–7.

45. Lilja H, Arulkumaran S, Lindecrantz K. Fetal ECG during labour; a presentation of a microprocessor based system. J Biomed Eng 1988;10:348–50.

46. Arulkumaran S, Lilja H, Lindecrantz K, Ratnam SS, Thavarasah AS, Rosen KG. Fetal ECG waveform analysis should improve fetal surveillance in labour. J Perinat Med 1990;187:13–22.

47. Neilson JP. Fetal electrocardiogram (ECG) for fetal monitoring during labour. Published online: 18 April 2012. Available at http://summaries.cochrane.org/CD000116/fetal-electrocardiogram-ecg-for-fetal-monitoring-during-labour

48. Westgate J, Harris M, Curnow JSH, Greene KR. Randomised trial of cardiotocography alone or with ST waveform analysis for intrapartum monitoring. Lancet 1992;2:194–8.

49. Amer-Wåhlin I, Hellsten C, Norén H, Hagberg H, Herbst A, Kjellmer I, et al. Cardiotocography only versus cardiotocography plus ST analysis of fetal electrocardiogram for intrapartum fetal monitoring: a Swedish randomised controlled trial. Lancet 2001; 358:534–8.

50. Westgren M, Kruger K, Ek S, Gruwevald C, Kublickas M, Naka K. Lactate compared with pH analysis at fetal scalp blood sampling. a prospective randomised study. Br J Obstet Gynaecol 1998;105:29–33.

51. Krüger K, Kublickas M, Westgren M. Lactate in scalp and cord blood from fetuses with ominous fetal heart rate patterns. Obstet Gynecol 1998;92:918–22.

52. Nordstrom L, Achanna S, Naka K, Arulkumaran S. Fetal and maternal lactate increase during active second stage of labour. Br J Obstet Gynaecol 2001;108:263–8.

53. Nordstrom L. Fetal scalp and cord blood lactate. Best Pract Res Clin Obstet Gynaecol 2004;18:467–76.

54. Kruger K, Hallberg B, Blennow M. Predictive value of fetal scalp blood lactate concentration and pH as a marker for neurologic disability. Am J Obstet Gynecol 1999;181:1072–8.

55. East CE, Leader LR, Sheehan P, Henshall NE, Colditz PB. Use of fetal scalp blood lactate for assessing fetal well-being during labour. Published online: 17Oct 2012. Available at http://summaries.cochrane.org/CD006174/use-of-fetal-scalp-blood-lactate-for-assessing-fetal-well-being-during-labour

56. Badawi N, Kurinczuk JJ, Keogh JM, Alessandri LM, O'Sullivan F, Burton PR, et al. Intrapartum risk factors for newborn encephalopathy: the Western Australian case–control study. BMJ 1998;317:1554–8.

57. Fusi L, Steer PJ, Maresh MJ, Beard RW. Maternal pyrexia associated with the use of epidural analgesia in labour. Lancet 1989;1:1250–2.

58. Impey L, Greenwood C, MacQuillan K, Reynolds M, Sheil O. Fever in labour and neonatal encephalopathy: a prospective cohort study. Br J Obstet Gynaecol 2001;108:594–7.

59. Grether JK, Nelson KB. Maternal infection and cerebral palsy in infants of normal birth weight. JAMA 1997;278:207–11.

60. Ten Years of Maternity Claims – An Analysis of NHS Litigation Authority Data. Published by NHS Litigation Authority, 2nd Floor, 151 Buckingham Palace Road, London, SW1W 9SZ, UK. © NHS Litigation Authority 2012.

61. Confidential Enquiry into Stillbirths and Deaths in Infancy. 4th Annual Report. London: Maternal and Child Health Research Consortium, 1997.

62. Hagberg B, Hagberg G, Beckung E, Uvebrant P. Changing panorama of cerebral palsy in Sweden. VII. Prevalence and origin in the birth year period 1991–1994. Acta Paediatrica 2001;90:271–7.

63. Electroninc Fetal monitoring. http://www.e-lfh.org.uk/projects/electronic-fetal-monitoring/

64. Arulkumaran S, Ingemarsson I, Montan S, Paul RH, Gibb D, Steer PJ, et al. Traces of you: fetal trace interpretation. Nederland: Philips Medical Systems; 2002. Ref. 4522 981 88671/862.

CHAPTER 7

Fetal Asphyxia

S Arulkumaran

'Abnormal parturition, besides ending in death or recovery, not infrequently had a third termination in other diseases ... a delay of only a few moments in the substitution of pulmonary for the ceased placental respiration would lead to the apprehension that even the want of a few breathings, if not fatal to the economy, may imprint a lasting injury upon it.'
  William John Little
  On the influence of abnormal parturition, difficult labours, premature birth, and asphyxia neonatorum, on the mental and physical condition of the child, especially in relation to deformities. Trans Obstet Soc London 1861–62; 3:293–344.

The National Health Service Litigation Authority (NHSLA) in the UK has recently published a 10-year review of maternity-related litigation.[1] For the period April 1995 to March 2011, of all medical litigation cases 20% were related to obstetrics and gynaecology; these accounted for 49% of the total pay-out, amounting to £5.2 billion. The largest sums within this were paid out for brain damage related to birth asphyxia. Detailed analysis revealed inability to interpret cardiotocograph (CTG) traces, failure to incorporate the clinical situation, delay in taking action and poor communication and team work. This is not a new phenomenon as these factors were identified in the 1997 Fourth Confidential Enquiry into Stillbirths and Deaths in Infancy (CESDI) that reported on intrapartum deaths of babies over 1500 g with no chromosomal or congenital malformation.[2] The latter inquiry found that 50% of deaths were avoidable and another 25% were potentially avoidable by a different action. Although only a small percentage of all births are affected by long-term neurological handicap or stillbirth they represent devastating outcomes for the parents and their family.

Since only a small percentage of cases of cerebral palsy are thought to be due to birth asphyxia whilst there are vast numbers of pathological CTGs which do not give rise to poor outcome, there is constant debate about whether an individual case is related to birth asphyxia. The advent of magnetic resonance imaging (MRI) and animal experimentation studying different types of hypoxia and induced brain injury have revealed that hypoxia at different stages of gestation results in injury of the part of the brain with the highest metabolic activity and growth at that stage of gestation. At term prolonged partial hypoxia causes injury to the motor cortical area whilst acute profound hypoxia causes injury to the thalamic, hypothalamic and basal ganglia regions.[3,4] The type of brain injury seen on MRI correlates with the type of cerebral palsy, i.e. motor cortical injury results in quadriplegic cerebral palsy whilst thalamic, hypothalamic, and basal ganglia injuries give rise to the athetoid or dyskinetic type of cerebral palsy. Based on such observations, a study from Sweden suggests that up to 28%[5] rather than the conventional 10% of cases[6] of cerebral palsy may be related to intrapartum asphyxia. In light of this information, this chapter examines the CTG patterns associated with injuries due to birth asphyxia and how birth asphyxia-related litigation may be reduced.

HYPOXAEMIA, HYPOXIA AND ASPHYXIA

In this chapter, the terms hypoxaemia, hypoxia and asphyxia are defined as follows: *hypoxaemia* refers to reduced oxygen in the blood and *hypoxia* refers to reduced oxygen in the tissues secondary to continuing hypoxaemia. *Asphyxia* is hypoxia and metabolic acidosis in the tissues. The fetus reacts to hypoxaemia by extracting more oxygen from the blood and this period is associated with reduced fetal movements and absence of fetal heart rate accelerations. With hypoxia there is a catecholamine surge causing vasoconstriction in non-essential organs (skin, muscle, bone, liver, intestines and kidneys), and an increase in cardiac output by raising the heart rate. This vascular redistribution mechanism maintains the oxygen requirements to the essential organs i.e. brain, heart and the adrenals. If the hypoxia is sustained, there is further deprivation of oxygen and the cells undertake anaerobic metabolism, converting glucose into lactic acid rather than CO_2 and water.

This state of hypoxia and metabolic acidosis results in asphyxia and is the final step before cellular and organ failure. The time needed to build up hypoxia and acidosis sufficient to cause asphyxia will vary from fetus to fetus depending on its 'physiological reserve' and also on the extent to which the blood supply to and from the placenta is disrupted. The disruption of oxygen supply may be a complete acute cessation due to placental abruption, or it may be intermittent in the form of cord compression in labour, or due to placental insufficiency. Lack of oxygen due to reduced placental perfusion associated with intrauterine growth restriction leads to hypoxaemic hypoxia, whilst that due to cord compression leads to ischaemic hypoxia, and these two mechanisms can co-exist. The different mechanisms of hypoxia that lead to acidosis and neurological injury have been studied by Myers[4] and are described below;

- Total asphyxia causes damage to the brainstem and thalamus
- Prolonged hypoxia with acidosis causes brain swelling and cortical necrosis
- Prolonged hypoxia without acidosis causes white matter damage
- Total asphyxia preceded by prolonged hypoxia with mixed acidosis causes damage to the cortex, thalamus and basal ganglia.

Based on the above, one should be able to identify the fetal heart rate (FHR) patterns associated with hypoxia and acidosis that may lead to neurological injury and these are discussed below.

FHR PATTERNS RELATED TO HYPOXIA AND ACIDOSIS

The features of the CTG (baseline rate, baseline variability, accelerations and decelerations) described in Chapter 6 may occur in various combinations in a given FHR trace. Beard et al showed that a fetus with FHR accelerations is unlikely to be acidotic.[7] Fleischer et al found that 50% of the fetuses may get acidotic in 90 minutes with late decelerations; in 120 minutes with variable decelerations; and in 190 minutes with reduced baseline variability.[8] By studying all four features of the FHR, certain patterns have been described that would suggest already existing hypoxia and neurological injury and others in which a rise in baseline rate and decelerations were prominent features before neurological injury occurred.[9] The evolution of acidosis is not an exact science, as the rate at

which acidosis develops depends on the type of FHR pattern and the 'physiological reserve' of the fetus. In the presence of similar pathological CTGs, those fetuses that are growth restricted, those with infection, or with scanty thick meconium-stained fluid develop hypoxia and acidosis at a faster rate than a fetus that is appropriately grown with a normal amount of clear amniotic fluid.[10,11]

The following patterns are described with adverse birth such as stillbirth or abnormal neurological outcome/cerebral palsy and may prove clinically useful in deciding the timing of intervention when taken in consideration with the clinical picture.

1. Acute hypoxia usually presents with prolonged bradycardia <80 bpm.[12]
2. Subacute hypoxia presents with steep decelerations reducing the FHR to <80 bpm and which last longer during the deceleration than the time the FHR is at the normal baseline rate.

The above two patterns usually present with acute clinical events such as placental abruption, cord prolapse or scar rupture, or in the late first or second stage of labour. At times the cause is not known and may be related to occult cord compression.

3. Gradually developing hypoxia may be manifest with the appearance of decelerations, absent accelerations, increasing tachycardia and finally marked reduction in baseline variability.
4. Longstanding hypoxia may show a pattern with reduced baseline variability and shallow late decelerations in a non-reactive trace.

Acute Hypoxia

Prolonged bradycardia or deceleration <80 bpm leads to acute hypoxia and if it is associated with placental abruption, cord prolapse and uterine scar rupture warrants immediate delivery. Uterine hyperstimulation causing bradycardia can be dealt with by acute tocolysis (see Chapter 28). Important considerations in other cases are the CTG prior to the bradycardia and potentially influencing associations such as thick meconium-stained amniotic fluid, intrauterine growth restriction (IUGR), infection and antepartum haemorrhage – in which acidosis can develop rapidly.

A FHR <80 bpm for longer than 6 minutes, i.e. prolonged bradycardia/prolonged deceleration, can lead to rapid acute hypoxia and acidosis. A prolonged deceleration <3 minutes is considered suspicious and >3 minutes as abnormal.[13]

Causes of transient bradycardia include hypotension (e.g. regional anaesthesia), dorsal position of the mother, uterine hyperstimulation, artificial rupture of the membranes and vaginal examination. In these cases remedial actions should be undertaken, such as maternal repositioning; correction of hypotension; stopping oxytocin and acute tocolysis for hyperstimulation with prostaglandins whilst awaiting recovery of the FHR. Pressure on the head at crowning with maternal bearing down in the second stage may also be associated with bradycardia, and if it does not recover within 6 minutes delivery should be expedited. At times the cause for bradycardia is not known and the FHR may not recover, despite the usual resuscitative measures, necessitating immediate delivery. The longer the bradycardia the greater is the chance for fetal acidosis.[12] The pH is likely to decline more rapidly in high-risk clinical situations such as thick meconium, oligohydramnios, IUGR, intrauterine infection and in cases where the CTG was suspicious or pathological before the onset of bradycardia. In such cases, if the bradycardia does not recover by 6 to 7 minutes, delivery should be undertaken immediately.

The placenta acts as the lungs for the fetus in utero. Carbon dioxide is eliminated and oxygen is absorbed through the placenta. For optimal gas exchange there should be adequate circulation on the maternal and fetal sides of the placenta. With the normal FHR of about 140 bpm for 10 minutes there are 1400 circulations through the placenta that help transfer carbon dioxide out of the fetal circulation and absorb adequate oxygen for the fetus. When the FHR is 80 bpm there will be only 800 circulations in 10 minutes and the fetus will miss 600 circulations. The amount of carbon dioxide excreted becomes less and accumulates within the fetus, leading to the formation of carbonic acid with a decline in pH – respiratory acidosis. With increasing duration of bradycardia the oxygen transferred to the fetus is also reduced, leading to anaerobic metabolism and accumulation of metabolites giving rise to metabolic acidosis within the cell with the drop of the pH. This has an additive effect to the already existing respiratory acidosis. Acidosis causes malfunction of the intracellular metabolic process, e.g. the Na^+/K^+ pump that maintains the cell wall integrity. This leads to influx of fluid and cell oedema that causes cell malfunction and finally death if the injury is not reversed in time.

If the FHR returns to normal within a short period of time the number of circulations through the placenta will normalize, allowing the respiratory acidosis to be corrected by transferring the carbon dioxide to the maternal circulation. This is a quick process whilst reversal of metabolic acidosis takes longer. If conservative measures fail, and the FHR does not return to normal within 6–9 minutes, delivery of the fetus and establishing neonatal respiration will quickly reverse the respiratory acidosis and, with time, the metabolic acidosis.

Subacute Hypoxia

Prolonged decelerations with the FHR below the baseline for a longer time than at the normal baseline rate lead to subacute hypoxia, i.e. the development of hypoxia and acidosis, but less rapidly compared with acute and prolonged bradycardia/deceleration. When such FHR decelerations are frequent and profound the evolution of hypoxia and acidosis can be rapid. It is difficult to quantify the duration for which the FHR should be below the baseline rate and the duration for which it should be at the correct baseline to prevent hypoxia and acidosis. It will depend on the 'physiological reserve' of each fetus. One could consider that the build up of hypoxia and acidosis is likely to be greater if the duration of the FHR at the normal baseline rate is one-third or less of the duration of deceleration. Initially this will result in slow elimination of carbon dioxide leading to respiratory acidosis, but as time passes, oxygen transfer will be critically reduced and metabolic acidosis will ensue with its consequences as explained above.

The series of traces in Figures 7-1–7-5 show the subacute hypoxia pattern with atypical variable decelerations and the final outcome in a fetus with severe metabolic acidosis. The end of the trace was bradycardia for 10 minutes and the baby was delivered at that stage by forceps (Fig 7-5).

Gradually Developing Hypoxia

In gradually developing hypoxia decelerations appear, followed by absence of accelerations, a rise in the baseline rate (with catecholamine surge) and a reduction in baseline variability. As always, one should consider the clinical picture of parity, cervical dilatation, rate of progress and high-risk factors and institute conservative measures (e.g. stopping oxytocin, hydration, change of maternal position), or perform fetal blood sampling (FBS), or consider delivery.

Figures 7-6–7-8 exhibit the pattern seen with gradually developing hypoxia: first the decelerations appear and accelerations disappear, then the depth and duration of the decelerations

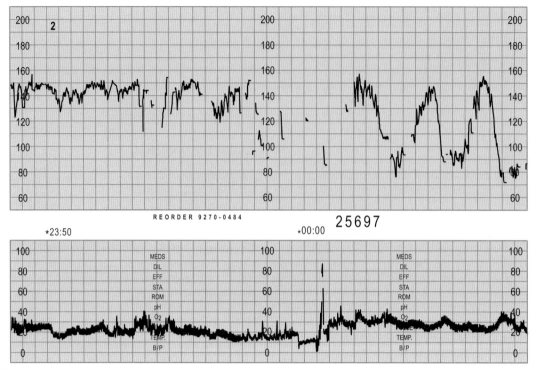

25697

FIGURE 7-1 ■ Decelerations start as shallow and then get steeper and wider lasting for 2 minutes and recovering to the baseline rate of 140 bpm for only 30 seconds.

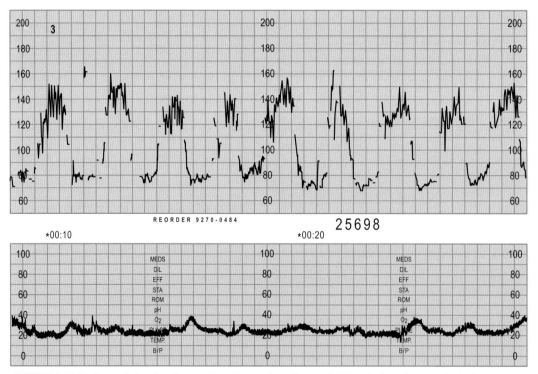

25698

FIGURE 7-2 ■ Prolonged decelerations with saltatory baseline variability during short period of recovery.

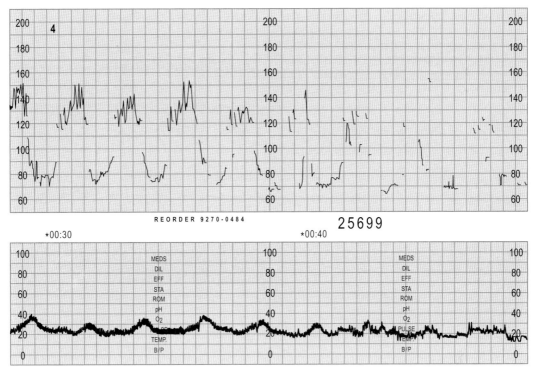

FIGURE 7-3 ■ The baseline rate drops from 150 bpm to 120 bpm with prolonged decelerations.

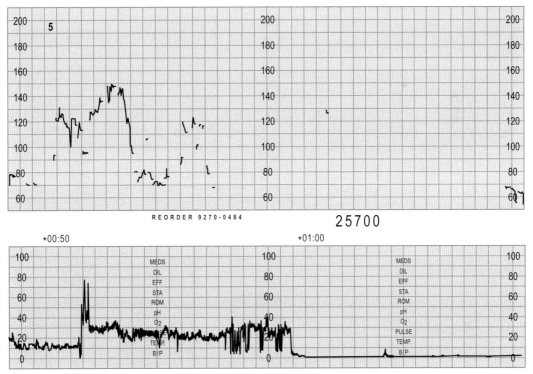

FIGURE 7-4 ■ Prolonged bradycardia following decelerations.

progressively become greater, along with a rise in the baseline rate due to the catecholamine surge due to hypoxic stress, and finally a reduction of the baseline variability when hypoxia affects the autonomic nervous system. The decelerations seen are variable, suggestive of cord compression as the mechanism that causes the hypoxia.

Longstanding Hypoxia

In cases with longstanding hypoxia there are no accelerations, the baseline variability is markedly reduced and there are shallow late decelerations, often <15 bpm. These characteristic features of hypoxia are seen even though the fetus may have a normal baseline rate. The absence of accelerations and 'cycling' suggests that the fetus may have already sustained asphyxial injury, or is hypoxic, or is affected by some other insult such as infection. Figure 7-9 is a FHR trace with features suggestive of longstanding hypoxia. This does not mean that the fetus has suffered neurological injury. Although numbers are not known, many may be born in poor condition but do well with no or minimal neurological injury. Hence there is an imperative to deliver these fetuses early if such a trace is identified. Many of these cases would have additional clinical features to suggest possible compromise, such as absent fetal movements, maternal pyrexia suggestive of infection, thick scanty meconium or bleeding. Additional exposure to uterine contractions may cause the condition of the fetus to deteriorate without any

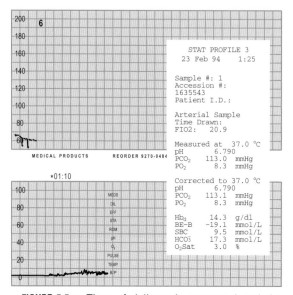

FIGURE 7-5 ■ Time of delivery is annotated and the strip shows a low pH and high base excess.

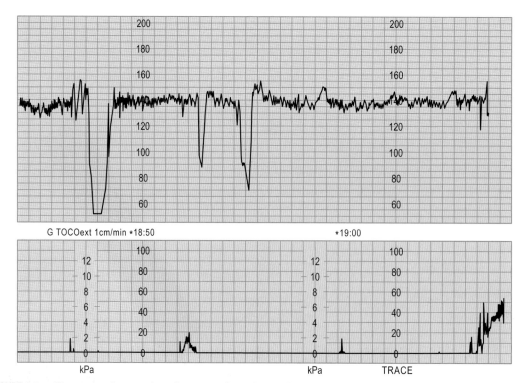

FIGURE 7-6 ■ The trace shows a baseline rate of 140 bpm with simple variable decelerations, normal baseline variability and accelerations. It has been misinterpreted as early decelerations.

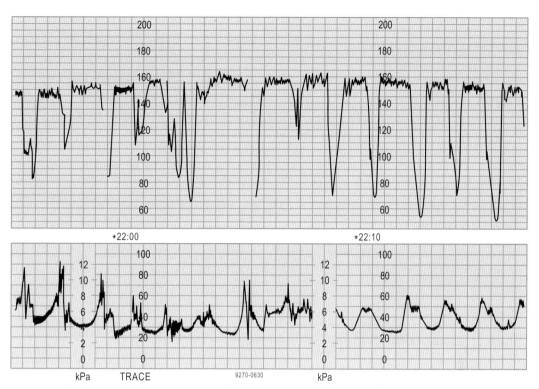

FIGURE 7-7 ■ Rise in baseline rate to 150 bpm, reduced baseline variability and no accelerations.

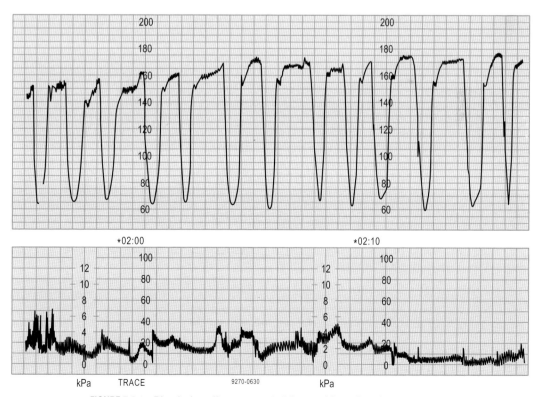

FIGURE 7-8 ■ Rise in baseline rate to 170 bpm with no baseline variability.

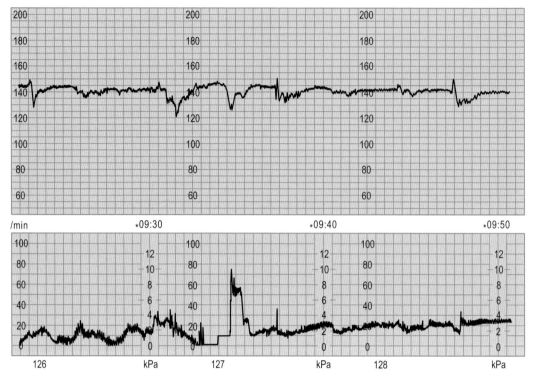

FIGURE 7-9 ■ A CTG with the baseline rate in the normal range, with no accelerations, minimal baseline variability and shallow decelerations suggestive of pre-existing hypoxia.

changes in the CTG – other than the terminal bradycardia.

Vascular Ischaemic Injury

A cerebral vascular injury such as haemorrhage or thrombosis can give rise to neurological deficits. A vascular ischaemic injury of the brain may take place due to vascular malformation in the brain vessels associated with pressure on the fetal head. At times a vascular thrombosis may form due to coagulation disorders. In many the cause is unknown. The time of this occurrence may be recognizable on the CTG as a sudden rise in the baseline rate with absence of accelerations and reduced variability of the FHR.[14] These infants may present with hemi-paretic cerebral palsy although the baby may show normal pH and blood gases at birth.[14,15]

In cases of prolonged bradycardia, if the FHR recovers, returns to the normal baseline rate, and shows reactivity with accelerations and cyclicity, then ischaemic or hypoxic neurological injury is unlikely. On the other hand, if the FHR does not recover at the time of delivery it may show signs of hypoxia. If it had recovered but has attained a higher baseline rate with reduced baseline variability and no reactivity or cyclicity, then it is suggestive of a vascular injury of a localized area.

The typical hypoxic injury with acute bradycardia is in the thalamic, hypothalamic and basal ganglia region of the brain.[4]

In cases of ischaemic injury the neonate may have convulsions several hours after birth. The CT or MRI scan may show a segmental or localized infarct in the brain. Injuries in the cortical or in the basal ganglia region are features of intermittent (prolonged partial) or acute (acute profound) asphyxial injury respectively. Radiological and epidemiological studies on these types of cerebral palsy are available in the literature.[16,17]

When the fetus is subjected to hypoxaemia there is a preferential redistribution of blood perfusion to the essential organs of heart, brain and adrenals in preference to skin, muscle and other viscera like the gut and kidneys.[18,19] Animal experimentation has shown that when there is severe mechanical compression of the head, as in some cases of the second stage of labour, there may be hardly any blood flow to the brain.[20] Similar findings have been shown in human fetuses with the use of near infrared spectroscopy, which shows reduction in oxyhaemoglobin in relation to deoxyhaemoglobin.[21] If these episodes are prolonged it may give rise to asphyxial brain injury with low Apgar scores and subsequent neurological disorders, including cerebral palsy. In such situations there is no generalized metabolic acidosis and the cord pH at birth may be normal as the insult is confined to the brain.

CORRELATION OF CTG PATTERNS WITH OBSERVED BRAIN INJURY

Animal experimental models have been used to correlate the different types of asphyxial injuries seen in the MRI with the resultant neurological outcome seen in the infant.[4] Severe fetal brady-cardia (acute hypoxia CTG pattern) leads to poor circulation, causes fetal asphyxia and renders the whole brain ischaemic. Different tissues have varying susceptibility to hypoxia-asphyxia based on their metabolic demands. Animal experiments suggest that there is damage to the putamina and lentiform nuclei within 10 minutes of profound lack of perfusion; to the central gyri, hippocampus and calcarine regions in 20–30 minutes; and to the whole cerebrum by 30 minutes – if the animal fetus is resuscitated before death.[22]

Unlike complete circulatory obstruction and ischaemia, if there is partial ischaemia and hypoxia, autoregulation results in vasodilatation to maintain cerebral blood flow. However, the border zones, which are the distal regions of the blood flow, may become underperfused and be damaged if unable to maintain the metabolic needs. It is estimated that neurons in this region may become irreversibly damaged in 30 minutes. Because of the preferential autoregulation mechanism the vital regions of the brain will not be ischaemic whilst the border zones are affected. The period for which the autoregulation process can continue, without affecting the rest of the brain, before final collapse is estimated to be 30–60 minutes.

Intermittent reduction in blood flow leading to increasing hypoxaemia and hypoxia is likely with profound intermittent deceleration seen with the subacute hypoxic CTG pattern, and during the terminal stages of gradually developing hypoxic patterns. In the sheep model, carotid artery occlusion for 30–40 minutes results in ischaemia and necrosis in the parasagittal cortex, basal ganglia and thalamus.[4] Parasagittal cortical injury similar to the watershed damage seen in human newborns can be produced by prolonged gradual obstruction of the carotid artery for periods of 1–2 hours. The experiment showed some variation from animal to animal, but in general there needed to be at least 30 minutes of partial asphyxia for parasagittal damage, and the damage was greater if the process continued for >60 minutes. Basal ganglia lesions were common with bradycardia lasting 30 minutes. When this period was longer than 30 minutes white matter damage in the watershed areas was seen. The odds of damage in the watershed area were significantly increased when prolonged bradycardia of 1 hour was compared with a period of less than 1 hour. Animal experiments have shown that 50 minutes of partial asphyxia, followed by 3–4 minutes of total asphyxia, results in cortical and basal ganglia damage. The MRI pictures of brain damage after prenatal, perinatal and post-natal asphyxia have been well described.[23]

FETAL ASPHYXIA AND MEDICOLEGAL IMPLICATIONS

To establish negligence, *causation* and *liability* have to be proven. The following features are sought for evidence of causation: pathological CTG, low Apgar score, low cord arterial pH, need for assisted ventilation, admission to neo-natal intensive care unit (NICU), hypoxic ischae-mic encephalopathy (HIE) and subsequent neurological damage. However, several metabolic disorders may cause neurological disability and a pathological CTG and inappropriate management may be coincidental. The following list of essential and additional criteria has been proposed to help determine whether birth asphyxia can be considered causative:[24]

Essential criteria:
- Evidence of metabolic acidosis in cord umbilical artery (UA) or early neonatal (NN) samples: pH <7.0 and base deficit >12 mmol/L
- Early onset of severe or moderate neonatal encephalopathy in infants >34 weeks
- Cerebral palsy of a spastic quadriplegic or dyskinetic type.

Additional criteria:
- A sentinel hypoxic event occurring immediately before or during labour
- A sudden rapid sustained deterioration in FHR pattern
- Apgar score <7 for more than 5 minutes
- Early evidence of multisystem involvement
- Early imaging evidence of acute cerebral involvement.

> 'One has to consider that the anomaly of the birth process, rather than being the causal etio-logical factor, may itself be the consequence of the real perinatal etiology'.
> Sigmund freud
> Die infantile cerebrallähmung. Vienna, 1897

The above criteria emphasize the need to cor-relate the neurological outcome described by the

transducer by listening to the fetal heart using a Pinard stethoscope or Doptone before application of the ultrasound transducer. Alternatively, the ECG signal can be monitored via the scalp electrode. On the ultrasound mode the monitor can record the maternal heart rate by picking up the pulsations of maternal vessels and also can double count the rate. Slippage of the ultrasound transducer from tracking the fetal heart to the maternal pulse during labour can occur on rare occasions.[28] This is more common in the second stage of labour.[29] If the heart rate accelerates corresponding to the onset and offset of the contractions in the second stage of labour, it is highly suspicious and needs to be verified by checking the maternal pulse by palpation or by using a pulse oximetry probe on the mother. With the fetal ECG electrode, accidental recording of maternal ECG has been reported when the fetus was dead. The whole CTG should be reviewed periodically to observe for sudden changes in the rate. Care should be taken when monitoring the second twin after delivery of the first twin as mistakes are made due to the ultrasound transducer recording the maternal heart rate. To overcome this problem some companies have produced a superficial pulse oximetry probe within the toco transducer called 'smart pulse', which records the maternal pulse on the CTG paper when the toco transducer is applied (Fig 7-10).

When the trace is technically unsatisfactory it is important to auscultate and record the findings in the notes or on the CTG paper. If feasible, a scalp electrode should be used to get a trace of better technical quality. Attention should be paid to monitoring the uterine contraction pattern at all times but especially when the FHR is pathological or if the mother is on oxytocin infusion.

Record Keeping

CTGs are recorded on thermosensitive paper that tends to fade after 3–4 years. CTG traces tend to go missing, especially if there was an adverse outcome. In a study of obstetric accidents 18 of 64 cases of possible litigation had lost FHR traces.[30] In another six cases the CTG could not be interpreted. Legally these traces need to be kept for 25 years. The fetal monitoring companies produce systems that have automatic online download of the CTG on servers. The archived cases on the server are valuable for teaching CTG and for research and audit. These systems come with overview monitors that can be kept at a central station. This facility helps the staff to discuss the cases outside the room without disturbing the women. It also acts as a 'neighbourhood watch'; another midwife or doctor at the central station may pick up a pathological CTG of concern that is missed by the immediate care giver in the room. This will facilitate discussion and appropriate action with the midwife outside the room.

Education and Training

The need for education and training is emphasized in the CESDI report and is required by the NHSLA for getting CNST (Clinical Negligence Scheme for Trusts) insurance rebates. Several books, CDs and websites are available. In-house training with review of the unit's own cases is the best way of reinforcing knowledge, in addition to regular education programmes.

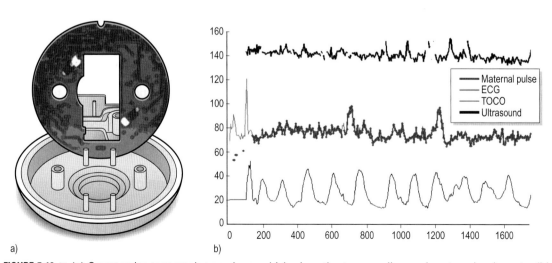

a)   b)

FIGURE 7-10 ■ (a) Smart pulse tocograph transducer which gives the toco reading and maternal pulse rate; (b) using a superficial oximetry module within the transducer (with permission from Philips).

The most junior doctors and midwives may be on the labour ward outside regular working hours. All staff cannot be released at the same time for face to face teaching and hence the electronic teaching and assessment system produced by the RCOG/RCM and e-learning for Health would be extremely useful.

Immediate attention is needed to evaluate the trace if it is pathological and to take necessary action. Hence, a senior person with adequate knowledge of CTG should be available to allay anxiety, to educate, to take appropriate action and to avoid unnecessary operative delivery. In some countries a consultant is available on the labour ward floor for 24 hours each day. In the UK attempts are made to provide consultant cover for 24 hours – at least in larger units.

Incident Reporting and Audit

Incident reporting of adverse outcomes and audit of poor outcome – low Apgar scores, low cord arterial pH, need for assisted ventilation, admission for neonatal intensive care and HIE – are essential to find out whether there is a system failure such as education and training, induction of personnel, supervision and inadequate staffing levels. All potential litigation cases need to be thoroughly evaluated by a risk management team. Findings of the risk management team and their recommendations need to be disseminated to all staff to prevent further recurrence.

CONCLUSIONS

Fetal asphyxia resulting in fetal or neonatal death or injury, especially at term, is a major tragedy for the women, their families and the staff. Staff do not make mistakes intentionally, yet it happens due to lack of knowledge and lack of senior staff for consultation. An inevitable consequence is litigation when there is a stillbirth or neurological injury. The couple want to know what happened and why, and whether the lessons learned can be applied to prevent recurrence. Rarely they sue thinking that the staff involved should account for their actions. Parents with handicapped children sue to recover the expenses in managing the child and for pain and suffering in addition to costs of future care. Obstetric litigation is distressing to all involved. Parents of a handicapped child would always prefer to have a normal child rather than considerable financial remuneration given for childcare. Their life is stressful and sad watching the child suffering. We have to do everything possible to eliminate or reduce such occurrences. There is no conflict between improving clinical care, minimizing clinical error and reducing obstetric litigation. They are complementary and can be achieved by research, audit, education and training and risk management – the components of clinical governance to improve healthcare.

REFERENCES

1. Ten Years of Maternity Claims: An Analysis of NHS Litigation Authority Data. Published by NHS Litigation Authority; 2nd Floor 151 Buckingham Palace Road, London, SW1W 9SZ. © NHS Litigation Authority, 2012.
2. Confidential Enquiry into Stillbirths and Deaths in Infancy. 4th Annual Report. London: Maternal and Child Health Research Consortium; 1997.
3. Pasternak JF. Hypoxic-ischemic brain damage in term infant – lessons from the laboratory. Pediatr Clin North Am 1993;40:1061–72.
4. Myers RE. Four patterns of perinatal brain damage and their conditions of occurrence in primates. Adv Neurol 1975;10:223–32.
5. Hagberg B, Hagberg G, Beckung E, Uvebrant P. Changing panorama of cerebral palsy in Sweden. VII. Prevalence and origin in the birth year period 1991–1994. Acta Paediatrica 2001;90:272–7.
6. Blair E, Stanley FJ. Intrapartum asphyxia: a rare cause of cerebral palsy. J Pediatr 1988;12:515–9.
7. Beard RW, Filshie GM, Knight CA, Roberts GM. The significance of the changes in the continuous fetal heart rate in the first stage of labour. J Obstet Gynaecol Br Commw 1971;78:865–81.
8. Fleischer A, Schulman H, Jagani N, Mitchell J, Randolph G. The development of fetal acidosis in the presence of an abnormal fetal heart rate tracing. I. The average for gestational age fetus. Am J Obstet Gynecol 1982;144:55–60.
9. Phelan JP, Kim JO. Fetal heart rate observations in the brain-damaged infant. Semin Perinatol 2000;24:221–9.
10. Lin CC, Mouward AH, Rosenow PJ, River P. Acid-base characteristics of fetuses with intrauterine growth retardation during labor and delivery. Am J Obstet Gynecol 1980;137:553–9.
11. Steer PJ. Fetal distress. In: Crawford J, editor. Risks of labour. Chichester: John Wiley; 1985. p. 11–31.
12. Ingemarsson I, Arulkumaran S, Ratnam SS. Single injection of terbutaline in term labor. Effect on fetal pH in cases with prolonged bradycardia. Am J Obstet Gynecol 1985;153:859–64.
13. National Institute of Clinical Excellence. Intrapartum care: Care of healthy women and their babies during childbirth. This guideline is an update of 'Electronic fetal monitoring: the use and interpretation of cardiotocography in intrapartum fetal surveillance' (Guideline C) issued in May 2001. Clinical guideline 55 – 2007: http://publications.nice.org.uk/intrapartum-care-cg55
14. Schifrin BS. The CTG and the timing and mechanism of fetal neurological injuries. Best Pract Res Clin Obstet Gynaecol 2004;18:467–78.
15. Micahelis R, Rooschuz B, Dopfer R. Prenatal origin of congenital spastic hemiparesis. Early Hum Dev 1980;4:243–55.
16. Rosenbloom L. Dyskinetic cerebral palsy and birth asphyxia. Dev Med Child Neurol 1994;36:285–9.
17. Stanley FJ, Blair E, Hockey A, Patterson B, Watson L. Spastic quadriplegia in Western Australia: a genetic epidemiological study. I. Case population and perinatal risk factors. Dev Med Child Neurol 1993;35:191–201.

18. Berger R, Garnier Y, Lobbert T, Pfeiffer D, Jensen A. Circulatory responses to acute asphyxia are not affected by the glutamate antagonist lubeluzole in fetal sheep near term. J Soc Gynecol Invest 2001;8:143–8.

19. Richardson BS, Carmichael L, Homan J, Johnston L, Gagnon R. Fetal cerebral, circulatory, and metabolic responses during heart rate decelerations with umbilical cord compression. Am J Obstet Gynecol 1996;175: 929–36.

20. O'Brien WF, David SE, Grissom MP, Eng RR, Golden SM. Effect of cephalic pressure on fetal cerebral blood flow. Am J Perinatol 1984;1:223–6.

21. Aldrich CJ, D'Antona D, Spencer JA, Wyatt JS, Peebles DM, Delpy DT, et al. The effect of maternal pushing on fetal cerebral oxygenation and blood volume during the second stage of labour. Br J Obstet Gynaecol 1995;102:448–53.

22. Williams CE, Gunn AJ, Synek B, Gluckman PD. Delayed seizures occurring with hypoxic-ischemic encephalopathy in the fetal sheep. Pediat Res 1990;27: 561–8.

23. Sie LT, van der Knapp MS, Oosting J, de Vries LS, Lafebar HN, Valk JMR. Patterns of hypoxic-ischaemic brain damage after prenatal, perinatal and postnatal asphyxia. Neuropaediatrics 2000;31:128–36.

24. McLennan A. A template for defining a causal relation between acute intrapartum events and cerebral palsy: international consensus statement. BMJ 1999;40: 13–21.

25. Electronic fetal monitoring. http://www.e-lfh.org.uk/projects/electronic-fetal-monitoring/

26. National Collaborating Centre for Women's and Children's Health – Commissioned by the National Institute for Health and Clinical Excellence. Caesarean section. November 2011. Available at http://www.nice.org.uk/nicemedia/live/13620/57162/57162.pdf

27. Ingemarsson I, Arulkumaran S, Ratnam SS. Single injection of terbutaline in term labor. 2. Effect on uterine activity. Am J Obstet Gynecol. 1985;153:865–9.

28. Gibb DMF, Arulkumaran S. Fetal monitoring in practice. 2nd ed. Oxford: Butterworth Heinemann; 1997. p. 10–9.

29. Nurani R, Chandraharan E, Lowe V, Ugwumadu A, Arulkumaran S. Misidentification of maternal heart rate as fetal on cardiotocography during the second stage of labor: the role of the fetal electrocardiograph. Acta Obstet Gynecol Scand 2012;91:1428–32.

30. Ennis S, Vincent CA. Obstetric accidents: a review of 64 cases. BMJ 1990;300:1365–7.

CHAPTER 8

INDUCTION OF LABOUR

SJ Stock · AA Calder

'The spontaneous onset of labour is a robust and effective mechanism which is preceded by the maturation of several fetal systems, and should be given every opportunity to operate on its own. We should only induce labour when we are sure that we can do better.'

ALEC TURNBULL, 1976

HISTORICAL BACKGROUND

The first reliable technique to be used widely in obstetric practice for induction of labour was amniotomy or artificial rupture of the membranes. It first entered the medical literature in 1756 when Thomas Denman (1733–1815) of the Middlesex Hospital of London wrote extolling its virtues. As a result it became known within Europe as the 'English method'.

Another mechanical method was devised in 1861 by Robert Barnes (1817–1907) of London, using a hydrostatic bag placed through the cervix and filled with water.[1] A similar approach was later taken by Camille Champetier de Ribes (1848–1935) in Paris[2] and by James Voorhees (1869–1929) in New York[3] which all preceded the understanding that the modus operandi was local release of prostaglandins.

However, it was not until oxytocin was made available for clinical application that any degree of reliability in labour induction could be achieved. Sir Henry Dale (1875–1968) made the first observation that posterior pituitary extract caused uterine contractions.[4] He gave samples to the obstetrician William Blair Bell (1871–1936) who began to use it for induction of labour.[5] Nevertheless, because the crude extracts of the posterior pituitary were of variable purity and potency, and because these were initially given as intramuscular injections with a poor degree of control, it was hardly surprising that there were instances of calamitous hyperstimulation of the uterus. It was not until the latter half of the 20th century that reliable preparations of oxytocin became available following its chemical characterization as an octapeptide and its synthetic elaboration.[6–8] There followed a period of controversy during which Geoffrey Theobald advocated a dilute intravenous infusion of oxytocin as a 'physiological drip',[9] motivated by the desire to maximize the safety of the drug, but actually reducing its potency and reliability. It was not until the late 1960s that Alec Turnbull and Anne Anderson advocated the more pharmacologically sound approach of oxytocin 'titration' whereby the dose rate was steadily increased until the uterus responded by contracting effectively, at which point the dose rate was held steady.[10] A significant new development in the practice of labour induction was the clinical availability of prostaglandins. First recognized in the 1930s, it took more than 30 years to reach the point of clinical application, largely as a result of work by Sune Bergstrom and his colleagues at the Karolinska Institute in Stockholm.[11] By 1975 it was clear that prostaglandins added an extra dimension to induction of labour, particularly since they not only provoked uterine contractions but also had a positive effect on cervical ripening.[12,13] As with oxytocin, a variety of different routes were explored before it was recognized that local delivery required a lower dose and greatly reduced unpleasant side effects. Simply introducing PGE_2 into the vagina has become the route of choice.[14]

More than a century after Barnes, Champetier de Ribes and Voorhees pioneered mechanical methods of induction of labour, things have come full circle, with increasing evidence that using a Foley catheter or cervical ripening balloon is an effective way of inducing labour, with lower rates of hyperstimulation than prostaglandin.[15]

INDICATIONS FOR INDUCTION OF LABOUR

Induction of labour is one of the most commonly performed obstetric interventions, with more than 20% of mothers in developed countries having their labour induced.[16] It is offered when it is believed that the outcome for mother or baby, or both, is better served by delivery than by allowing the pregnancy to continue. Each pregnancy should be assessed in respect of the 'obstetric balance' (Fig 8-1). The perceptive clinician will immediately recognize that such a view is unduly simple for two reasons. First, the risks of the process of induction of labour must be considered. There is no virtue in intervening by inducing labour to avoid a perceived risk if the nature of the labour which results risks greater jeopardy for either party. Second, an intervention which may be in the interests of one partner in the pregnancy may counter the interests of the other. For instance, induction of

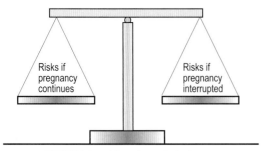

FIGURE 8-1 ■ The obstetric balance.

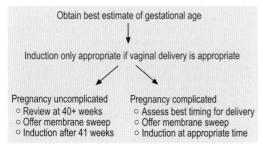

FIGURE 8-2 ■ A paradigm to be followed when the question of interruption of pregnancy arises.

labour in a mother with pre-eclampsia may be beneficial in reducing the risks which she faces, while at the same time exposing the offspring to the risks of prematurity.

When considering whether to offer induction of labour or not, each pregnancy must be considered individually, taking account of the risks and benefits to mother and baby deriving from specific complications and the risks of induction of labour. Importantly, the mother's preferences, values and perceptions of risk should be considered. Common indications for induction of labour are outlined below. Figure 8-2 outlines a paradigm to be followed when the question of interruption of pregnancy arises.

Prolonged Pregnancy

It is estimated that up to 10% of pregnancies continue beyond 294 days (42 weeks). Both mother and fetus are at increased risk when the pregnancy continues beyond term, with the risk of neonatal and postneonatal death significantly increased after 41 weeks.[17]

A Cochrane systematic review and meta-analysis of trials of induction of labour at or beyond term (37 weeks and beyond) found that compared with expectant management, a policy of labour induction was associated with fewer perinatal deaths (risk ratio 0.31, 95% confidence interval (CI) 0.12 to 0.88) and less meconium

aspiration in babies (risk ratio 0.50, 95% CI 0.34 to 0.73).[18]

Although it is commonly perceived that induction of labour can increase operative deliveries including caesarean section, it is important to note that there were actually fewer caesarean sections with induction of labour compared with expectant management (risk ratio 0.89, 95% CI 0.81 to 0.97).[19]

Pre-Eclampsia and Gestational Hypertension

Hypertensive disorders in pregnancy are associated with increased maternal and neonatal morbidity. In cases of severe pre-eclampsia, ending the pregnancy is the treatment of choice. In milder cases the risks and benefits of induction of labour are less clear cut. A randomized controlled trial of induction of labour (n=377) or expectant monitoring (n=379) for women with mild gestational hypertension or pre-eclampsia at 36 weeks or greater gestation found that fewer women randomized to induction of labour developed poor maternal outcome (relative risk 0.71, 95% CI 0.59–0.86, p<0.0001).[20] Neonates born to mothers randomized to induction of labour were lighter, but no differences in neonatal morbidity were seen. In cases of mild pre-eclampsia and gestational hypertension prior to 36 weeks' gestation, the potential risks of iatrogenic prematurity associated with induction of labour are higher and must be balanced against the risks of continuing the pregnancy.

Maternal Diabetes

Women with diabetes have higher risk of pregnancy complications including intrauterine death, macrosomia and birth trauma. There has been only one randomized-controlled trial of induction of labour in diabetic pregnancies, comparing induction of labour at 38 weeks' gestation to expectant management to 42 weeks. There was no difference in caesarean section rates between groups (relative risk 0.81, 95% confidence interval (CI) 0.52–1.26), but the risk of macrosomia was lower with induction of labour (relative risk 0.56, 95% CI 0.32–0.98).[20] The UK National Institute for Clinical Excellence (NICE) has reviewed the evidence for management of diabetic pregnancy and recommends that induction of labour (or caesarean section if indicated) is offered at 38 weeks' gestation to women with diabetes requiring insulin (NICE guideline Diabetes in Pregnancy (CG63)).

Twins and Multiple Pregnancy

Epidemiological data suggest that in twin pregnancies 'term' may be earlier than in singletons, and morbidity and mortality in twin pregnancies are the lowest in association with delivery at 36–38 weeks' gestation. Current NICE guidelines endorse elective delivery around 37 weeks for dichorionic twins and 36 weeks for monochorionic twins. There is not clear evidence from randomized trials that induction of labour improves outcomes for twins, but a recent randomized trial of elective delivery around 37 weeks' gestation compared to expectant management, did suggest that neonatal morbidity may be reduced, principally through a reduction in birth weight <3rd centile.[21] The trial thus supports observational data, and current national recommendations that women with uncomplicated twin pregnancy should be offered delivery around 37 weeks to optimize infant outcome.

Preterm Prelabour Rupture of the Membranes

When the fetal membranes rupture before the onset of labour the risks of intrauterine infection leading to neonatal and/or maternal sepsis with continuing pregnancy must be weighed against the risks of prematurity resulting from immediate delivery. At gestations remote from term the risks of prematurity are considerable, and expectant management with monitoring of maternal and fetal wellbeing appears to be preferable unless there are clear signs of impending maternal or fetal compromise. The results of the PPROMEXIL trial[22] suggest that even when prelabour rupture of membranes occurs closer to term expediting delivery by inducing labour does not confer any benefits. The paper, which also includes a meta-analysis of similar trials, found that overall rates of neonatal sepsis were low, and there was no reduction in risk of neonatal sepsis (relative risk of 1.06 (95% CI 0.64 to 1.76)) or caesarean section (relative risk 1.27 (95% CI 0.98 to 1.65)) with induction of labour compared to expectant management. It supports a 'watch and wait' approach, unless there is clear evidence of infection or other concerns for maternal or fetal wellbeing.

Intrauterine Growth Restriction

When there is an inadequate oxygen or nutrient supply to the fetus, there are progressive alterations in the growth, metabolic, cardiovascular and behavioural parameters of the fetus, which represent increasing hypoxaemia and acidosis. When such fetal compromise is suspected, immediate delivery may decrease the risk of damage due to intrauterine hypoxia. However, it may also increase the risks of prematurity. The Growth Restriction Intervention (GRIT) trial[23] aimed to assess the effects of immediate delivery and delayed delivery of the preterm fetus (24–36 weeks) with suspected growth restriction. Overall there were no differences in neurodevelopment impairment or death and disability at or after 2 years, but more babies in the immediate delivery group were ventilated for more than 24 hours (relative risk 1.54, 95% CI 1.20 to 1.97), and more women in the immediate delivery group had caesarean delivery (relative risk 1.15, 95% CI 1.07 to 1.24). A Cochrane review of immediate or deferred delivery for the preterm fetus with suspected fetal compromise concluded that more research is needed, but where there is uncertainty whether or not to deliver, deferring delivery until test results worsen or increasing gestation favours delivery may improve the outcomes for mother and baby.[24]

There is also no clear evidence of benefit to induction of labour in cases of growth restriction identified at term. A randomized trial (DIGITAT) found no important differences in adverse outcomes between induction of labour and expectant monitoring in women with growth restriction greater than 36 weeks. The authors concluded that women who are keen on non-intervention can safely choose expectant management with intensive maternal and fetal monitoring; however, it is rational to choose induction to prevent possible neonatal morbidity and stillbirth.[25]

Elective Induction of Labour

Elective induction of labour (i.e. in the absence of a recognized medical complication) may be offered for maternal or physician preference or social and geographical considerations (e.g. availability of partner, distance from hospital). A population based cohort study found that perinatal mortality and maternal complications were lower and vaginal delivery rates higher in association with elective induction of labour around term, when compared to expectant management.[26] However, induction of labour was associated with higher rates of neonatal unit admission. Other studies have found a reduction in caesarean delivery associated with elective induction of labour when compared to expectant management.[27] Although these findings are from observational studies, they can be used to help counsel women about management options for delivery.

METHODS OF INDUCTION

It is recognized that some labours can be induced with ease while others may prove extremely resistant to induction. It is likely that the biggest single factor is the proximity to the spontaneous onset of labour. Because the transition from the state of pregnancy maintenance to established labour is a gradual one (see Chapter 1), it is obvious that if a particular woman is programmed to be in labour tomorrow, labour induction today is likely to be simple. In contrast if, even at or beyond term, spontaneous labour remains a distant prospect then induction is almost inevitably fraught with difficulty. The most useful predictor of this is the degree of cervical ripening. Indeed, the original study on which Bishop based his cervical scoring system correlated the score to the interval before spontaneous labour began.[28] A high score presaged a short delay before the onset of labour; a low score indicated that it remained a distant prospect. The former was shown to be favourable for induction of labour, the latter unfavourable.

In practice, the application of a scoring system based on Bishop's concept provides a reliable prediction of how successful labour induction is likely to be, but also of what method is most suitable (Fig 8-3). If the cervical score (Table 8-1) is high, labour is imminent and can usually be successfully induced by amniotomy alone, with or without oxytocin to stimulate uterine contractions. In cases where the cervix is unfavourable, cervical ripening is indicated before amniotomy and oxytocin. A variety of techniques have been in and out of vogue in the past 50 years. Although some of these may now seem primitive or bizarre, those which enjoyed any success had in common the provocation of those substances, especially oxytocin or prostaglandins, which participate in spontaneous labour. Thus, breast stimulation (which causes release of oxytocin), castor oil, enema, Foley catheters, Bougies, membrane sweeping and even sexual intercourse have had their advocates. All of the latter provide or provoke the release of prostaglandins.

Membrane Sweeping

This technique, which by necessity is only possible once the cervix has ripened sufficiently to allow the passage of a finger, is also dependent on the release of endogenous prostaglandins but in this instance from those tissues which are normally associated with the generation of labour stimuli.[29] Its particular virtue lies in its simplicity and its comparative lack of risk and that with

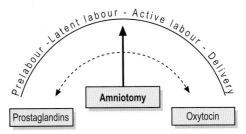

FIGURE 8-3 ■ A scheme for labour induction. Prostaglandins may be used to greatest advantage in prelabour and latent labour, prior to amniotomy. Oxytocin is most effective following amniotomy. The best timing for amniotomy is after latent labour has begun.

Cervical Feature	Pelvic Score			
	0	1	2	3
Bishop Score[28]				
Dilatation (cm)	0	1–2	3–4	5–6
Effacement (%)	0–30	40–60	60–70	80+
Station* (cm)	−3	−2	−1/0	+1/+2
Consistency	Firm	Medium	Soft	−
Position	Posterior	Mid-posterior	Anterior	−
Modified Bishop Score[44]				
Dilatation (cm)	< 1	1–2	2–4	> 4
Length of cervix (cm)	> 4	2–4	1–2	< 1
Station* (cm)	−3	−2	−1/0	+1/+2
Consistency	Firm	Average	Soft	−
Position	Posterior	Mid; Anterior	−	−

TABLE 8-1 **Cervical Scoring Systems**

*In both systems, station is measured in cm relative to the ischial spines.

maintenance of the integrity of the membranes the labour may follow a more natural pattern of onset.

Prostaglandins

Intravaginal prostaglandins are the most common method of induction of labour.[11] They are effective at cervical ripening and hastening delivery, and are commonly administered as a gel, or a slow release pessary. A potential drawback of administered prostaglandins is that they affect both cervical ripening and contractions simultaneously, which is not what happens physiologically, when the cervix ripens before myometrial contractions start. Contractions occurring before the cervix is ripe are not effective in progressing labour and increase the risk of uterine hyperstimulation with fetal heart rate changes. However, in nulliparous women or women with previous vaginal deliveries, there is no evidence that prostaglandin-induced uterine hyperstimulation is associated with substantial harm, since prostaglandins do not increase the risk of caesarean section or neonatal unit admission.

Nitric Oxide Donors

It has been proposed that the ideal strategy for induction of labour would be administration of a cervical ripening agent which does not stimulate contractions, decreasing the need for fetal monitoring during ripening (enabling outpatient use) and reducing the risk of uterine rupture. Nitric oxide donors induce cervical ripening without inducing uterine contractions, but trials of their use for induction of labour have been disappointing, as they do not hasten the onset of delivery or reduce the need for additional agents when used for induction of labour.[30]

Transcervical Foley Catheter

A recent randomised control trial (PROBAAT) has shown that induction of labour with an intracervical Foley catheter[31] induces cervical ripening without inducing uterine contractions and is as successful as prostaglandin for induction of labour, according to the number of failed inductions and caesarean section rates. In a meta-analysis, Foley catheter induction is similar to prostaglandin induction for caesarean section rate but significantly reduces rates of hyperstimulation (odds ratio 0.44, 95% CI 0.21–0.91) and postpartum haemorrhage (0.60, 0.37–0.95). Although women's views of the Foley catheter were not formally assessed, 74% of eligible women approached agreed to participate in the trial, and less than 0.5% declined when allocated to the Foley catheter, implying high pretreatment acceptability. There was no evidence of increased infection for either mothers or babies with Foley catheter use. The low cost of the Foley catheter could make it particularly useful in resource-limited settings.[31]

COMPLICATIONS OF INDUCTION OF LABOUR

Induction of labour is not an intervention to be embarked upon lightly. Indeed, the complications of induction can exceed the putative risks of the condition for which the induction was performed. The main complications are as follows:

Fetal Immaturity

A fundamental requirement before embarking on induction is confirmation of gestational age. The use of ultrasound in early pregnancy has improved gestational age assessment. Although outcomes for babies born after 34 weeks are generally favourable, it is important to recognize that 'late preterm births' (34–36+6 weeks), which constitute more than 70% of preterm births, are more likely to have long-term neurodevelopmental problems than those born at term, and have higher infant mortality.[32] These authors also showed that 'early term' births (37+0 to 38+6 weeks) are associated with an increased risk of significant complications when compared to those born after 39 weeks. The injudicious use of induction of labour at late preterm or early term gestations can thus have a significant negative impact on the wellbeing of babies, their families and long-term health outcomes.

Uterine Hyperstimulation

Although hypertonic uterine action can be seen in labour of spontaneous onset, it is natural to blame induction agents if their administration is followed by evidence of uterine hyperstimulation. This should be rare if protocols for administration of oxytocic agents are carefully followed but can occur within such guidelines, and may require acute tocolysis (see Chapter 28). Women of high parity (≥4) are at special risk and they merit particularly close monitoring.

Amniotomy

Amniotomy may lead to cord prolapse or abruptio placentae when there is polyhydramnios. It is important to take particular care to control the slow release of liquor from the uterus in these cases, otherwise the cord may be washed down and the sudden reduction in volume of the uterus may cause placental separation. With the most marked degrees of polyhydramnios it may be justified to carry out amniocentesis and reduce the liquor volume before amniotomy. Even without polyhydramnios, if the fetal head is free at the pelvic brim the risk of cord prolapse can be increased. With a normal amount of amniotic fluid and the fetal head settled into the pelvic brim, the risk of cord prolapse with amniotomy is not increased over spontaneous rupture of the membranes.

Complications Specific to Oxytocin

Prolonged administration of concentrated oxytocin accompanied by large volumes of diluents carries the risk of water intoxication which has, in rare circumstances, led to maternal death. If protocols for dose rates and concentrations of this agent are followed this is not a risk. An association between administration of oxytocin during labour induction and an increased rate of neonatal jaundice has been proven, although this is rarely of important clinical significance.[33]

Unsuccessful Induction of Labour

The definition of unsuccessful induction is where the intervention does not lead to effective and progressive labour.[34] Some women resist all efforts to ripen the cervix with prostaglandins or to go into labour with prostaglandins and/or oxytocin. The reasons for this remain obscure. There may be a biological defect such as placental sulphatase deficiency[35] which prevents the sensitization of the uterus to oxytocic agents, or perhaps these women lack some essential cytokine or other factor (see Chapter 1). The constellation of failed induction, dystocia and atonic postpartum haemorrhage in women with prolonged pregnancy might lead one to speculate about a possible intrinsic myometrial dysfunction which predisposed them to failure to go into spontaneous labour, poor response to induction and postpartum uterine atony.

The challenge for the obstetrician is recognizing cases in which vaginal delivery is unlikely to be safely achieved, and performing timely caesarean section to avoid complications in these cases. Maternal characteristics that have been associated with increased risk of unsuccessful induction of labour include nulliparity, advanced maternal age, short stature, increased weight and high body mass index, while unfavourable fetal characteristics include macrosomia and low gestational age.[36] Unfortunately, none is strong enough to be used as an individual predictor of success. Favourability of the cervix at the start of induction is an important predictor, with the most important element of the Bishop score being dilatation. Other predictors, including transvaginal ultrasound and biochemical markers (including fetal fibronectin) have been suggested but have no advantage over digital cervical assessment.[36]

A SYSTEMATIC APPROACH TO INDUCTION OF LABOUR

The following stepwise approach to labour induction is recommended.

Phase I

The following questions should be addressed:
- What is the gestational age of the pregnancy based on the most reliable available evidence?
- What is the state of health of the mother and what risks does she face?
- What is the state of health of the fetus and the evidence of current and potential compromise?
- Are there any special features in the history which require consideration? These include previous uterine surgery, precipitate delivery, difficult vaginal delivery, birth injury or stillbirth.
- What is the state of the uterus and its contents?
  - are the fetal membranes ruptured or intact?
  - what is the situation of the fetus: estimated weight, presentation and level of the presenting part?
  - is the myometrium responsive? (In practice this can really only be determined by observing its response to oxytocic drugs)
  - what is the degree of cervical ripeness? (see Table 8-1).

Phase II

Once the above information has been assembled the clinician should discuss delivery options with the mother. Management should take into account women's preferences and needs, and women should have the opportunity to make informed choices about their care and treatment in partnership with healthcare professionals.

Induction of labour and communication of risk are key areas identified by women as priorities for healthcare research, indicating the importance that women place on decision-making about induction of labour, and their perception that this could be improved.[37]

There are three possible outcomes to this consultation:

1. Pregnancy continues with appropriate surveillance
2. Delivery by caesarean section
3. Induction of labour.

Phase III

When the decision is that labour should be induced the following approach is recommended:

If the cervix is unripe it may be appropriate to follow a protocol for 'priming' or 'ripening' as a prelude to labour induction *per se*. This has the important advantage of removing from both the mother and the clinical attendants the expectation that labour will be instantly established, thus reducing the likelihood that either party becomes disillusioned or disheartened by slow progress. Time taken to prepare the cervix so that the active phase of induced contractions will be effective is a worthwhile investment.

The usual three methods at the obstetrician's disposal to achieve successful labour and delivery are prostaglandins, amniotomy and oxytocin. However, as discussed above, mechanical methods of induction of labour such as transcervical Foley catheter may also be used. The order in which these are listed here is intentional since prostaglandins are effective in ripening, effacing and dilating the cervix to the extent required for amniotomy to be appropriate, and oxytocin is largely ineffective before amniotomy. So the appropriate sequence of use is prostaglandin or transcervical Foley catheter→ amniotomy→ oxytocin (see Fig 8.3).

To emphasize the importance of this approach it should be stressed that amniotomy achieved with a struggle when the cervix is still long, firm and closed does little but condemn the woman to a long and usually unsuccessful labour[38] (Table 8-2). It is our belief that the optimal timing of membrane rupture in labour, spontaneous or induced, is when the cervix is fully effaced and ≥3 cm dilated. When such a policy is followed intravenous oxytocin may not be necessary, but it is our experience that over 70% of nulliparous women undergoing cervical ripening require oxytocin augmentation of contractions.

SPECIAL SITUATIONS

Previous Caesarean Section

Although previous caesarean is a relative contraindication to labour induction, each case must be considered individually. If the prospects of vaginal delivery are small and the prospects of a prolonged non-progressive labour are high, then it is prudent to recommend repeat caesarean section. That said, appropriate selection will lead to successful vaginal delivery in nearly 70% of cases, although complications rates are higher than with caesarean section. This topic is covered in Chapter 14.

Late Intrauterine Fetal Death

Amniotomy should be avoided in cases of intrauterine fetal death because of the increased risks of sepsis within the necrotic intrauterine tissues. Consequently prostaglandins are preferable, with or without preceding antigestagen such as mifepristone (200 mg orally). Induction of labour in women with late intrauterine death using a combination of mifepristone and misoprostol appears to reduce the delivery interval by approximately 7 hours compared with published regimens not including mifepristone, with an average duration of labour of 8 hours.[39] Vaginal misoprostol for induction of labour appears

TABLE 8-2 **Outcome of 125 Consecutive Labour Inductions[38] by Amniotomy and Intravenous Oxytocin Titration in Primigravid Women at Term, According to the Degree of Cervical Ripeness (Modified Bishop Score[42])**

Modified Bishop Score	Number	Induction–Delivery Interval (Mean)	Caesarean Section Rate	Depressed Apgar Score
0–3: unripe	31	14.9 h	32%	23%
4–7: intermediate	69	8.9 h	4%	6%
8–11: ripe	25	6.4 h	0	0
All cases	125	9.9 h	10.4%	8.8%

TABLE 8-3   **Protocols and Dosages for the Appropriate Use of Prostaglandins and Oxytocin[42]**

Intact Membranes

PGE$_2$ vaginal tablets 3 mg 6–8 hourly to maximum of 6 mg or PGE$_2$ vaginal gel – Nulliparas Bishop
  Score 4 or less – 2 mg

All other patients 1 mg, repeat 6 hourly to maximum 4 mg

Ruptured Membranes

(Either spontaneous or artificial) Intravenous infusion **oxytocin*** 30 international units in 500 ml
  normal saline = 60 milliunits per ml

∴ 1 ml per hour represents 1 milliunits/minute

Time (minutes)	0	30	60	90	120	150	180	210	240	270
Dose rate (milliunits/min)	1	2	4	8	12	16	20	24	28	32

*Oxytocin infusion delivered via syringe driver or infusion pump with non-return valve.
12 milliunits/minute adequate for most women. Maximum dose 32 milliunits/minute rarely required.
Oxytocin should not be commenced within 6 hours of last PGE$_2$ dose.

equally effective as gemeprost or prostaglandin E2, but is much cheaper, and NICE recommended that misoprostol is used for induction in cases of late intrauterine fetal death, with dose adjustment according to gestational age (100 μg 6-hourly before 26 weeks; 25–50 μg 4-hourly at 27 weeks or more). Similar regimes are recommended for induction of labour in cases where termination of pregnancy is indicated due to congenital anomaly or pregnancy complication. Vaginal misoprostol appears to be as effective as oral therapy but associated with fewer adverse effects.[40]

High Parity

As already mentioned, mothers of high parity have a higher risk of uterine hyperstimulation in response to induction. We therefore advocate a policy of amniotomy alone if conditions are favourable. If contractions do not become established, continuous administration of oxytocin is appropriate but this should be reduced or discontinued once contractions are established. If the cervix is unripe, mechanical methods may be preferable due to their lower risk of hyperstimulation.[15]

Prelabour Rupture of the Membranes

Spontaneous rupture of the membranes presents hazards to both mother and fetus, principally from intrauterine sepsis – which increases the longer delivery is delayed. Except where, for reasons of fetal immaturity, continuation of the pregnancy is proposed the need for induction of labour may arise. Since a significant proportion of such cases will go into labour within a few hours it is appropriate to anticipate this happening but we advocate stimulating contractions if this has not occurred after 12–24 hours.[41] Clearly amniotomy is not generally required but the protocols for employing prostaglandins and oxytocin are otherwise the same. Table 8-3 outlines the protocols and dosages for the appropriate use of prostaglandins and oxytocin.[42]

Misoprostol

It is noteworthy that misoprostol, originally developed as a gastric cytoprotective agent, has over the past 15 years been very widely employed for induction of labour and abortion. This happened without the normal safety assessments and without the blessing of either the manufacturers or the regulatory authorities. Indeed a wide variety of routes of administration and dosage regimes were employed. The factor which drove this unusual situation to develop was undoubtedly the cost to the prescriber, since tablets usually given orally and expressly contraindicated in pregnancy could be employed for obstetric purposes at a tiny fraction of the cost of conventional prostaglandins.

It is a cause for surprise and relief that no serious complications appear to have accompanied this 'off-label' use of misoprostol and efforts are now in course to regularize this reality within the drug formularies.[43]

REFERENCES

1. Barnes R. On the indications and operations for the induction of premature labour and for the acceleration of labour. Trans Obstet Soc Lond 1861;3:132–9.
2. Champetier de Ribes CLA. De l'accouchement provoqué. Dilatation du canal genital (col de l'utérus, vagin et

vulve) a l'aide de ballons introduit dans la cavité utérine pendant la grossesse. Ann Gynéc 1888;30:401–38.

3. Voorhees JD. Dilatation of the cervix by means of a modified Champetier de Ribes balloon. Med Rec 1900; 58:361–6.

4. Dale HH. The action of extracts of the pituitary body. Biochem J 1909;4:427–47.

5. Bell WB. The pituitary body and the therapeutic value of infundibular extract in shock, uterine atony and intestinal paresis. BMJ 1909;2:1609–13.

6. Kamm O, Aldrich TB, Grote IW, Rowe LW, Bugbee EP. The active principles of the posterior lobe of the pituitary gland. I. The demonstration of the presence of two active principles. II. The separation of the two principles and their concentration in the form of potent solid preparations. J Am Chem Soc 1928;50:573–91.

7. DuVigneaud V, Ressler C, Swan JM, Roberts CW, Katsoyannis PG, Gordon S. The synthesis of an octapeptide with the hormonal activity of oxytocin. J Am Chem Soc 1953;75:4879–80.

8. Boissonas RA, Guttmann S, Jaquenand PA, Waller TP. A new synthesis of oxytocin. Helvetica Chimica Acta 1955;38:1491–5.

9. Theobald GW, Graham A, Campbell J, Gange PD, O'Driscoll WJ. The use of posterior pituitary extract in physiological amounts in obstetrics. BMJ 1948;2: 123–7.

10. Turnbull AC, Anderson AMB. Induction of labour: results with amniotomy and oxytocin titration. J Obstet Gynaecol Br Commonw 1968;75:32–41.

11. Baskett TF. The development of prostaglandins. Best Pract Res Clin Obstet Gynaecol 2003;17:703–6.

12. Karim SMM, Hillier K, Trussell RR, Patel RC, Tamusange S. Induction of labour with prostaglandin E₂. J Obstet Gynaecol Br Commonw 1970;77:200–4.

13. Calder AA, Embrey MP. Prostaglandins and the unfavourable cervix. Lancet 1973;2:1322–4.

14. MacKenzie IZ, Embrey MP. Cervical ripening with intravaginal PGE₂ gel. BMJ 1977;2:1369–72.

15. Jowziak M, Bloemenkamp KW, Kelly AJ, Mol BW, Irion O, Boulvain M. Mechanical methods for induction of labour. Cochrane Database Syst Rev 2012;3:CD001233.

16. Mealing NM, Roberts CL, Ford JB, Simpson JM, Morris JM. Trends in induction of labour, 1998–2007. Aust NZ J Obstet Gynaecol 2009;49:599–606.

17. Hilder L, Costeloe K, Thilaganathan B. Prolonged pregnancy: evaluating the gestation-specific risks. Br J Obstet Gynaecol 1998;105:169–73.

18. Gulmezoglu AM, Crowther CA, Middleton P, Heatley E. Induction of labour for improving birth outcomes at or beyond term. Cochrane Database Syst Rev 2012;6: CD004945.

19. Hannah ME, Hannah WJ, Hellnann J, Hewson J, Milner R, Willan A. Induction of labour compared with serial antenatal monitoring in post-term pregnancy. N Eng J Med 1992;326:1587–92.

20. Koopmans CM, Bijlenga D, Groen H, Vijgen SM, Aarnoudse JG, Bekedam DJ, et al. Induction of labour versus expectant monitoring for gestational hypertension or mild pre-eclampsia. Lancet 2009;374:979–88.

21. Dodd JM, Crowther CA, Haslam RR, Robinson JS. Elective birth at 37 weeks of gestation for twin pregnancy at term. BJOG 2012;119:964–73.

22. van der Ham DP, Vijgen SM, Nijheus JG, van Beek JJ, Opmeer BC, Mulder ALM, et al. Induction of labor versus expectant management in women with preterm prelabor rupture of membranes. PLoS Med 2012;9(4): e1001208.

23. Thornton JG, Hornbuckle J. Infant wellbeing at two years of age in the Growth Restriction Intervention (GRIT). Lancet 2007;364:513–20.

24. Stock SJ, Bricker L, Norman JE. Immediate versus deferred delivery of the preterm with suspected fetal compromise. Cochrane Database Syst Rev 2012;7: CD008968.

25. Boers KE, Vijgen SM, Beljenga R, Bekedam DJ, Kwee TW, Speuderman J. Induction versus expectant monitoring for intrauterine growth restriction at term (DIGITAT). BMJ 2010;341:c7087.

26. Stock SJ, Ferguson E, Duffy, A, Ford I, Chalmers J, Norman JE. Outcomes of elective induction of labour compared with expectant management. BMJ 2012; 344:e2838.

27. Caughey AB, Sundaram V, Kaimal AJ, Cheng YW, Gienger A, Little SE, et al. Systematic review: Elective induction of labor versus expectant management of pregnancy. Ann Intern Med 2009;151:252–63.

28. Bishop EH. Pelvic scoring for elective induction. Obstet Gynecol 1964;24:266–9.

29. Boulvain M, Stan C, Irion C. Membrane sweeping for induction of labour. Cochrane Database Syst Rev 2001;2:CD000451.

30. Kelly AJ, Munsom C, Minden L. Nitric oxide donors for cervical ripening and induction. Cochrane Database Syst Rev 2011;6:CD006901.

31. Norman JE, Stock S. Intracervical Foley catheter for induction if labour. Lancet 2011;387: 2054–5.

32. Spong CY, Mercer BM. Timing of indicated late-preterm and early-term birth. Obstet Gynecol 2011;118: 323–33.

33. Calder AA, Moar VA, Ounsted MK, Turnbull AC. Increased bilirubin levels in neonates after induction of labour by intravenous prostaglandin E₂ or oxytocin. Lancet 1974;2:1339–40.

34. MacVicar J. Failed induction of labour. J Obstet Gynaecol Br Commonw 1971;78:1007–10.

35. France JT, Sneddon RJ, Liggins CG. A study of a pregnancy with low oestrogen production due to placental sulphatase deficiency. J Clin Endocrinol Metab 1973; 36:1–3.

36. Crane JM. Factors predicting labor induction success. Clin Obstet Gynecol 2006;49:573–84.

37. Cheyne H, McCourt C, Semple K. Mother knows best: Developing a consumer led, evidence informed, research agenda for maternity care. Midwifery 2012 Aug 6 [Epub ahead of print].

38. Embrey MP, Calder AA. Induction of labour. In: Proceedings of the third study group. London: RCOG Press; 1975.

39. Wagaarachchi PT, Ashok PW. Medical management of late intrauterine death using a combination of mifepristone and misoprostol. BJOG 2002;109:443–7.

40. Royal College of Obstetricians and Gynaecologists. Late intrauterine fetal death and stillbirth. Green-top Guideline 55. London: RCOG; 2010.

41 Hannah ME, Ohlsson A, Farine D. Induction of labor compared with expectant management for prelabour rupture of the membranes at term. TERMPROM Study Group. N Engl J Med 1996;334:1005–10.

42. Induction of labour. Evidence based guideline No. 9. Royal College of Obstetricians and Gynaecologists. Clinical Effectiveness Support Unit. London: RCOG Press; 2001.

43 Calder AA, Loughney AD, Weir CJ, Barber JW. Induction of labour in nulliparous and multiparous women: a UK, multicentre, open-label study of intravaginal misoprostol in comparison with dinoprostone. BJOG 2008; 115:1279–88.

44. Calder AA, Embrey MP, Hillier K. Extra-amniotic prostaglandin E2 for the induction of labour at term. J Obstet Gynaecol Br Commonw 1974;81:39–46.

CHAPTER 9

PRETERM LABOUR

JE Norman

'The usual period of a woman's going with child is nine calendar months; but there is very commonly a difference of one, two or three weeks. A child may be born alive at any time from three months: but we see none born with powers of coming to manhood, or of being reared, before seven calendar months, or near that time. At six months it cannot be.'
William Hunter c. 1760
Cited by Thomas Denman. In Introduction to the Practice of Midwifery. New York: E. Bliss and E. White, 1825, p253

INTRODUCTION

Although preterm deliveries constitute a small proportion of all births, their contribution to serious complications, especially those leading to perinatal death and morbidity, is hugely disproportionate. In 2010 it is estimated that 14.9 million babies worldwide (around 11.1% of all births) were premature.[1] Globally, preterm birth is the single biggest cause of neonatal death.[2] Babies born at 'term' (conventionally considered to be 37–42 weeks of gestation) have consistently better outcomes than those born 'preterm', with the risk of neonatal mortality and morbidity rising exponentially as the gestation of delivery decreases. Preterm labour is the single biggest cause of preterm birth, so that effective 'treatment' of preterm labour could have a major impact on global perinatal health. Such treatments include those aimed at preventing or halting preterm labour and also those that improve outcomes for babies of women in preterm labour. After decades in which there were few effective therapies, some promising strategies are emerging, which improve outcomes in a subset of women and babies. Despite this, the global toll of the adverse effects of preterm birth continues to rise, with preterm labour remaining the single biggest cause of neonatal mortality and morbidity in resource rich countries.

DEFINITION

The definition of preterm birth is not without controversy. The ICD10 (International Statistical Classification of Diseases and Related Health Problems 10th Revision) definition of preterm labour is the onset (spontaneous) of labour before 37 weeks of gestation (http://apps.who.int/classifications/icd10/browse/2010/en#/O60), thus preterm birth under this definition is considered to be birth before 37 completed weeks of gestation. The lower gestational limit is not defined under this system, although the WHO recommends that all babies born with any signs of life should be considered live births (and hence would be included). The lack of a consensus about the lower limit of preterm birth causes problems in comparing data among countries, with many countries (including Scotland, the USA and Brazil) not defining their lower gestational limit, some (such as Switzerland and Denmark) using a lower limit of 22 weeks and others (including Australia and Canada) using 20 weeks as the lower gestational limit of preterm birth.[1] Thus a woman who delivers a baby at 21 weeks with no signs of life would be likely to be considered to have had a miscarriage in Switzerland and Denmark, and probably in the majority of countries with no defined lower limit, but would be considered to have had a stillbirth in Australia and Canada. The birth would be defined as a preterm birth in the latter two countries but not the former two. Comparisons are further complicated by the use in some countries of low birth weight as a surrogate for preterm birth: this is inappropriate because not all small babies are preterm, and not all preterm babies are small.[3] Lastly, due to the phenomenon of delayed ovulation, where ultrasound is used to estimate gestational age (as is common in many resource rich countries), the calculated mean duration of pregnancy is consistently shorter, and the rate of prematurity is around 20% higher, than when gestation is calculated from the date of the last menstrual period.[4]

A recent report by the Global Alliance to Prevent Prematurity and Stillbirth has highlighted that similar aetiologies (albeit in different proportions) are involved in a pregnancy loss in the second trimester and in the mid third trimester, and that the risk of adverse outcome for the neonate decreases progressively as gestation advances, even beyond 37 weeks' gestation.[5,6] They propose a new definition and classification system whereby preterm birth would be 'any birth (which includes stillbirths and pregnancy terminations) that occurs after 16 weeks' gestation and before term (i.e., 39 weeks' gestation). The complete population of preterm deliveries within the gestational range as described earlier includes live births, stillbirths, multiple pregnancies, pregnancy terminations, and newborn infants with congenital malformations'.[5] The recommendation from this group is that 'gestational age estimation should, whenever possible, be corroborated by an early, high quality ultrasound and the best obstetric estimate be used for all gestational age determinations'.

PRETERM LABOUR VERSUS PRETERM BIRTH

The focus of this chapter is preterm labour, although this is not the only pathway to preterm birth. A categorization of (spontaneous) preterm labour, preterm premature rupture of membranes and elective (induced) preterm birth has been widely used, with Scottish data suggesting that the proportions of each (amongst all singletons delivering preterm) are 62%, 15% and 23% respectively[7] (Fig 9-1). Villar proposes that preterm birth is defined by pathway to delivery (spontaneous or care giver initiated) AND signs of initiation of parturition (evidence of initiation of parturition (including preterm premature rupture of membranes) or no evidence of

initiation of parturition) AND the presence of significant fetal, maternal or placental pathological conditions.[5] Under this classification, both preterm labour and preterm premature rupture of membranes would be considered to have evidence of initiation of parturition, whereas elective (induced) preterm birth would not. The pathway to delivery would be spontaneous in women presenting in preterm labour and those with preterm premature membrane rupture (because oxytocin augmentation of contractions is also considered in the spontaneous category) but would be care giver initiated in women undergoing elective (induced) preterm birth.

INCIDENCE OF PRETERM BIRTH

The incidence of preterm birth continues to rise globally, although both Scotland and the USA have seen a modest downturn in rates over the last few years. In the USA, this has been attributed to one or more of the widespread use of progesterone prophylaxis for prevention of preterm birth, a reduction in elective late preterm births and a change in maternal risk factor profiles.[8] In Scotland, the reduction in preterm births has been attributed to the ban on smoking in public places which came into effect in 2006.[9]

AETIOLOGY AND MECHANISMS

The 'cause' of preterm labour is incompletely understood.[10] Preterm labour is often accompanied by one or more of the following pathologies: intrauterine infection, intrauterine inflammation, utero-placental ischaemia, utero-placental haemorrhage, uterine stretch and maternal stress. It is not possible to determine whether these events 'cause' preterm labour, although there is strong circumstantial evidence of the role of intrauterine infection and inflammation. This is firstly because, even using relatively insensitive culture techniques, around 25–40% of women in preterm labour have demonstrable intrauterine infection. The proportion rises progressively as gestational age of labour onset declines. Secondly, intrauterine infection/inflammation stimulates an inflammatory response, including production of prostaglandins, implicated in increasing cervical ripening and myometrial contractility. Lastly, in animal models, intrauterine injection of microorganisms or pro-inflammatory agents (such as lipopolysaccharide) is effective in stimulating preterm labour.

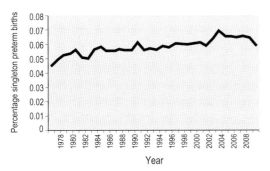

FIGURE 9-1 ■ Singleton preterm births in Scotland, expressed as a percentage of all singleton births, live and still, 1978 to 2010.[54]

TABLE 9-1   **Risk Factors for Preterm Labour**

Risk Factors for Preterm Labour, Adapted From Ref 10

Black ethnicity
Low socioeconomic group
Single marital status
Extremes of maternal age
Extremes of maternal BMI
Short interpregnancy interval
Previous preterm birth
Multiple pregnancy
Destructive treatments to cervix for cervical intra-epithelial neoplasia
Co-existent maternal systemic disease (e.g. diabetes mellitus)
Stress
Smoking
Drug use

TABLE 9-2   **Predictive Tests for Preterm Birth in Asymptomatic Women with Singleton Pregnancy**

	Positive LR	95% CI
Birth before 34 weeks' gestation:		
Cervicovaginal fluid fetal fibronectin[18]	7.65	3.93–14.68
Birth before 35 weeks' gestation:		
Cervical length measurement of <25 mm (at <20 weeks' gestation)[21]	4.31	3.08–6.01
Birth before 37 weeks' gestation:		
Cervicovaginal fluid fetal fibronectin[18]	3.40	2.29–5.05

CI, confidence interval; LR, likelihood ratio.

RISK FACTORS

The risk factors associated with preterm labour are listed in Table 9-1.

OUTCOMES

There is a clear dose–response relationship between gestation of preterm birth and risk of perinatal death, with outcomes being worst in babies born at earlier gestational ages, and the nadir not being reached until 40 weeks' gestation. For example, UK data show the combined rate of early neonatal, late neonatal and postneonatal death is 580 per 1000 babies born at 24 weeks, 98 per 1000 babies born at 28 weeks, 12 per 1000 for babies born at 34 weeks and 1 per 1000 for babies born at 40 weeks' gestation.[11] Babies who survive preterm birth also have a greater incidence of morbidity, and again this is inversely proportional to gestational age at delivery. For example, in the EPICure study (a prospective cohort of around 300 children who were born before 25 weeks' gestation in 1995, and who survived to reach the neonatal unit), 49% had neuromotor or sensory (sight or hearing) disability (with 23% of the total having severe disability) when assessed at 30 months of age, and the remainder had no disability according to the study criteria.[12] Subsequent studies have confirmed a 'dose dependent' effect of prematurity on long-term adverse health outcomes, which is inversely proportional to gestational age at delivery.[13–15] As with death, the nadir of 'prematurity' on educational attainment at school is not reached until birth at 40 weeks of gestation,[16] suggesting that even those who apparently have 'no disability' suffer long-term adverse consequences of prematurity.

PREDICTION

Although clinical risk factors for preterm labour have been identified, and predictive tests proposed, no strategy is sufficiently effective to be in widespread use in clinical practice. One of the most widely used clinical indicators, history of spontaneous preterm birth in a previous pregnancy, is associated with likelihood ratios of 4.62 (95% CI 3.28–6.52) and 2.26 (95% CI 1.86–2.74) respectively for birth before 34 and 37 weeks' gestation in a subsequent pregnancy.[17] The most widely used and the most effective tests for preterm labour prediction in asymptomatic women are detection of fetal fibronectin (fFN) in vaginal fluid and cervical length measurement.[17] The predictive ability of these strategies varies with the gestation of testing, the definition of a positive test (e.g. the length of the cervix or the quantitation of the fetal fibronectin) and the gestation of delivery being predicted. Typical summary likelihood ratios from meta-analyses of a range of studies are shown in Table 9-2. There is some evidence that fFN testing reduces the risk of preterm birth, with odds ratios of 0.54 (95% CI 0.34–0.87), although no benefit in terms of reduction in adverse outcomes was seen.[18] Newer tests are continually being proposed and evaluated – each of cervico-vaginal fluid prolactin and proteome profile and matrix metalloproteinase-8 in amniotic fluid shows promise, but they require further studies to define their efficacy.[19]

DIAGNOSIS

Preterm labour is a diagnosis that can confidently be made only in established labour. Many women present with symptoms suggestive of preterm labour (e.g. uterine contractions) but are found to have a closed cervix on examination. A proportion of such women will labour and deliver within a short space of time, but it is often very difficult for both women and their care givers to identify those who are, and those who are not, in the early stages of preterm labour. Again, cervicovaginal fluid fibronectin and cervical length measurements are amongst the best tests. In this scenario, the negative likelihood ratio (i.e. the effect of a negative test on the confidence with which preterm labour can be *excluded* as a diagnosis) is often the most helpful. For birth within 7–10 days of testing, fetal fibronectin has a negative likelihood ratio (i.e. a negative test reduces the risk of preterm birth) of 0.36 (95% CI 0.28–0.47),[18] and cervical length measurement of <15mm has a negative likelihood ratio of 0.026 (95% CI 0.0038–0.182)[20] in singleton pregnancies.

MANAGEMENT

Treatment with the object of reducing the incidence, risks and complications of preterm labour falls into three principal categories:

- Measures aimed at preventing preterm labour including early recognition and treatment of infection, cervical cerclage, progesterone prophylaxis and risk modification such as cessation of smoking and drug abuse.
- Tocolysis to try to abolish or arrest preterm labour.
- Obstetric interventions aimed at minimizing the complications of preterm delivery.

PREVENTION OF PRETERM LABOUR

Reducing Infection

Given the known link between intrauterine infection and preterm birth, with ascending infection from the vagina as the most likely route of entry, it is perhaps disappointing that antibiotics appear to be ineffective at preventing preterm birth, even in settings with a high prevalence of infective morbidity.[21,22] There is controversy about treatment of bacterial vaginosis, with some meta-analyses suggesting that early treatment, particularly with clindamycin, might reduce the risk of late but not early preterm birth.[23,24] Despite the emerging link between periodontitis and preterm birth, periodontal treatment does not appear to reduce the risk of preterm birth.[25]

Mechanical Methods of Maintaining Cervical Length

The procedure of cervical cerclage is discussed elsewhere in this book. For women with a singleton pregnancy, a previous history of preterm birth and a short cervix on ultrasound (<25 mm at <24 weeks' gestation), cerclage reduces both preterm birth *and* perinatal mortality and morbidity, with a relative risk (95% CI) for this latter outcome of RR (relative risk) 0.64 (95% CI 0.45–0.91).[26,27] Importantly, in women with a singleton pregnancy and a previous preterm birth, screening with ultrasound followed by selected cerclage in those with a short cervix appears as effective as routine cerclage insertion based on history alone.[28] Cerclage is ineffective at preventing preterm birth in women with a twin pregnancy – indeed, it appears harmful in this scenario.[26] An alternative mechanical method is the Arabin pessary, a device which covers the cervical os. A recent randomized trial of 385 women showed a marked reduction of risk of preterm birth before 34 weeks in women with a short cervix (<25mm) who were 'treated' with the pessary.[29] Further studies are probably required to determine the place of the Arabin pessary in routine clinical practice.

Progesterone

Several large studies and a meta-analysis have suggested that progesterone reduces the risk of preterm birth in women with a singleton pregnancy and a history of preterm birth[30,31] and in women with a short cervix on ultrasound.[32–34] Some studies have shown a reduction in neonatal morbidity.[31,33] There is an absence of significant evidence on any longer-term benefit for the baby – addressing this evidence gap is the focus of the OPPTIMUM study currently underway in the UK and Europe.[35] Again, twins respond differently, with progesterone failing to reduce rates of preterm birth in twin pregnancy.[36]

TOCOLYSIS TO ABOLISH OR ARREST PRETERM LABOUR

An array of drugs have been used to try to abolish or arrest preterm labour, including β sympathomimetics (ritodrine), oxytocin antagonists (atosiban), calcium channel blockers (nifedipine), prostaglandin synthase inhibitors (indomethacin) and nitric oxide donors (nitroglycerine). None has been shown to improve neonatal mortality or morbidity in women presenting in preterm labour, leading the Royal College of Obstetricians and Gynaecologists in the UK to conclude 'In the absence of clear evidence that tocolytic drugs improve outcome following preterm labour, it is reasonable not to use them'.[37] Calcium channel blockers such as nifedipine have some evidence of benefit in terms of reducing delivery within 7 days of receiving treatment (RR 0.76; 95% confidence interval (CI) 0.60 to 0.97) and prior to 34 weeks' gestation (RR 0.83; 95% CI 0.69 to 0.99).[38] It is possible that the combination of a tocolytic agent such as nifedipine with either corticosteroids to improve fetal lung maturation and/or magnesium sulphate to reduce perinatal brain injury might be more effective than the latter alone, but such strategies have not been subjected to large randomized trials. Importantly, the maternal side effects of treatment with tocolytic agents are becoming increasingly clear, with use of multiple agents being particularly problematic.[39] Any decision to give tocolysis should be carefully considered by both mother and clinician.

MINIMIZING THE COMPLICATIONS OF PRETERM DELIVERY

Corticosteroids

In contrast to the unproven effects of tocolytic agents on improving neonatal outcome, there is overwhelming evidence that prenatal steroids are of benefit to babies destined to be born preterm. A single course of antenatal corticosteroids (dexamethasone, betamethasone or hydrocortisone) reduces neonatal death (RR 0.69; 95% CI 0.58 to 0.81), cerebroventricular haemorrhage (RR 0.54; 95% CI 0.43 to 0.69) and necrotizing enterocolitis (RR 0.46; 95% CI 0.29 to 0.74)[40] in preterm babies. Enthusiasm for the beneficial effects of corticosteroids and difficulties about the diagnosis of preterm labour have led to many babies being exposed to multiple doses of corticosteroids before birth. Studies of the effect of such a strategy have come to differing conclusions, with the Cochrane review suggesting that multiple doses were beneficial in the short term, with a significant reduction in respiratory distress syndrome (RR 0.83; 95% CI 0.75–0.91) and serious neonatal morbidity (RR 0.84; 95% CI 0.75–0.94)[41] whereas a single large trial (n > 2000 babies) has shown a dose-dependent reduction in birth weight in association with antenatal corticosteroids.[42] Until the long-term effects are clearer a single dose of steroids should be the standard of care for babies likely to be born preterm.

Magnesium Sulphate

This agent is widely used for seizure prophylaxis in women with pre-eclampsia and for the treatment of eclampsia. Emerging evidence from a number of studies suggests that its antenatal administration may also reduce hypoxic ischaemic cerebral damage in babies destined to be born preterm. Antenatal magnesium sulphate reduces both cerebral palsy (RR 0.68; 95% CI 0.54–0.87) and gross motor dysfunction in premature infants (RR 0.61; 95% CI 0.44–0.88). Demonstrable benefit is currently restricted to babies born before 30 weeks' gestation. An ongoing study (Magenta – http://www.adelaide.edu.au/arch/research/clinical_trials/) will determine whether antenatal administration also improves outcome in babies delivered from 30 to 34 weeks' gestation. The optimal regimen is uncertain: a simple strategy endorsed by an expert consensus group suggests that women under 30 weeks' gestation who are likely to deliver within the next 24 hours should be given a 4 g loading dose of magnesium sulphate (slowly over 20–30 minutes) followed by a 1 g per hour maintenance dose via the intravenous route.[43]

Routine Antibiotics

The lack of efficacy of antibiotics to prevent preterm labour has been described above. An alternative strategy has been to give antibiotics to women who present in preterm labour, in the hope that they will delay delivery and improve outcome for the baby. In women with intact fetal membranes, such a strategy is singularly unsuccessful, with no short-term beneficial effect of either co-amoxiclav or erythromycin for the neonate.[44] Additionally, a comprehensive follow-up study has suggested that routine antibiotic administration to women in preterm labour is actually harmful, with increased rates of cerebral palsy in the offspring exposed to prenatal antibiotics, with some evidence of a dose-dependent effect.[45] Thus there is no justification to give antibiotics routinely to women presenting with preterm labour and intact fetal membranes. Antibiotic prophylaxis against group B streptococcal infection for women in preterm labour is <u>not</u> now recommended routinely, and should be restricted to women who are known to be colonized with the infection.[46]

PRETERM PREMATURE MEMBRANE RUPTURE

Diagnosis

The diagnosis of pPROM is made by a combination of history from the woman, followed by a sterile speculum examination to visualize amniotic fluid in the vagina. The false positive rates of the nitrazine test (to identify pH change) and identification of 'ferning' on a slide are such that these tests are not routinely recommended in clinical practice.[47] Ultrasound examination can be helpful if it confirms a decrease in amniotic fluid volume.

Prognosis and Management

Women with pPROM are at increased risk of spontaneous labour, with the average latency period being less than 3 days.[48] In view of the risk of preterm delivery, most authorities recommend that such women should be given corticosteroid prophylaxis.[47] Women with pPROM are also at increased risk of ascending infection leading to chorioamnionitis. A common practice, endorsed by national guidelines in the UK, is to offer induction of labour to women with pPROM once they reach 34 weeks' gestation.[47] However, a recent trial and updated meta-analysis suggests that the benefits of expediting delivery are minimal, with no effect of early delivery on neonatal sepsis (RR of 1.06; 95% CI 0.64 to 1.76) or caesarean section (RR 1.27; 95% CI 0.98 to 1.65), when compared with expectant management.[49] The reduction in histologically confirmed chorioamnionitis in the early delivery group in the van den Ham study (RR 0.69; 95% CI 0.49 to 0.96) and the lack of adverse effect on respiratory distress in the updated meta-analysis (RR 1.03; 95% CI 0.8–1.32) may be a justification to continue a policy of early delivery (from 34 weeks' gestation) for women and their care givers who prefer this option.[49]

If expectant management is planned, antibiotic prophylaxis with erythromycin is recommended by some authorities[47] as it is associated with an improvement in a composite neonatal outcome in the short term[50] with no evidence of harm in the long term.[51] Given the known harmful long-term effects of antibiotics to women in preterm labour with *intact* fetal membranes,[45] antibiotics should be withheld if there is any uncertainty about fetal membrane rupture. Tocolysis is not indicated.

MODE OF DELIVERY FOR PRETERM INFANTS

The optimal mode of delivery of the preterm infant is unknown. The greater vulnerability of the preterm infant might lead some clinicians and pregnant women to wish to avoid vaginal delivery. Randomized trial evidence on this issue is extremely limited, with only four studies of 116 women in total being considered of an adequate standard for a systematic review.[52] Not surprisingly, given the small sample size, there is no evidence from these trials of either caesarean section or vaginal delivery being superior in terms of avoiding birth trauma, perinatal death or neonatal intensive care admission. A recent observational study of over 4000 babies has shown that, in babies from 24 to 32 weeks' gestation, attempted vaginal delivery is safe and likely to be achieved in babies presenting by the vertex.[53] For babies presenting by the breech, there was an increased risk of death for babies between 24 and 32 weeks, and an increased risk of the combination of death and asphyxia for those between 24 and 27 weeks when vaginal delivery was attempted. Less than 30% of pregnancies presenting by the breech in which vaginal delivery was allowed between 24 and 32 weeks' gestation actually managed to deliver vaginally. Although multivariate analysis was used, the risk of confounding remains. Nevertheless, in women delivering preterm, these data support a practice of attempting vaginal delivery for babies presenting by the vertex. For babies presenting by the breech, it would appear that the strategy of planned caesarean section, as recommended for babies at term with persistent breech presentation, may have advantages.[53]

CONCLUSION

Preterm labour remains the biggest contributor to adverse neonatal outcome in both resource rich and resource poor settings. A number of interventions, including antenatal corticosteroid and magnesium sulphate prophylaxis have now been shown to improve outcome for the neonate. Prevention of preterm delivery remains the goal, but it is essential that any agent used for this indication is shown to improve long-term childhood outcomes, and does not merely change the gestation of delivery. Given intensive lobbying by many groups, including the Gates Foundation and the March of Dimes in the USA, and Tommy's the Baby Charity and Action Medical Research in the UK, together with support from governmental bodies, it is to be hoped that novel interventions to prevent preterm birth will be identified over the next few decades.

REFERENCES

1. Blencowe H, Cousens S, Oestergaard MZ, Chou D, Moller AB, Narwal R, et al. National, regional, and worldwide estimates of preterm birth rates in the year 2010 with time trends since 1990 for selected countries: a systematic analysis and implications. Lancet 2012; 379:2162–72.
2. Lawn JE, Cousens S, Zupan J. 4 million neonatal deaths: when? Where? Why? Lancet 2005;365:891–900.
3. Lawn JE, Gravett MG, Nunes TM, Rubens CE, Stanton C. Global report on preterm birth and stillbirth (1 of 7): definitions, description of the burden and opportunities to improve data. BMC Pregnancy Childbirth 2010; 10(Suppl. 1):S1.
4. Yang H, Kramer MS, Platt RW, Blondel B, Breart G, Morin I, et al. How does early ultrasound scan estimation of gestational age lead to higher rates of preterm birth? Am J Obst Gynecol 2002;186:433–7.
5. Villar J, Papageorghiou AT, Knight HE, Gravett MG, Iams J, Waller SA, et al. The preterm birth syndrome: a prototype phenotypic classification. Am J Obstet Gynecol 2012;206:119–23.
6. Goldenberg RL, Gravett MG, Iams J, Papageorghiou AT, Waller SA, Kramer M, et al. The preterm birth syndrome: issues to consider in creating a classification system. Am J Obstet Gynecol 2012;206:113–18.
7. Norman JE, Morris C, Chalmers J. The effect of changing patterns of obstetric care in Scotland (1980–2004) on rates of preterm birth and its neonatal consequences: perinatal database study. PLoS Med 2009;e1000153.
8. Norwitz ER, Caughey AB. Progesterone supplementation and the prevention of preterm birth. Rev Obstet Gynecol 2011;4:60–72.
9. Mackay DF, Nelson SM, Haw SJ, Pell JP. Impact of Scotland's smoke-free legislation on pregnancy complications: retrospective cohort study. PLoS Med 2012;9: e1001175.
10. Goldenberg RL, Culhane JF, Iams JD, Romero R. Epidemiology and causes of preterm birth. Lancet 2008; 371:75–84.
11. Moser K, Macfarlane A, Chow YH, Hilder L, Dattani N. Introducing new data on gestation-specific infant mortality among babies born in 2005 in England and Wales. Health Stat Q 2007;35:14–27.
12. Wood NS, Marlow N, Costeloe K, Gibson AT, Wilkinson AR. Neurologic and developmental disability after extremely preterm birth. EPICure Study Group. New Eng J Med 2000;343: 378–84.
13. Boyle EM, Poulsen G, Field DJ, Kurinczuk JJ, Wolke D, Alfirevic Z, et al. Effects of gestational age at birth on health outcomes at 3 and 5 years of age: population based cohort study. BMJ 2012;344:e896.
14. Shapiro-Mendoza CK, Tomashek KM, Kotelchuck M, Barfield W, Nannini A, Weiss J, et al. Effect of late-preterm birth and maternal medical conditions on newborn morbidity risk. Pediatrics 2008;121:e223–32.
15. Mwaniki MK, Atieno M, Lawn JE, Newton CR. Long-term neurodevelopmental outcomes after intrauterine and neonatal insults: a systematic review. Lancet 2012; 379:445–52.
16. MacKay DF, Smith GC, Dobbie R, Pell JP. Gestational age at delivery and special educational need: retrospective cohort study of 407,503 schoolchildren. PLoS Med 2010;7:e1000289.
17. Honest H, Forbes CA, Duree KH, Norman G, Duffy SB, Tsourapas A, et al. Screening to prevent spontaneous preterm birth: systematic reviews of accuracy and effectiveness literature with economic modelling. Health Technol Assess 2009;13:1–627.
18. Berghella V, Hayes E, Visintine J, Baxter JK. Fetal fibronectin testing for reducing the risk of preterm birth. Cochrane Database Syst Rev 2008;4:CD006843.
19. Conde-Agudelo A, Papageorghiou AT, Kennedy SH, Villar J. Novel biomarkers for the prediction of the spontaneous preterm birth phenotype: a systematic review and meta-analysis. BJOG 2011;118:1042–54.
20. Tsoi E, Fuchs IB, Rane S, Geerts L, Nicolaides KH. Sonographic measurement of cervical length in threatened preterm labor in singleton pregnancies with intact membranes. Ultrasound Obstet Gynecol 2005;25: 353–6.
21. Simcox R, Sin WT, Seed PT, Briley A, Shennan AH. Prophylactic antibiotics for the prevention of preterm birth in women at risk: a meta-analysis. Austral N Z J Obstet Gynaecol 2007;47:368–77.
22. van den Broek NR, White SA, Goodall M, Ntonya C, Kayira E, Kafulafula G, et al. The APPLe study: a randomized, community-based, placebo-controlled trial of azithromycin for the prevention of preterm birth, with meta-analysis. PLoS Med 2009;6:e1000191.
23. McDonald H, Brocklehurst P, Parsons J. Antibiotics for treating bacterial vaginosis in pregnancy. Cochrane Database Syst Rev 2005;1:CD000262.
24. Lamont RF, Nhan-Chang CL, Sobel JD, Workowski K, Conde-Agudelo A, Romero R. Treatment of abnormal vaginal flora in early pregnancy with clindamycin for the prevention of spontaneous preterm birth: a systematic review and metaanalysis. Am J Obstet Gynecol 2011; 205:177–90.
25. Chambrone L, Pannuti CM, Guglielmetti MR, Chambrone LA. Evidence grade associating periodontitis with preterm birth and/or low birth weight: II: a systematic review of randomized trials evaluating the effects of periodontal treatment. J Clin Periodontol 2011;38: 902–14.
26. Berghella V, Odibo AO, To MS, Rust OA, Althuisius SM. Cerclage for short cervix on ultrasonography: meta-analysis of trials using individual patient-level data. Obstet Gynecol 2005;106:181–9.
27. Berghella V, Rafael TJ, Szychowski JM, Rust OA, Owen J. Cerclage for short cervix on ultrasonography in women with singleton gestations and previous preterm birth: a meta-analysis. Obstet Gynecol 2011;117: 663–71.
28. Berghella V, Mackeen AD. Cervical length screening with ultrasound-indicated cerclage compared with history-indicated cerclage for prevention of preterm birth: a meta-analysis. Obstet Gynecol 2011;118: 148–55.
29. Goya M, Pratcorona L, Merced C, Rodo C, Valle L, Romero A, et al. Cervical pessary in pregnant women with a short cervix (PECEP): an open-label randomised controlled trial. Lancet 2012;379:1800–6.
30. da Fonseca EB, Bittar RE, Carvalho MH, Zugaib M. Prophylactic administration of progesterone by vaginal suppository to reduce the incidence of spontaneous preterm birth in women at increased risk: a randomized

placebo-controlled double-blind study. Am J Obstet Gynecol 2003;188:419–24.

31. Meis PJ, Klebanoff M, Thom E, Dombrowski MP, Sibai B, Moawad AH, et al. Prevention of recurrent preterm delivery by 17 alpha-hydroxyprogesterone caproate. New Eng J Med 2003;348:2379–85.

32. Fonseca EB, Celik E, Parra M, Singh M, Nicolaides KH, Thornton S, et al. Progesterone and the risk of preterm birth among women with a short cervix. New Eng J Med 2007;357:462–9.

33. Romero R, Nicolaides K, Conde-Agudelo A, Tabor A, O'Brien JM, Cetingoz E, et al. Vaginal progesterone in women with an asymptomatic sonographic short cervix in the midtrimester decreases preterm delivery and neonatal morbidity: a systematic review and metaanalysis of individual patient data. Am J Obstet Gynecol 2012; 206:124 e1–19.

34. Dodd JM, Flenady VJ, Cincotta R, Crowther CA. Progesterone for the prevention of preterm birth: a systematic review. Obstet Gynecol 2008;112:127–34.

35. Norman JE, Shennan A, Bennett P, Thornton S, Robson S, Marlow N, et al. Trial protocol OPPTIMUM – Does progesterone prophylaxis for the prevention of preterm labour improve outcome? BMC Pregnancy Childbirth 2012;12:79.

36. Norman JE, Mackenzie F, Owen P, Mactier H, Hanretty K, Cooper S, et al. Progesterone for the prevention of preterm birth in twin pregnancy (STOPPIT): a randomised, double-blind, placebo-controlled study and meta-analysis. Lancet 2009;373: 2034–40.

37. Royal College of Obstetricians and Gynaecologists. Tocolysis for women in preterm labour. RCOG 2011.

38. King JF, Flenady V, Papatsonis D, Dekker G, Carbonne B. Calcium channel blockers for inhibiting preterm labour; a systematic review of the evidence and a protocol for administration of nifedipine. Austral NZ J Obstet Gynaecol 2003;43:192–8.

39. de Heus R, Mol BW, Erwich JJ, van Geijn HP, Gyselaers WJ, Hanssens M, et al. Adverse drug reactions to tocolytic treatment for preterm labour: prospective cohort study. BMJ 2009;338:b744.

40. Roberts D, Dalziel S. Antenatal corticosteroids for accelerating fetal lung maturation for women at risk of preterm birth. Cochrane Database Syst Rev 2006;3: CD004454.

41. McKinlay CJ, Crowther CA, Middleton P, Harding JE. Repeat antenatal glucocorticoids for women at risk of preterm birth: a Cochrane Systematic Review. Am J Obstet Gynecol 2012;206:187–94.

42. Murphy KE, Willan AR, Hannah ME, Ohlsson A, Kelly EN, Matthews SG, et al. Effect of antenatal corticosteroids on fetal growth and gestational age at birth. Obstet Gynecol 2012;119:917–23.

43. Antenatal Magnesium Sulfate for Neuroprotection Guideline Development Panel. Antenatal magnesium sulfate prior to preterm birth for neuroprotection of fetus, infant and child. Adelaide, Australia: Australian Research Centre for Health of Women and Babies; 2010.

44. Kenyon SL, Taylor DJ, Tarnow-Mordi W. Broad-spectrum antibiotics for spontaneous preterm labour: the ORACLE II randomised trial. ORACLE Collaborative Group. Lancet 2001;357:989–94.

45. Kenyon S, Pike K, Jones DR, Brocklehurst P, Marlow N, Salt A, et al. Childhood outcomes after prescription of antibiotics to pregnant women with spontaneous preterm labour: 7-year follow-up of the ORACLE II trial. Lancet 2008;372:1319–27.

46. Royal College of Obstetricians and Gynaecologists. The prevention of early-onset neonatal group B streptococcal disease. Green-top Guideline no 36. London: RCOG; 2012.

47. Royal College of Obstetricians and Gynaecologists. Preterm prelabour rupture of membranes. London: RCOG; 2010.

48. Simhan HN, Canavan TP. Preterm premature rupture of membranes: diagnosis, evaluation and management strategies. BJOG 2005;12(Suppl. 1):32–7.

49. van der Ham DP, Vijgen SM, Nijhuis JG, van Beek JJ, Opmeer BC, Mulder AL, et al. Induction of labor versus expectant management in women with preterm prelabor rupture of membranes between 34 and 37 weeks: a randomized controlled trial. PLoS Med 2012;9:e1001208.

50. Kenyon SL, Taylor DJ, Tarnow-Mordi W. Broad-spectrum antibiotics for preterm, prelabour rupture of fetal membranes: the ORACLE I randomised trial. ORACLE Collaborative Group. Lancet 2001;357: 979–88.

51. Kenyon S, Pike K, Jones DR, Brocklehurst P, Marlow N, Salt A, et al. Childhood outcomes after prescription of antibiotics to pregnant women with preterm rupture of the membranes: 7-year follow-up of the ORACLE I trial. Lancet 2008;372:1310–18.

52. Alfirevic Z, Milan SJ, Livio S. Caesarean section versus vaginal delivery for preterm birth in singletons. Cochrane Database Syst Rev 2012;6:CD000078.

53. Reddy UM, Zhang J, Sun L, Chen Z, Raju TN, Laughon SK. Neonatal mortality by attempted route of delivery in early preterm birth. Am J Obstet Gynecol 2012;207:117 e1–8.

54. Information Services Division, NHS National Services Scotland. Births in Scottish hospitals (year ending 31 March 2010). 2011.

CHAPTER 10

ASSISTED VAGINAL DELIVERY

TF Baskett

There is no chapter in the history of obstetrics that is more central to the development of the clinical art of obstetrics than the invention and evolution of the obstetric forceps. Indeed, there are few surgical instruments that remain in use, albeit modified, more than three centuries after their introduction. In contrast, the other instrument used to assist vaginal delivery, the vacuum extractor, while having its origins some 150 years ago, has really only been developed in practical clinical terms over the past half century. Because assisted vaginal delivery was and remains an essential clinical obstetrical skill its history and evolution over almost four centuries will be recorded here. Indeed, to a large extent it was the development of the obstetric forceps in the hands of the 'man-midwife' that allowed the physician access to the birth chamber, formerly almost the sole purview of the midwife.

HISTORICAL BACKGROUND

Four important events mark the evolution of the obstetric forceps: (1) the invention, (2) the introduction of the pelvic curve, (3) the introduction of axis-traction devices, (4) the return to a modified 'straight' forceps for application to the low, transversely placed head.

THE INVENTION OF THE FORCEPS

On 3 July 1569 there disembarked at Southampton a Huguenot refugee family by the name of Chamberlen (Chamberlayne, Chamberlaine and Chamberlin are other spellings). The family consisted of William the father (whether he ever practised medicine or was qualified to do so has not been determined), his wife and three children. Two other sons were born a year and 3 years, respectively, after the family had settled in England. The eldest and the youngest son were both named Peter and are referred to by obstetric historians as 'Peter the older' and 'Peter the younger'. To add to the confusion there was a third Peter, a son of Peter the younger, known under the designation 'Dr Peter Chamberlen' because he was Doctor of Medicine at Padua (1619), Oxford (1620) and Cambridge (1621) and a Fellow of the College of Physicians (1628); while the father and uncle were of the Barber Surgeons Company (date of admission round about the years 1596–8). Further reference to these three Peters will be under the respective numbers I, II and III which some historians have very wisely adopted for the purpose of distinguishing them.

For many years the invention was attributed to Peter III (Dr Peter Chamberlen), who was born in 1601 and died in 1683. This impression, however, is almost certainly refuted by his own statement:[1] 'My Fame begot me envie and secret enemies which mightily increased when my Father added to me the knowledge of "Deliveries and the Cures of Women".' There is therefore every justification for concluding that the inventor of the obstetric forceps was either Peter I or Peter II, or possibly both.

Peter I (1560?–1631) attained the greater distinction and his rise to fame was as dramatic as it was rapid. He attended Anne of Denmark, Queen Consort of James I and other notable women in society in their confinements. And for so doing as a Barber Surgeon he was arraigned before the College of Physicians in 1612 and incarcerated in Newgate Prison. By the intervention of the Queen and the Archbishop of Canterbury, the President and Censors of the College were prevailed upon to permit his release.

Peter II (1572–1626), the brother, some 10 or 12 years younger, was also interested in midwifery and he was the first to suggest the creation of an Incorporation of Midwives, a project with which Peter III, his son, was more particularly identified.

The probability is that Peter I was the inventor and that the date of the invention was shortly before or shortly after 1600. There is of course the other remote possibility that if 'Old Father William' did practise medicine, as some historians thought was the case, he may have been the actual inventor of the instrument.[2]

The secret was kept in the family for 100 years or more. But many attempts were made – presumably the secret was beginning to leak out – to trade the instrument in Paris and Amsterdam by Hugh Chamberlen Senior (son of Peter III), who possessed all his father's combativeness and business instincts, coupled with his ability to retain a position at Court and amongst numerous clients in the highest social scale. Historical was his encounter with the great obstetrician Francois Mauriceau (1637–1709) in Paris in 1670 when, to test the value of the forceps, Mauriceau gave him a rachitic dwarf (who had been many days in labour) to deliver. Of course, Chamberlen failed and Mauriceau chuck-

HISTORICAL BACKGROUND (Continued)

led! Yet, like all commercial travellers, so little was he abashed by his failure that within 6 months we find him again in Paris, on this occasion attempting to sell the invention to the French Government.[3,4]

It was not until the 18th century was well advanced that the secret of the forceps became known. It was first announced by Edmund Chapman (1680?–1756), the obstetrician of Essex and London, who publicly made known the forceps used by the Chamberlens.[5]

Space does not permit, nor is the occasion suitable, to pursue here the story of this most remarkable family and its doings; nor to describe the schemes – medical, political and commercial – which they sponsored. Fortunately, in Aveling's historic volume[1] we possess a complete record of all these details and of what perhaps was the crowning event in the romance of the forceps, the discovery in 1818 of a number of the Chamberlens' instruments (Fig 10-1) in a well-concealed chest in Woodham Mortimer Hall, Essex, which had been purchased by Peter III round about 1630 and continued in the possession of the family until 1715.

On the death in 1728 of Hugh (Junior), son of Hugh (Senior) and grandson of Peter III, the male line of the Chamberlens became extinct. He too was a popular obstetrician and physician and carried on a most successful practice amongst the highest classes of society of London. As far as can be judged, he shed the aggressive enthusiasm, commercial instincts and timely sanctimoniousness of his forebears. He mellowed, was popular with the fellows and was three times elected a Censor of the College of Physicians. He is commemorated in the cenotaph in the north aisle of the choir in Westminster Abbey erected by the son of his patron the Duke of Buckingham, no doubt at the instigation of the Duchess, with whom he lived on intimate terms following the death of the Duke. Thus is the story of the family rounded off by these events!

The forceps of the Chamberlens – admittedly those illustrated here were early patterns – was simple in design and possessed only a cephalic curve, and in this form they remained for well over 100 years (1600?–1747).

THE INTRODUCTION OF THE PELVIC CURVE

To André Levret (1703–1780) is attributed this improvement, which he brought to the notice of the Paris Academy in 1747. As is often the case, other individuals came up with the same idea at about the same time. Benjamin Pugh (1715–1798), an obstetrician in Chelmsford, Essex, claimed, in the preface of his 1754 Treatise of Midwifery, 'The curved forceps I invented upwards of 14 years ago…'[6] It is likely that about the same time William Smellie (1697–1763) independently conceived the same modification, but in respect of the design of the forceps it is mainly for the simplification of the lock ('English lock') that we are indebted to him. The lock Chapman designed was simply a slot in each blade and not nearly so secure as Smellie's lock.

Incidentally, we would mention here that Smellie was the first to recommend forceps for the delivery of the after-coming head in breech extractions and it was largely because he found the straight forceps unsuitable that he invented a long double-curved forceps.[7]

With the addition of this new pelvic curve the instrument was obviously more suitable for extracting a fetal head arrested high in the pelvis, but it still suffered from one of the chief faults of the long straight forceps: namely that when applied to a high head much of the traction force (a third to a half) was expended by pulling the head against the pubes.

THE INTRODUCTION OF AXIS-TRACTION DEVICES

Etienne Stéphane Tarnier (1828–1897) will ever be honoured as the inventor of axis-traction forceps.[8] But long before Tarnier described his instrument in 1877 it had been fully appreciated that, even with the long double-curved forcep, traction in the axis of the pelvis was impossible and that a great deal of the force exerted by the operator was lost by the head being pulled against the anterior pelvic wall. Levret, Smellie and Baudelocque, for example, in order to obviate this, gave directions how traction

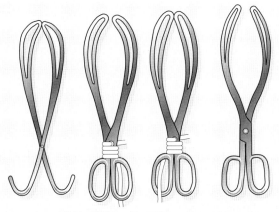

FIGURE 10-1 ■ Chamberlen's forceps.

Continued on following page

HISTORICAL BACKGROUND (Continued)

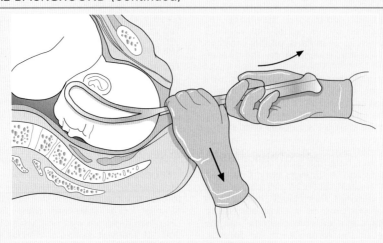

FIGURE 10-2 ■ Pajot's manoeuvre.

was to be made as far back as possible. Charles Pajot (1816–1896) of Paris popularized the manoeuvre to assist this posteriorly directed traction (Fig 10-2). Although known as Pajot's manoeuvre it was first described by the Danish obstetrician Mathias Saxtorph (1740–1800).[9]

With the object of obtaining traction in the axis of the pelvis, many alterations and additions to the ordinary double-curved forceps were suggested in times past. One of the earliest – that of Saxtorph – was the use of bands through the fenestrae of the blades. A century later this suggestion reappeared in the recommendation of Poullet to pass cords through holes made immediately below the fenestrae of the blades; in more recent times Haig Ferguson once again recommended this primitive device.[10]

As far as can be ascertained, the suggestion of having special traction handles was made first by Hermann of Berne in 1844.[11] But the rods in Hermann's forceps were employed on the same principle as that by which Saxtorph and Pajot effected their manoeuvres. Hermann's device seems to have been forgotten, if, indeed, it ever became very generally known.

An important step in the evolution of the instrument was Hubert's traction bar, described in 1860, for by it traction could undoubtedly still be exerted in the axis of the pelvis. Still later, the ends of the handles were bent backwards in a wide perineal curve. Alternatively, a detachable traction handle incorporating a perineal curve was applied to either the upper or the lower ends of the handles – some patterns recently employed (Neville-Barnes, Haig Ferguson) have the latter arrangement. It is perfectly evident to everyone that, in employing the ordinary forceps with the head at the brim, a large amount of force is dissipated against the anterior pelvic wall: Tarnier estimated that nearly half the traction force was lost. With axis-traction forceps this is avoided in greater part. The mechanics of axis-traction forceps were very carefully considered by Tarnier[8] and by Milne Murray.[12] To those interested in this now historical subject

we would commend the writings of those two authorities.

THE INTRODUCTION OF STRAIGHT FORCEPS FOR ROTATION OF THE FETAL HEAD

The Norwegian obstetrician, Christian Kielland (1871–1941), designed straight forceps without a pelvic curve to facilitate delivery from the mid-pelvis in cases of malrotation with occipito-transverse and occipito-posterior positions of the fetal head.[13] In fact, William Smellie had used the same principles of rotation almost two centuries before.[14] Kielland laid down very precise rules for the use of his forceps which could be more correctly applied than forceps with a pelvic curve to the incompletely rotated fetal head in the mid or upper pelvis.[15] In 1928, Lyman Barton (1866–1944), a rural general practitioner in New York State, developed straight forceps with a hinged anterior blade to facilitate application to the fetal head arrested in the transverse position at the pelvic brim.[16] Arvind Moolgaoker later modified the Kielland forceps to incorporate a distance-spacing wedge between the handles to maintain the parallel positions of the forcep blades around the fetal head.[17] Kielland's forceps enjoyed considerable use in the middle part of the 20th century and continue to be applied in some hospitals for arrested occipito-posterior and occipito-transverse positions in the low–mid-pelvis.

THE VACUUM EXTRACTOR

The history of the vacuum extractor is much shorter but its use is increasing, so that a majority of assisted vaginal deliveries are now performed using this instrument as opposed to the obstetric forceps. The vacuum principle was probably first applied in medicine with a cupping-glass to treat depressed skull fractures in infants and adults.[18] The first attempted obstetrical application was in 1705 by James Yonge, surgeon to the Naval Hospital in Plymouth, England. He unsuccessfully attempted to deliver a fetus 'by a cupping-glass fixt to the scalp with an air pump'.[19] Neil Arnott (1788–1874), a Scot who received his education in Aberdeen and

HISTORICAL BACKGROUND (Continued)

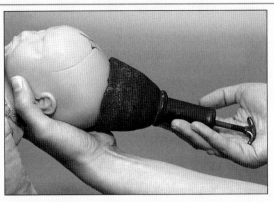

FIGURE 10-3 ■ Simpson's air tractor. This early attempt to develop an instrument was hampered by an inability to produce sufficient negative pressure. The piston was of metal, the cup of wood and the rim was lined with leather which when wet allowed an airtight seal with the presenting part of the fetus. (Property of the Department of Obstetrics and Gynaecology, University of Edinburgh).

London, practised medicine in London and outlined the principles of a pneumatic tractor.[20] There is no evidence that Arnott used his tractor for clinical purposes but he did propose its application in obstetrics: 'Now it seems peculiarly adapted to the purpose of obstetric surgery, viz, as a substitute for the steel forceps in the hands of men who are deficient in manual dexterity, whether from inexperience or natural inaptitude'.[20]

Some 20 years later James Young Simpson of Edinburgh (1811–1870), acknowledging the work of Arnott, developed a practical suction-tractor[21] (Fig 10-3). After his initial publications Simpson wrote no more on the subject and in the same year developed the obstetric forceps that bear his name and continue in use 150 years later.

The next century saw a number of attempts to apply the vacuum principle to assist vaginal delivery, but none achieved clinical utility.[18] Tage Malmström of Sweden (1911–1995) was the father of the modern extractor. His unique contribution was a metal cup with an in-curved rounded margin. Thus, the peripheral margin of the cup attached to the fetal scalp had a narrower diameter than the upper margin, thereby producing a 'chignon' and effectively increasing the total surface area of application and reducing the risk of cup detachment during traction. Malmström introduced his prototype in 1953 with refinements culminating in 1957.[22,23] Malmström's cup had the suction and traction portions attached by one port in the centre of the cup. The English obstetrician Geoffrey Bird (1922–2001), who worked in Kenya, Australia and Papua New Guinea, made the next significant contribution to development of the vacuum extractor. He separated the traction and suction ports and emphasized the importance of accurate cup placement over the flexion point of the fetal head to minimize the presenting diameter.[24] In order to facilitate placement of the cup over the flexion point in deflexed occipito-transverse and occipito-posterior positions Bird further modified the cup so that the suction port originated from the lateral margin. This so-called 'posterior cup' facilitated placement over the flexion point in the deflexed fetal head.[25]

In the 1970s, in an attempt to reduce scalp trauma attributed to the metal cups, vacuum cups were manufactured with soft material. These softer cups did reduce the superficial scalp trauma but were associated with a much higher failure rate of achieving delivery, up to 25%, compared to a failure rate of <5% with the metal cups.[18] By the end of the 20th century, due to this high failure rate, vacuum cups were manufactured with harder plastic, and these continue in widespread use.[26]

GENERAL CONSIDERATIONS

Assisted vaginal delivery of cephalic presentations involves the use of either forceps or vacuum to achieve delivery of the fetal head. These instruments allow the operator to apply extraction forces along the pelvic curve. In the case of the vacuum this is achieved by applying suction and traction to the fetal scalp, while the forceps cradle the parietal and malar bones of the fetal skull and, in addition to applying traction, laterally displace maternal tissue. The second stage of labour is one of the most dramatic occasions in a woman's life and the decision to intervene and use instrumental delivery of the fetal head is a significant one. From the obstetrician's point of view assisted vaginal delivery is the application of the art of obstetrics in stressful circumstances. The spectre of litigation looms and the level of expectation is high. In an increasing number of areas in obstetrics evidence-based data are available, but for assisted vaginal delivery this is very limited and the outcome depends more on the judgement, training and experience of the obstetrician.

The rates of assisted vaginal delivery vary from country to country and within countries from hospital to hospital. In broad terms the range varies between 5 and 20% and it is commonly about 10–12% of all deliveries.[27] Similarly, there are variations in obstetric practice worldwide which influence the choice of forceps and vacuum for assisted vaginal delivery. These variations depend on operator choice, clinical indications, local policies and, occasionally, maternal choice. However, the last 10–15 years have seen an almost universal increase in the frequency of use of vacuum extraction and a decline in the use of forceps assisted delivery.[28] There is no evidence to support improved safety of either instrument over the other. A Cochrane systematic review[29] showed that compared with forceps the vacuum extractor is:

- more likely to fail to achieve vaginal delivery
- more likely to be associated with cephal-haematoma and retinal haemorrhage
- more likely to be associated with maternal worries about the baby
- less likely to be associated with significant maternal perineal and vaginal trauma
- no more likely to be associated with low 5-minute Apgar scores or the need for phototherapy.

The vacuum extractor has been favoured by many because of the reduction in maternal pelvic floor injury compared with forceps delivery. Although this is the case in the short term, a 5-year follow up of women in one randomized-controlled trial showed no difference in long-term maternal pelvic floor function between the two instruments.[30] A potential drawback to the use of the vacuum extractor is the higher rate of failed delivery compared with forceps. This then raises the dilemma of the sequential use of forceps following failed vacuum, with potentially increased risk to mother and infant; this will be discussed later in this chapter. We will not further debate in detail the comparative merits of the two instruments as the well-trained obstetrician should be adept with both and should select the one best suited to the woman's individual circumstances.

UTERO-FETAL-PELVIC RELATIONSHIPS

A number of these principles have been reviewed in Chapter 5 but the main elements will be emphasized here. The interaction between uterine work, descent of the fetal head and the pelvic architecture should be viewed as a dynamic relationship rather than a set of mathematical measurements. Factors to be assessed are: uterine work; maternal effort; fetal head, including: presentation, position, attitude (flexed/deflexed), synclitism, station, caput and moulding; and the bony pelvis.

Uterine Work

Before considering operative vaginal delivery one should ensure that there has been adequate uterine action to provide maximum descent of the fetal head by propulsion before resorting to traction. This is particularly important in the nulliparous woman and in those with epidural analgesia. It is important to recognize that in normal spontaneous labour there is an increase in the endogenous production of oxytocin in the second stage. Thus, nature actively manages the second stage of labour with increased oxytocin production to augment uterine action and aid descent of the presenting part.[31] Epidural analgesia blocks Ferguson's reflex so that this normal endogenous surge of oxytocin in the second stage of labour does not occur.[32] This is particularly evident in the nulliparous woman in whom the addition of oxytocin in the second stage of labour will, to some extent, offset the increased need for operative vaginal delivery associated with epidural analgesia.[33] This is much less often required in the multiparous woman but, occasionally, and after careful appraisal to rule out cephalopelvic disproportion, oxytocin augmentation may be necessary for the multiparous woman with epidural analgesia in the second stage of labour.

Maternal Effort

It is essential that the resource of maternal effort should be guided appropriately.[34] During the second stage of labour the fetal head descends, flexes and rotates anteriorly. These cardinal movements are accomplished by effective uterine action and maternal expulsive efforts. From the aspect of maternal effort there are two phases to the second stage of labour. In the first, *passive phase*, uterine action causes descent of the fetal head to the pelvic floor. At this point maternal effort will be productive and should be added as the *active phase*. In the multiparous woman the passive phase may be very brief as the head often descends rapidly to the pelvic floor after full cervical dilatation. In the nulliparous woman, however, the fetal head is often only at the level of the ischial spines at full dilatation and time, aided by effective uterine action, is required to allow descent to the pelvic floor before enlisting maternal effort and entering the active phase of the second stage.

As with the first stage of labour the progressive nature of the second stage is more important than a fixed time limit. A working definition of arrest of progress in the second stage is no descent after 30 minutes in the multiparous woman and 60 minutes in the nulliparous woman. Protracted progress is <2 cm/hour descent in multipara and <1 cm in nullipara. Protracted progress in the second stage of labour is much more common in the nulliparous woman than in multipara. In the nulliparous woman it is reasonable to encourage no maternal effort for 1 hour after full cervical dilatation. In about half of nulliparous women the descent of the fetal head will be quite rapid during this time and descent to the pelvic floor will be obvious – productive maternal effort can then be encouraged. In the remaining half, however, progress is protracted and after 1 hour oxytocin augmentation should be started. This can be administered for another hour, after which maternal effort is encouraged as the oxytocin augmentation is continued. The virtue of this approach is that it reduces the likelihood of exhausting the mother in achieving fetal descent through the mid-pelvis, which is more appropriately accomplished by uterine contractions. Although individual women's stamina varies considerably, 1 hour of full maternal effort is usually the most productive. Thus, with the above guiding principles, by 3 hours of the second stage one should be in a position to decide whether vaginal delivery is imminent with continued maternal effort, or whether assisted vaginal delivery may be necessary. If there is continued arrest of descent in the mid-pelvis then caesarean section may be more appropriate (Fig 10-4).

Fetal Head

There are a number of characteristics of the fetal head that can be assessed to evaluate its accommodation by the bony pelvis and pelvic floor.

Position

The position may be occipito-anterior, occipito-transverse or occipito-posterior. Usually the head descends to the mid-pelvis in the transverse position. The normal progression is for the head to rotate anteriorly as it descends to the pelvic floor. Such rotation is favoured by the available space and the tone of the pelvic floor

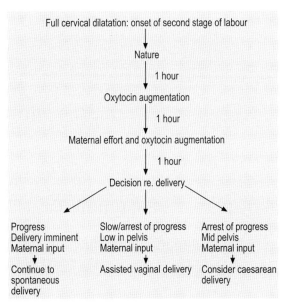

FIGURE 10-4 ■ Guideline for arrest/protraction of second stage of labour in nullipara.

musculature, a benefit which may be lost with regional anaesthesia. If the pelvic floor muscle tone is not maintained the forward and medial sloping nature of the pelvic floor is lost, favouring deflexion and malrotation of the fetal head. Posterior rotation is less advantageous as it presents a larger diameter to the pelvis.

Attitude

The attitude of the fetal head may be flexed (smaller diameter) or deflexed (larger diameter).

Synclitism

Synclitism is the parallel relationship between the planes of the fetal head and of the pelvis. This is assessed by feeling the sagittal suture of the fetal head and its relationship to the transverse plane of the pelvic cavity. When both parietal bones present equally and neither precedes the sagittal suture, the head is synclitic. Anterior asynclitism, which is normal, occurs when the anterior parietal bone is felt more easily because it precedes the sagittal suture which is further back in the transverse plane of the pelvis. In posterior asynclitism, a sign of cephalopelvic disproportion, the posterior parietal bone occupies more of the transverse plane and it precedes the sagittal suture which is more anterior (Fig 10-5).

Station

The station of the fetal head is the relationship of the foremost bony part of the fetal head to the

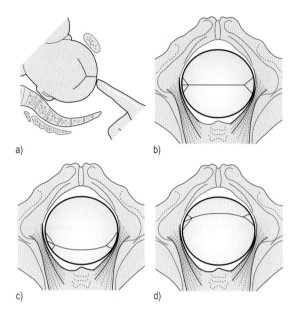

a)   b)

c)   d)

FIGURE 10-5 ■ Synclitism and asynclitism. (a) Detection of asynclitism, estimating how far from the symphysis the sagittal suture lies. (b) LOT normal synclitism, both parietal bones present equally. (c) LOT anterior asynclitism, anterior parietal presentation. (d) LOT posterior asynclitism, posterior parietal presentation.

ischial spines. When this is at the level of the ischial spines the station is zero; levels above and below the ischial spines are designated –1 cm to –5 cm and +1 cm to +5 cm respectively.

Caput Succedaneum

Caput succedaneum is the oedematous swelling formed on the presenting portion of the fetal scalp during labour. This is a serous effusion which overlies the aponeurosis. The assessment of caput is rather subjective but is expressed as none, +, ++, or +++. One+ or two+ is quite compatible with normal spontaneous delivery. Three+ may also be compatible with normal or easy assisted vaginal delivery, but in general is more indicative of a tighter fit between the fetal head and the pelvis.

Moulding

Moulding is the change in shape of the fetal head as it adapts to the pelvic canal. This is associated with compression of the bones of the skull and the relationship of the edges of these bones to each other is how moulding is classified. Depending on accessibility to the examining finger, this is usually assessed by the relationship of the two parietal bones at the sagittal suture or the occipital and parietal bones in the area of the posterior fontanelle. In this regard the parietal bones always over-ride the occipital bone. This point is a guide to identification of the posterior fontanelle. The classification of moulding is as follows: none = bones normally separated; + = bones touching; ++ = bones overlapping but

easily separated with digital pressure; +++ = bones overlapping and not separable with digital pressure (Fig 10-6). The + and ++ degrees of moulding are compatible with normal vaginal delivery. Three+, however, is more likely to denote relative cephalopelvic disproportion, particularly if it exists at both the sagittal suture and the posterior fontanelle.

DESCRIPTION OF THE PELVIC DIAGONAL CONJUGATE

'With the tip of my finger I could hardly reach the jutting forward of the last vertebra of the loins and upper part of the sacrum; from which circumstances I understood the pelvis at that part was not above half or three-quarters of an inch narrower than those that are well formed'.
    William Smellie
    A Treatise on the Theory and Practice of Midwifery. London: D. Wilson, 1752

Bony Pelvis

X-ray pelvimetry has a limited, if any, role in modern labour management. Ultrasound has been used as an aid to documenting the position and station of the fetal head and the extent of overlap of the fetal cranial bones.[35] This application of ultrasound has not found widespread clinical application on the labour floor.

Clinical pelvimetry has limitations but is still a worthwhile endeavour. If one carries this out in every patient managed during labour a useful bank of clinical experience will be obtained. By measurement of your own fingers and fist you should be able to assess the following points:

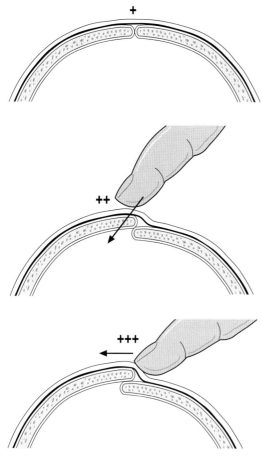

FIGURE 10-6 ■ Degrees of moulding. + Parietal bones together but not overlapped. ++ Parietal bones overlap but are reduced by digital pressure. +++ Parietal bones overlap but are not reducible by digital pressure.

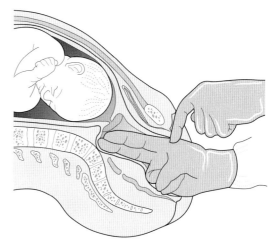

FIGURE 10-7 ■ Measurement of the diagonal conjugate.

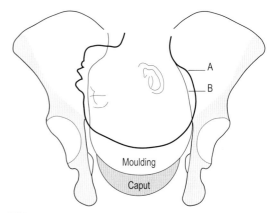

FIGURE 10-8 ■ Caput and moulding may give a false sense of fetal descent. A: Fetal head before descent without caput and moulding. B: Fetal head after descent with caput and moulding.

- diagonal conjugate – at least 12 cm (Fig 10-7)
- curve of the sacrum – should be curved and the lower end should not be inclined anteriorly
- pelvic sidewalls – should be parallel and not converge
- ischial spines – blunt and not prominent
- sacrospinous ligaments – should accept two finger-breadths (>4 cm)
- subpubic arch – not narrowed, should accommodate two fingers
- inter-tuberous diameter – should hold the closed fist (at least 10 cm).

ASSESSMENT FOR ASSISTED VAGINAL DELIVERY

In assessing suitability for assisted vaginal delivery, it is essential that a combined abdominal and vaginal examination be performed to accurately establish the level of descent of the fetal head. In this context vaginal examination can be misleading because of the difficulty in assessing the contribution of caput and moulding to the true level of descent (Fig 10-8). It is here that careful abdominal palpation following the principles laid down by Crichton is most helpful.[36] He proposed a clinical estimation of descent of the fetal head in fifths, as palpable above the pelvic brim (Fig 10-9). The occiput and sinciput should be carefully palpated. In general, if only the sinciput is palpable the head is one-fifth above the pelvic brim and this corresponds to the lowest part of the fetal bony skull being at the level of the ischial spines. With vaginal examination alone and a moderate or major degree of moulding the bony part of the fetal skull may appear to be

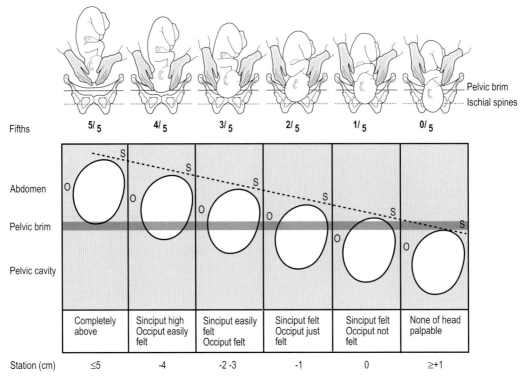

Fifths

	5/5	4/5	3/5	2/5	1/5	0/5

Pelvic brim
Ischial spines

Abdomen

Pelvic brim

Pelvic cavity

	Completely above	Sinciput high Occiput easily felt	Sinciput easily felt Occiput felt	Sinciput felt Occiput just felt	Sinciput felt Occiput not felt	None of head palpable

| Station (cm) | ≤5 | -4 | -2 -3 | -1 | 0 | ≥+1 |

FIGURE 10-9 ■ Clinical estimation of the fetal head in fifths palpable above the pelvic brim, and the relationship to station.

much lower. If none of the fetal head can be palpated above the pelvic brim then it has descended to at least spines +1 to +2 cm. In modern obstetrics it is rarely indicated to assist vaginal delivery at a level higher than this. Thus, abdominal palpation is in many ways the critical and decisive component of the combined abdominal–vaginal assessment. As Chassar Moir (1964) noted in a previous edition of this book:

> 'It is a good working rule never to apply the forceps if the sinciput can still be felt per abdomen. This should be remembered when examining the patient that has been long in labour, for the extreme moulding of the head and the considerable size of the caput succedaneum may give a false impression to the examining vaginal fingers to the degree of descent already achieved.'

In addition to accurately determining the level of descent of the fetal head, the position and attitude of the fetal head are very important. These can be ascertained by identifying the sagittal suture and the anterior and posterior fontanelles. In this context the occipital and frontal bones always ride under the parietal bones with moulding. By identifying the posterior fontanelle of the fetal head the position (occipito-anterior (OA), occipito-transverse (OT), occipito-posterior (OP)) can be readily ascertained. If the posterior fontanelle is easily palpable the head must be well flexed, which presents the smallest diameter to the pelvis.

If, however, the posterior fontanelle cannot be felt, move in the opposite direction along the sagittal suture to see if the anterior fontanelle is palpable. Normally, with a well-flexed fetal head the anterior fontanelle is difficult to feel as it is much deeper in the pelvis towards the sinciput. If it is easily palpable the head is usually considerably deflexed, which presents a larger diameter to the pelvis. If, due to caput, there is difficulty in identifying the sutures one should feel anteriorly for the fetal ear. Feel for the pinna and canal, as the ear can be folded forward to give a false impression of the true position. The ear as a landmark can be useful in assessing the level of the head as it is just below the maximum biparietal diameter. Thus, if it is easily felt during maternal bearing-down effort, there is unlikely to be significant disproportion.[37] The acquisition of these clinical skills requires the proverbial 'long apprenticeship at the bedside of women in labour'; indeed, many of the necessary skills could be described as 'obstetric braille'.

INDICATIONS FOR OPERATIVE VAGINAL DELIVERY

Most indications for assisted vaginal delivery are relative and fall into three categories: maternal, fetal and non-progressive labour/dystocia.[38,39]

Maternal

The mother's medical condition may limit the desirability or ability for maternal effort, e.g. cerebrovascular disease, severe pre-eclampsia/eclampsia, and cardiac disease. Maternal fatigue and exhaustion may lead to unproductive, non-progressive and demoralizing effort. This may culminate in maternal request for assisted vaginal delivery.

Fetal

Presumed fetal compromise as manifest by non-reassuring fetal heart rate pattern is a common indication for assisted vaginal delivery. Here again, the indication is often relative and dependent upon the interpretation of the fetal heart rate abnormality, the presence or absence of meconium, and the availability of fetal scalp blood sampling (see Chapter 6). In these circumstances, in the second stage of labour, the fetus can often be delivered more rapidly by assisted vaginal delivery than by caesarean section. However, it is essential to be sure that assistance with either forceps or vacuum is straightforward as the combination of hypoxia and trauma is potentially damaging to the fetal brain.

Non-Progressive Labour/Dystocia

In a prolonged, non-progressive second stage of labour the indication to assist delivery is usually based on a combination of maternal and fetal reasons. The mother may be exhausted and demoralized that her efforts are not productive. Prolonged second stage of labour may damage the maternal pelvic floor.[40] The fetal contribution to a non-progressive second stage of labour may be due to macrosomia or an unfavourable position and attitude of the fetal head presenting a wider diameter to the pelvis. Most commonly this occurs with a deflexed occipito-transverse or occipito-posterior position of the fetal head, with the larger diameter resulting in relative cephalopelvic disproportion. Skilfully performed, assisted vaginal delivery can correct the unfavourable position and flex the fetal head allowing safe and easy vaginal delivery. A prolonged, non-progressive second stage of labour

may cause the potentially lethal combination of trauma and hypoxia to the fetal brain; with the third potentially damaging component being fetal infection, manifest by chorioamnionitis. The following guidelines have been suggested for time limits in the second stage of labour, at which point consideration should be given to assisted delivery:[41]

- nullipara: 2 hours without regional anaesthesia and 3 hours with regional anaesthesia
- multipara: 1 hour without regional anaesthesia and 2 hours with regional anaesthesia.

Although these are reasonable guidelines no rigid time limits should be applied; however, maternal and perinatal morbidity are increased when the second stage of labour exceeds 3 hours.[42,43] It is also inappropriate to have a laissez-faire, open-ended approach which can lead to an indefinite, indecisive and interminable second stage. Of relevance is the duration of the active phase with maternal effort, as this has the most potential for negative effects on the fetal head and the maternal pelvic floor. The appropriate time for intervention is based upon a combination of the fetal and maternal factors noted above, a careful appraisal of the feto-pelvic relationships and the mother's wishes.

CLASSIFICATION OF ASSISTED VAGINAL DELIVERY

The American College of Obstetricians and Gynecologists has been the organization that has most consistently defined the types of operative vaginal delivery.[41] Other speciality organizations have adopted this classification[38,39] (Table 10-1).

PREREQUISITES FOR ASSISTED VAGINAL DELIVERY

Indication and Assessment

The indication should be clearly established and documented. The essentials of the feto-pelvic relationship should be confirmed and these include: full cervical dilatation and membranes ruptured; vertex presentation; the exact position and attitude of the head should be known; the head should be ≤ one-fifth palpable per abdomen and the pelvis should be deemed adequate. As mentioned previously, it should be rare that operative vaginal delivery is undertaken with the head even one-fifth palpable above the pelvic

TABLE 10.1	**Types of Operative Vaginal Delivery**[41]
Mid	Fetal head is ≤ one-fifth palpable per abdomen
	Leading point of the skull is above station +2 cm (0 => +1 cm) but not above the ischial spines
	Two subdivisions:
	(a) rotation ≤45°
	(b) rotation >45°
Low	Leading point of the skull (not caput) is at station ≥ +2 cm and not on the pelvic floor
	Two subdivisions:
	(a) rotation ≤45°
	(b) rotation >45°
Outlet	Fetal scalp visible without separating the labia
	Fetal skull has reached the pelvic floor
	Sagittal suture is in the antero-posterior diameter, or right or left occiput anterior, or occiput posterior position (rotation ≤45°)
	Fetal head is at or on the perineum

brim. The bladder should be emptied by straight catheterization and if an indwelling catheter is in place, the bulb should be deflated and the catheter removed just before the procedure to reduce the risk of urethral or bladder damage.

Informed Consent

Genuinely informed consent can be difficult to obtain in the stressful environment surrounding the second stage of labour. However, the options generally include waiting, assisted vaginal delivery or caesarean section – and these should be discussed with the woman and her partner. In some circumstances the course of action is quite clear, e.g. acute fetal bradycardia with the head at the pelvic outlet requiring only easy assistance with forceps or vacuum. On other occasions the head may be arrested in the low–mid-pelvis and a more detailed outline of the options and answers to the woman's questions are more appropriate.

Analgesia

If the assistance required is in the low or outlet portion of the pelvis, infiltration of the perineum with local anaesthetic may be all that is required. Alternatively, pudendal block is effective for most low assisted deliveries. In general, more analgesia is required for forceps than for vacuum

assisted deliveries. If the fetal head is in the low–mid-pelvis, and particularly if rotation is required, then epidural or spinal anaesthesia is optimum.

Training

The potential for maternal and fetal trauma with assisted vaginal delivery performed by inexperienced operators is considerable. Obstetricians in training should have adequate supervised experience with spontaneous vaginal delivery and low and outlet assisted vacuum and forceps delivery. The judgement and technical skills required for assisted vaginal delivery in the low–mid pelvis, particularly with rotation, are considerable and more senior obstetrical staff with experience should directly supervise juniors in the acquisition of these skills.[44,45] This is an area of obstetrics fraught with risks of poor clinical outcome and litigation. The two go hand-in-hand and it is not acceptable for inadequately trained staff to be unsupervised in the performance of these procedures.

TRIAL OF ASSISTED VAGINAL DELIVERY

> 'Knowledge is more than equivalent to force.'
> Samuel Johnson, 1709–84.

To the experienced obstetrician it is usually clear that the head is in the low or outlet pelvis and that assisted vaginal delivery can be accomplished with ease in the delivery room. However, in cases where the fetal head is arrested in the low–mid pelvis, particularly at spines +1 cm to + 2 cm, the potential for difficulty is greater and it is usually prudent to declare a trial of forceps or trial of vacuum. This is a long-established principle in obstetrics, well articulated on both sides of the Atlantic ocean, and remains relevant.[15,46–48]

It entails moving the woman to the operating theatre so that either an assisted vaginal delivery or caesarean section can be undertaken. This is explained to the woman and her partner, as well as to the anaesthetist and nursing staff, and they are told that if the forceps or vacuum delivery proceeds smoothly then vaginal delivery will be accomplished with safety. However, if there are any difficulties then the attempt at vaginal delivery will not be sustained and the obstetrician can immediately back off and proceed to caesarean section. In this way any pressure on the obstetrician to persist with attempted vaginal delivery when difficulty is encountered is removed. In most instances vaginal delivery is achieved with ease and safety, but on other occasions difficulty is encountered and caesarean section can be promptly undertaken with minimal risk of damage to mother or fetus. This was nicely summarized by Chassar Moir (1964) in a previous edition of this book:

> '*Although seemingly simple, the conception of trial forceps is a most important advance in policy, and is the logical outcome of the increased safety of the modern caesarean operation … I have on several occasions deliberately pursued this policy and believe that by so doing I have acted in the best interest of both the mother and child, avoiding an unnecessary caesarean section in some cases, and a mutilating vaginal delivery in others*'.

and by Ian Donald in his emphasis on the difference between a failed forceps delivery, undertaken without preparations for immediate caesarean section if necessary, and a failed trial of forceps:

> '*Trial of forceps, advisedly undertaken, however comes into a completely different class. Here, one recognizes all the difficulties in advance and has made due preparations for them … The decision to abandon forceps and to proceed to caesarean section must not be regarded as a matter of "failed forceps" but as an enlightened step in recognition of the hazards, particularly to the baby of persisting with vaginal delivery*'.
> PRACTICAL OBSTETRIC PROBLEMS. 5TH ED.
> LONDON: LLOYD-LUKE, 1979, P654

FORCEPS ASSISTED DELIVERY

The ambivalent attitude of the medical profession towards obstetrics forceps is exemplified by the different viewpoints expressed by two of the great obstetricians of the 18th century, Edmund Chapman and William Hunter.

> 'I can, from my own experience, affirm it to be a most excellent instrument, and so far from hurting or destroying, that it frequently saves the mother's life, and that of the child … All I can say in praise of this noble instrument, must necessarily fall short of what it justly demands'.
> Edmund Chapman. A treatise on the improvement of midwifery. Chiefly with regard to the operation. 2nd ed. London: Brindley Clarke and Corbett, 1735.

> 'To a poor woman that is quite exhausted, forceps may be of considerable service – but I wish to God they had never been contrived … I am convinced the forceps has killed three, I may say ten women to one that it has saved, and therefore we should never use it on any occasion but where it is absolutely necessary.'
> William Hunter, c.1760

Almost three centuries later medical and lay opinion remains divided about the role of forceps in modern obstetric practice, although not quite to the extreme views expressed above. Nevertheless, if assisted vaginal delivery was to be abandoned then some 5–20% of women currently delivered by this method would only have two options: either delivery by caesarean section or a return to days before forceps when some women would labour for many hours and even days in the second stage of labour, with disastrous consequences for them and their infant.

The construction and anatomy of the forceps is shown in Figure 10-10. Over three centuries more than 700 types of forceps have been invented and new ones continue to be produced. In clinical terms there are the classical forceps exemplified by Simpson's and similar types such

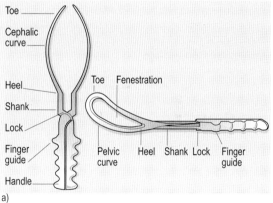

a)

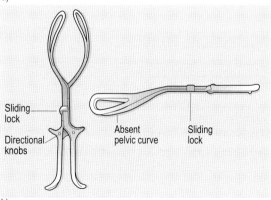

b)

FIGURE 10-10 ■ Anatomy of the forceps. (a) Simpson's classical forceps. (b) Kielland's rotation forceps.

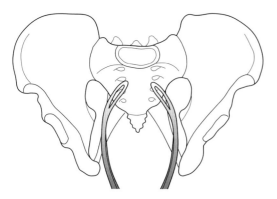

FIGURE 10-11 ■ The ideal position of the forceps blades relative to the maternal pelvis.

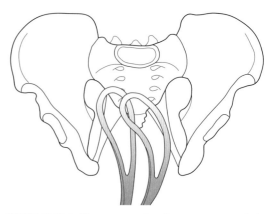

FIGURE 10-12 ■ The range of safe movement of the forceps blades relative to the pelvis.

as Neville–Barnes, Haig Ferguson and Tucker–MacLean, which has solid blades. The two right and left branches are composed of blades, shanks and handles. The cephalic curve of the blade relates to the fetal head and the pelvic curve to the maternal pelvis. The blades are usually locked at the junction of the shanks and handles. Forceps designed for rotation, most commonly Kielland's forceps, have a cephalic curve but minimal pelvic curve of the blades. This allows rotation within the pelvis and helps avoid trauma to the maternal soft tissues by narrowing the rotational arc of the toes of the blades. When using rotation forceps it is common to encounter asyncliticism so these forceps have a sliding lock which allows for its correction. Individual obstetricians have their favourite make of forceps, usually depending on their training and familiarity. In clinical terms one needs to be familiar with a pair of classical forceps such as Simpson's, and a rotational forceps, such as Kielland's. Those interested in details of the various types of forceps available should consult the bibliography at the end of this chapter.

CLASSICAL FORCEPS

Once the indications for assisted forceps delivery have been established and the prerequisites mentioned have been fulfilled the woman is placed in the lithotomy position with appropriate leg supports. The blades of classical forceps are so constructed that they are in perfect position transversely in the pelvis (Fig 10-11) with a safe range of movement of approximately 45° on either side from the transverse: these limits are between the iliopectineal eminence and the sacroiliac joint behind (Fig 10-12). The forceps blades should be placed as a cephalic application

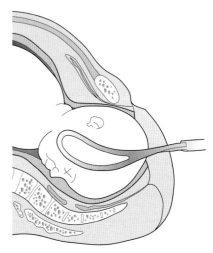

FIGURE 10-13 ■ The ideal biparietal bimalar application of the forceps blades to the fetal head.

along the side of the head covering the space between the orbits and the ears (Fig 10-13). This cephalic application is biparietal and bimalar. As such the pressure is evenly distributed to the least vulnerable areas. If the cephalic application is asymmetrical – such as a brow-mastoid application – the subsequent compression and traction forces are also asymmetrically applied to the underlying falx cerebri and tentorium, risking intracranial haemorrhage.

'Branche gauche à la main gauche, à gauche la première: tout doit être gauche, sauf l'accoucheur ...'
    'Left blade in the left hand, to the left at first; all is gauche, except the skill of the obstetrician ...'
    Charles Pajot
    Travaux d'obstetrique et de gynécologue précédés d'elements de practique obstetricale. Paris: H. Lauwereyns, 1882

Once the precise position of the fetal head has been ascertained – either direct occipito-anterior (OA) or left or right occipito-anterior (LOA, ROA) – the forceps are placed together and lined up as a ghost or phantom application holding the forceps in front of the perineum in the same orientation as they will be applied to the fetal head. The left blade is held in the left hand and inserted to the left side of the pelvis just in front of the left ear of the fetus. In doing this the fingers of the right hand are placed just inside the vagina and the thumb of the right hand against the heel of the blade. The left hand holding the handle is then rotated down in an arc while the fingers and thumb of the right hand guide the blade into the correct position (Fig

10-14a). Changing hands, the same procedure is used to insert the right blade (Fig 10-14b). Most forceps have the 'English lock' in which the right handle fits into the lock on the left shank. Thus, there is no need to manipulate one handle above the other as they just lock in naturally. The above description is for the direct OA position. For LOA and ROA positions the procedure is the same, taking care to line up the blades and their application to the oblique orientation of the fetal head. No force should be required to apply or lock the blades of the forceps. Unless they can be applied and locked easily one should stop and recheck the position of the fetal head. One of the more common reasons for difficulty is an unsuspected occipito-posterior position.

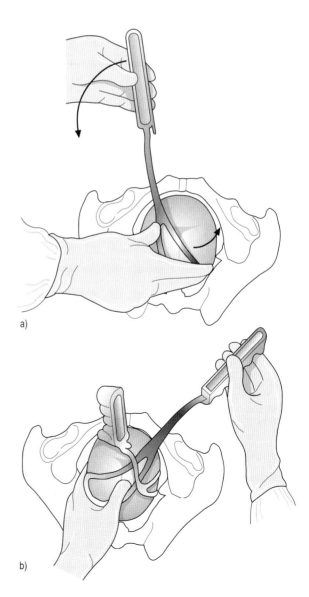

a)

b)

FIGURE 10-14 ■ (a) Insertion of left blade. The fingers and thumb of the right hand guide the blade into correct position while the left hand rotates the handle in a downward arc. (b) The same procedure is carried out for insertion of the right blade using the opposite hands.

Once the handles have locked satisfactorily check that the application is correct by the following:

- The posterior fontanelle should be located midway between the sides of the blades with the lambdoidal suture lines equidistant from the forcep blades.
- The posterior fontanelle should be one finger-breadth above the plane of the shanks. If the fontanelle is more than one finger-breadth above this plane, traction will tend to deflex the head, presenting a larger diameter to the pelvis.
- The sagittal suture should be perpendicular to the plane of the shanks throughout their length. If the shanks run obliquely to the sagittal suture the application is asymmetrical – towards a brow–mastoid orientation.
- The amount of palpable fenestration of each of the blades should be equal on each side. In fact, there should be barely any fenestration felt and at most one finger should be able to be inserted between it and the head (Fig 10-15).

Unless all the above checks are fulfilled the forceps will need to be manipulated or reapplied.

The compression forces of the forceps are the least desirable aspect. These can be kept to a minimum if the operator grasps and applies traction via the finger guards which are placed close to the lock so that the least compression force is applied, as opposed to squeezing the handles at their end. This is best achieved using an underhand grip with the index and middle fingers on the finger guards while the other hand is placed on the shanks of the forceps to help apply downward traction (Pajot's manoeuvre) to ensure that the traction is in the curve of the pelvis and not dissipated against the pubic arch (Fig 10-16).

Traction is applied during a uterine contraction and, aided by maternal effort, should be carefully directed along the pelvic curve – the curve of Carus. During traction the obstetrician can be seated or standing and the arms should be flexed at the elbows. It is difficult to teach how much traction is appropriate – obviously the least required is the best. A recent study using an isometric strength testing unit shows that junior obstetricians can be trained to reproduce and not exceed the 'ideal' traction forces of 30–45 lb.[49] Muscular obstetricians, of both sexes, are capable of applying considerable and undesirable force with forceps. The guiding principle is that mild to moderate traction, which admittedly is in the eye of the beholder, should cause progressive descent when co-ordinated with each uterine contraction. Generally it is clear whether there is descent of the fetal head or not with the first pull. There is an unyielding feel to obstructed cases that dictates that the trial of forceps should be abandoned. Strong traction should not be applied or necessary for safe assisted vaginal delivery.

As the head descends to the perineum and the occiput passes under the symphysis the direction of traction is gradually changed forwards and upwards to end up about 45° above the horizontal. As the head extends over the perineum the handles are elevated to about 75° above the horizontal, and one hand is removed from the forceps to guard the perineum or perform episiotomy if necessary. Once the head is almost delivered the forceps blades can be removed by reversing the manoeuvres used for their insertion. Usually the right blade is removed first. If too much force is required to remove the blades then the head can be gently eased out with the blades in position.

When the head is LOA or ROA, after the blades have been appropriately placed and checked, rotation through the 45° towards the midline should be performed in a gradual and gentle manner without traction. This is carried out by slightly elevating the handles and rotating slowly through an arc, allowing the maternal tissues and fetal head to adapt to the changing position. Once the rotation is completed the position of the blades should be checked again

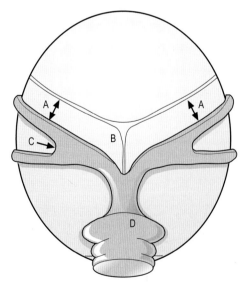

FIGURE 10-15 ■ Checks for correct position of forceps relative to the head. A: Blades equidistant from lambdoidal sutures. B: Posterior fontanelle one finger-breadth above plane of shanks. C: At most one finger-breadth between fenestra and head. D: Shanks perpendicular to sagittal suture.

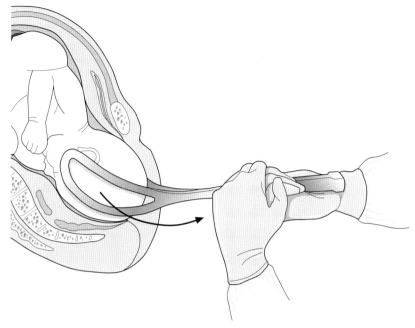

FIGURE 10-16 ■ Appropriate grip for traction which should be directed along the pelvic curve.

to make sure that they have not slipped during rotation.

OCCIPITO-POSTERIOR DELIVERY

If the fetal head has descended and arrested low in the pelvis (*spines ≥+3 cm*) with the head in the direct OP position, or a few degrees to either side of direct OP, it may be best to assist delivery in this position, 'face-to-pubes', rather than attempt rotation. In most of these cases it seems that the fetal head fits the pelvis best in the direct OP position. This is more likely in the anthropoid type of pelvis with a longer anteroposterior diameter compared with the transverse dimensions. In these cases the head descends low in the pelvis and, if the pelvis is large and the fetus small, delivery will be spontaneous in the face-to-pubes position. In those cases in which arrest occurs low in the pelvis it may be necessary to assist the delivery with forceps, although this entails a greater risk of perineal trauma compared with the OA position.

The technique for insertion and application of the forceps is the same as for the OA position, but the pelvic curve of the blades is reversed in its relationship to the sides of the fetal head. The toes of the blades, rather than facing towards the ears as in the OA application, curve toward the mouth (Fig 10-17). In checking the application of the forceps to the landmarks of the skull, the shanks should be parallel to the sagittal suture

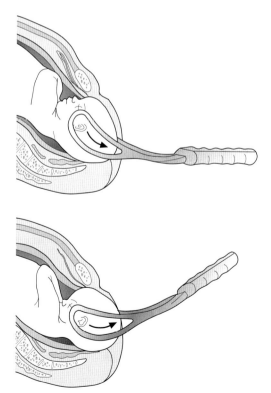

FIGURE 10-17 ■ Relationship of forceps blades to the fetal head in occipito-posterior position.

but the posterior fontanelle will be one finger-breadth below, rather than above the shanks as in the OA check. Traction is downwards and backwards initially but the occiput will distend the perineum more than the sinciput does in the OA position. Thus, a mediolateral episiotomy is usually required. As the occiput distends the perineum, traction is progressively directed upwards to flex the occiput over the perineum. Excessive downward traction in the initial phase will tend to deflex the fetal head and increase the diameter presenting to the perineum.

DELIVERY WITH ROTATION

Assisted vaginal delivery involving rotation of OT and OP positions of the fetal head requires some of the finest clinical judgement in obstetrics. For it is in these situations that the risk of maternal trauma and, particularly, fetal trauma is highest. The reader is referred again to the earlier parts of this chapter and the prerequisites for assisted vaginal delivery. For any assisted vaginal delivery involving rotation it is sensible to encapsulate these considerations by asking oneself the question 'why am I not doing a caesarean section?'. Having said that, in many instances of malrotation of the fetal head, deflexion is involved, presenting a larger diameter of the fetal head to the pelvis. If rotation and flexion of the fetal head can be safely and successfully achieved the diameter of the fetal head is reduced, and often light traction is all that is required to effect delivery. In contrast, the arrested fetal head in the OA position already has the narrowest diameter presenting so that more traction may be required to effect delivery.

In addition to the risks of intracranial trauma, rotation procedures carry the extremely rare but potentially catastrophic risk of cervical spinal cord trauma – at its worst producing quadriplegia.[50] This risk is probably due to a combination of reasons. Usually there has been a prolonged labour, the amniotic fluid has drained and the uterus 'hugs' the fetus. Under these circumstances, if the fetal head is rotated the shoulders (which are grasped by the uterus) may not rotate, making the cervical spine vulnerable. If, in addition, there is a degree of fetal hypotonia associated with hypoxia there may be no protection of the cervical spinal column from the hypotonic fetal neck and shoulder muscles. Thus, rotation procedures should be avoided in the presence of fetal hypoxia. It is also logical that any rotational manoeuvre of the fetal head should be accompanied by concomitant rotation of the fetal shoulders.

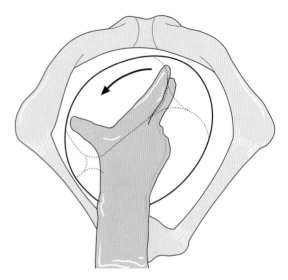

FIGURE 10-18 ■ Digital rotation.

Digital Rotation

In some cases of LOT and ROT positions it is possible to rotate the occiput anterior with digital pressure alone. This will allow the use of the classical OA forceps to aid delivery. For the LOT position, the tips of the index and middle fingers of the right hand are placed against the elevated edge of the anterior parietal bone along the lambdoidal suture and close to where it joins the posterior fontanelle (Fig 10-18). Using counterclockwise and downward pressure during a uterine contraction, with or without maternal bearing-down effort, the head can often be rotated to LOA or even direct OA. This obviates the need to use rotational forceps. Once the head has been rotated the fingers of the right hand remain against the left parietal bone to counteract any tendency for the occiput to rotate back to LOT. With the head thus held in the OA position the right blade of the forceps can be applied. The fingers can then be withdrawn and while the right blade steadies the position of the head in the OA position the left blade can be applied. For ROT positions the left hand is used and the manoeuvres are carried out in the opposite direction.

Manual Rotation

If digital rotation is unsuccessful the manual technique can be used. However, if the head is deeply impacted in the pelvis it may be difficult to get a good enough grasp of the head to achieve manual rotation. The fully supinated hand is inserted into the vagina – the left hand for right occipito-posterior (ROP) and the right hand for

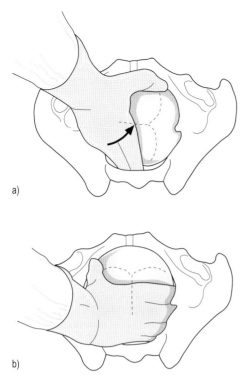

FIGURE 10-19 ■ Manual rotation. (a) LOT head grasped with right hand. (b) LOT rotated to OA.

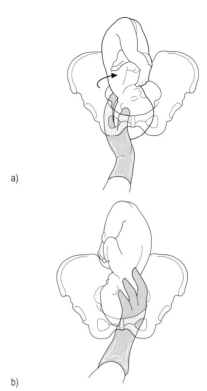

FIGURE 10-20 ■ Manual head and shoulder rotation: Pomeroy's manoeuvre. (a) ROP: left hand grasps head with fingers behind the anterior shoulder. (b) Head and shoulders rotated from ROP to LOA.

left occipito-posterior (LOP) positions. The head is grasped with the fingers high and widespread on one side of the head, and the thumb high on the other; the occipital region should now be well in the palm of the hand. The head is elevated only enough to allow flexion and rotation such that the sinciput comes round to the position previously occupied by the occiput (Fig 10-19). Thus, one tends to overcorrect the rotation. Simultaneously with this rotation the other hand is placed on the maternal abdomen behind the shoulder pulling it towards the midline. In some cases, if the vaginal hand can reach high enough to the posterior shoulder this is also dislodged from one side of the sacral promontory to the other, again while the external hand on the maternal abdomen puts concomitant rotational pressure on the anterior shoulder. This is sometimes known as Pomeroy's manoeuvre (Fig 10-20).[51]

In some cases, provided the head remains OA after the rotation, oxytocin augmentation may help bring the head down to spontaneous delivery. In most instances, however, forceps delivery from the OA position will be required following the manual rotation.

Regional anaesthesia and an adequately relaxed uterus are necessary for satisfactory manual rotation. Epidural and spinal anaesthesia provide good pain relief but, if the uterus is firmly contracted around the fetus, tocolysis with intravenous nitroglycerine may have to be given. Most of the large series with successful manual rotation were carried out in the days when general anaesthesia with profound uterine relaxation was used.

Forceps Rotation

If digital or manual rotation of the head is not feasible, forceps rotation can be considered. Although a number of forceps have been used for this purpose there is greatest experience with those devised by Kielland in 1915. He designed his forceps without a pelvic curve so that rotation of the fetal head arrested in the transverse position could be achieved without the trauma to maternal tissues that is incurred by the wide excursion of the toes of forceps that have a pelvic curve. In many hospitals, forceps rotation has been abandoned but there are still units where the skill with this instrument has been retained.[52,53] The main indication is the deflexed fetal head arrested in the transverse or posterior position. In modern obstetrics this is often associated with epidural analgesia and, while the head may be low (≥+2 cm), the deflexed and malrotated head presents a larger diameter. If the head can be safely rotated and flexed the presenting diameter is reduced and often mild traction will safely effect delivery.

> 'If the head is in the pelvic cavity, rotation can be completed with the forceps ... the head is rotated 90° from the transverse into the exact anteroposterior diameter before its extraction through the pelvic narrows is begun. In such a case rotation is carried out without simultaneous traction. The forceps, held tightly closed, are turned about the axis of the handles'.
> Christian Kielland
> Eine neue form und einführungsweise der geburtszange, stets biparietal an den kindlichlen schädel gelagt. Munchen Med Wchnscr 1915; 62:923

In order to allow for correct application and manoeuvre of Kielland's forceps the woman's perineum should protrude slightly over the edge of the delivery table. Before application the Kielland forceps are assembled and held outside the pelvis in the position to which they will be applied to the fetal head (Fig 10-21a). The directional knobs on the shanks should be towards the fetal occiput. The obstetrician then takes the anterior blade and there are three techniques by which this can be applied – classical, wandering and direct.

The *classical* or inversion technique was that originally described by Kielland for use when the fetal head was higher in the pelvis than would be acceptable for forceps delivery today. It will be described here, largely for historical interest, as it is associated with a small risk of perforation of the lower uterine segment and entanglement of the fetal hand, forearm or umbilical cord. The middle and index fingers of one hand are inserted under the symphysis with the palmar surface up. The anterior blade is held in the other hand at an angle of about 45° above the horizontal with the cephalic surface up (Fig 10-21b). The toe of the blade is guided over the finger tips and the handle is pressed down and the blade passed up until it occupies the space in the lower uterine segment between the anterior shoulder and the side of the fetal head. The shank is now lying over the anterior parietal bone. The blade is then rotated through 180° and fits down over the parietal bone (Fig 10-21b). Throughout these manoeuvres extreme gentleness should be exercised. If there is any resistance the technique should be abandoned.

The *wandering* technique has less potential for trauma to the maternal tissues than the classical technique. Nonetheless, great care has to be exercised or trauma to the vaginal vault can occur with the toe of the blade. The anterior blade is inserted posteriorly into the vagina and the fingers guide the blade around the sinciput and face of the fetus while the other hand rotates the blade in a downward arc. Once again this move must be gentle and no force should be necessary (Fig 10-21c). If the head is very deflexed the face may present an obstruction to this manoeuvre. In this case it may be best to use the reverse wandering technique over the occiput.

If the fetal head is low, and particularly if there is anterior asyncliticism, the *direct* technique can be used. The middle and index fingers of one hand are inserted palmar surface down between the anterior parietal bone and the maternal symphysis. The other hand guides the blade directly over the parietal bone to the correct cephalic application (Fig 10-21d).

The posterior blade is inserted into the hollow of the sacrum. A protective hand is placed as high as possible posteriorly and the blade guided between that and the posterior parietal bone of the fetal head. The tips of the fingers should guide the toe of the blade around the fetal head and away from the vaginal tissues overlying the sacrum and sacral promontory. This is aided by depression on the handle with the other hand (Fig 10-21e). Most junior obstetricians are surprised at how much depression of the handle is required to guide the toe of the blade around the fetal head. Once both blades have been appropriately placed the operator often finds that there is more of the shank of the anterior blade protruding than there is of the posterior blade. This may be due to incorrect application but is usually due to anterior asyncliticism. Thus, provided the obstetrician is secure in the parietal application of each blade, they are locked. The sliding lock allows one to, at least partially, correct the asyncliticism. However, much of the asyncliticism will not be corrected until rotation has occurred. The relationship of the blades to the sagittal suture and posterior fontanelle should be checked. Before rotation it is helpful to try and flex the fetal head. This can be achieved, after the correct application has been confirmed, by moving the handles towards the sinciput.

Rotation should be gentle and easy. If it is not then one should check the application very carefully and consider again whether forceps delivery is safely feasible. With the hand in the supine position the index and middle fingers and the thumb grasp the finger guides and the handles are depressed posteriorly. Rotation should occur slowly and gently with pronation of the hand (Fig 10-21f). At the same time the other hand, or that of an assistant, applied to the abdomen should guide the anterior shoulder around in the same direction as the occiput. Provided one has an assistant to manipulate the shoulder it is useful for the obstetrician to use the other hand to retract the vaginal wall so that the rotation of the fetal head can be observed directly. This ensures that the forceps remain properly applied, rather than just rotating around the surface of the head. Once rotation is achieved the correct application of the forceps is checked again.

Traction with Kielland's forceps should take account of the reduced pelvic curve. Thus, the appropriate position for the obstetrician is on one knee. One hand with the index and middle fingers below the finger grips applies traction and the heel of the other hand applies downward traction on the shanks (Pajot's manoeuvre). The head is guided downwards and backwards and as the occiput appears below the symphysis the handles are slowly elevated to the horizontal position (Fig 10-21g). There are some obstetricians who will use the Kielland's only to rotate the fetal head and then remove the blades and apply a pair of classical forceps with a pelvic curve for traction and final delivery of the head. There is no doubt that safe use of Kielland's forceps

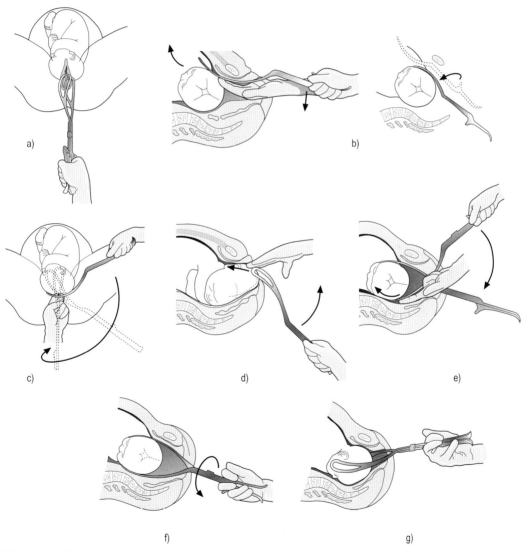

FIGURE 10-21 ■ Kielland's forceps: left occipito-transverse. (a) Orientation of forceps, directional buttons towards occiput. (b) Classical (inversion) application of anterior blade. (c) Wandering technique of applying anterior blade. (d) Direct application of anterior blade. (e) Introduction of posterior blade. (f) Gentle rotation from LOT to OA. (g) Traction with Kielland's forceps.

requires considerable training and supervision. In many training programmes this is not now available.

FLEXION AND VACUUM ASSISTED DELIVERY

'The large amount of force apparently required in some cases is because it is misdirected. The head is not properly flexed, and traction is exerted in a direction that would tend to pull the occiput through the pubic symphysis, instead of under the pubic arch'.

Peter McCahey

Atmospheric tractor: a new instrument and some new theories in obstetrics. Med Surg Rep (Philadelphia) 1890; 43:619–623

VACUUM ASSISTED DELIVERY

In recent years obstetricians have moved from using forceps to the vacuum for the majority of assisted vaginal deliveries. There are those who feel that the training and experience required to perform safe forceps delivery is more than that for vacuum assisted delivery. There is an element of truth in this supposition, but it is a potentially dangerous assumption. The 'suck-it-and-see' school of vacuum assisted delivery assumes that placing the vacuum device on the fetal head and applying traction is a safe and simple option to overcome dystocia. Nothing could be further from the truth and the potential for fetal damage with the vacuum is as great as it is with the forceps. The predelivery assessment and prerequisites discussed earlier in this chapter should be just as stringent for vacuum assisted as for forceps assisted deliveries.

Vacuum assisted delivery does have a lower risk of maternal vaginal and perineal trauma compared with forceps. In addition, it can often be performed with less profound anaesthesia: local infiltration or pudendal block, compared to epidural or spinal.

There are many different varieties of vacuum cups and devices, but they fall into two main categories – rigid cup and soft cup. The original rigid cups were metal and usually the Malmström or the Bird modification of the Malmström. More recently, rigid plastic cups have been manufactured.[26] In the 1970s cups were developed with softer material in an attempt to reduce scalp trauma attributed to the hard cups. The first of these was the Kobayashi Silastic cup[54] and there have been many other soft cups developed since that time. In general the soft cups do reduce superficial scalp trauma but have a higher failure-to-deliver rate than the hard cups.[55,56] The principles of use with all of the cups, however, are the same and will be reviewed here.

The first and most essential piece of information is the identification of the *flexion point*.[25] This is situated approximately 3 cm in front of the posterior fontanelle. If traction is directed from this point the fetal head is flexed to the narrowest suboccipito-bregmatic diameter (9.5 cm). Most of the vacuum cups are 5 or 6 cm in diameter. Thus, if the cup is applied so that the rear edge is just at the posterior fontanelle it should be over the flexion point. The other way of assessing this is to gauge the relationship of the leading edge of the cup to the anterior fontanelle. The distance between the anterior fontanelle and the flexion point is approximately 6 cm. Thus, when the cup is correctly placed there should be about 3 cm (two finger-breadths) between the leading edge and the anterior fontanelle (Fig 10-22). In addition to correct flexion of the head one wants to avoid asyncliticism, which will also increase the diameter of the fetal head presenting to the pelvis. The biparietal diameter is 9.5 cm and this assumes no asyncliticism. If the cup is applied off the central sagittal

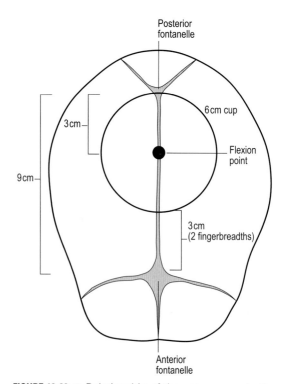

FIGURE 10-22 ■ Relationship of the vacuum cup to the flexion point.

suture, this paramedian application will cause asyncliticism during traction and increase the presenting diameter of the fetal head. Thus, there are four possible applications of the vacuum cup (Fig 10-23):

- flexing median – which provides the optimum and narrowest suboccipito-bregmatic and biparietal diameters
- deflexing median – which produces the wider occipito-frontal diameter
- flexing paramedian – which produces a wider paramedian diameter
- deflexing paramedian – which provides the worst combination of wider diameters with the occipito-frontal and paramedian diameters.

It has been shown that the amount of fetal scalp trauma is least with the correct flexing median cup application.[57]

The above rationale dictates the correct placement of the vacuum cup in a median position over the flexion point. Once the cup has been applied the vacuum is created to about 0.2 kg/cm^2 and the index finger carefully run around the periphery of the cup to ensure that no maternal tissue has been included. If all is clear the vacuum is increased to 0.8 kg/cm^2 (600 mmHg). There is no need to increase the vacuum in increments and, other than a delay of a minute or two while one carefully checks its application and the exclusion of maternal tissues,

waiting several minutes for the 'chignon' to develop is unnecessary.

Both the metal and rigid plastic cups have an in-curved margin. Thus, the peripheral margin of the cup attached to the fetal scalp has a narrower diameter than the upper curved margin and it is this that produces the chignon. In addition to the atmospheric pressure on the cup against the vacuum created, this has the effect of reducing the risk of cup detachment and also adds to the effective diameter of the cup, such that a 5 cm cup effectively becomes a 6 cm cup.

The traction force needed to detach the vacuum cup will depend on the diameter of the cup and the vacuum created. The calculation of the force needed to detach the cup ('pop-off') when the cup is pulled in a perpendicular direction is given in Table 10.2.

Traction force is the maximum theoretical force possible based on the vacuum holding over the given cross-sectional area of the cup and pulling at right angles to the cup surface seal. There is additional force added from the trapping of the tissue that wedges itself into the cup. One can use 760 mmHg vacuum as the upper limit as that is as close to pure vacuum as one can get at sea level. The force calculation assumes a perpendicular traction force pulling out from the back surface of the cup ignoring frictional effects. Traction angled off the perpendicular will be modified by the vector angle.

Clinically, traction is carried out in conjunction with the uterine contractions and maternal effort. If the traction is carried out at an angle off the perpendicular the force required to pull off the edge of the cup can be quite low (Fig 10-24). It is essential that the axis of traction be perpendicular to the cup – the best guiding rule is that the direction of pull should never go

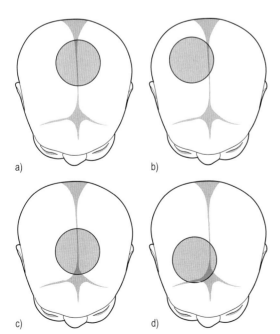

FIGURE 10-23 ■ The four potential vacuum cup applications. (a) Flexing median. (b) Flexing paramedian. (c) Deflexing median. (d) Deflexing paramedian.

TABLE 10.2	**Force Needed to Detach the Vacuum Cup**		
Cup Diameter (mmHg)	Vacuum (kg/cm^2)		Traction Force (lb)
5 cm	500	0.65	29
	600	0.80	35
	700	0.96	41
	760	Atmospheric	45
6 cm	500	0.65	42
	600	0.80	51
	700	0.95	59
	760	Atmospheric	64

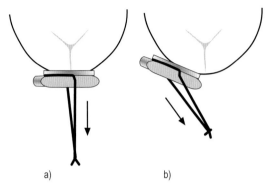

a)   b)

FIGURE 10-24 ■ Cup placement and traction. (a) Correct perpendicular traction within the circumference of the cup diameter. (b) Oblique traction and/or paramedian application predispose to cup detachment.

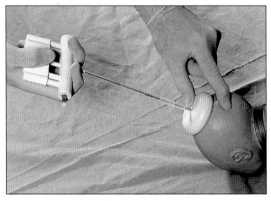

FIGURE 10-25 ■ Technique of vacuum extraction.

outside the circumference of the cup. Traction should be with the index and middle fingers on the traction bar and the thumb of the other hand should be placed on the surface of the cup with the forefinger placed against the scalp and underlying bone. This allows one to detect what Bird called 'negative traction', in which the scalp is drawn away from the skull but the bony skull does not descend.[25]

Repeated negative traction may result in fluctuations of pressure within the cranium and increase the risk of scalp and intracranial haemorrhage. Therefore, the thumb applies countertraction to reduce the chance of cup detachment and the index finger assesses whether the scalp is just being pulled off the bone or the bone is descending appropriately. Thus, the two hands work in combination with the finger and thumb of the left hand, keeping the cup pressed to the surface of the scalp and the index finger assessing descent, while the right hand ensures that the traction is in the perpendicular plane to the cup (Fig 10-25). This co-ordinated effort between

the two hands and fingers should be practised on manikins.

Some of the vacuum delivery devices, such as the commonly used OmniCup, have traction force indicators.[58] In clinical use most vacuum deliveries are achieved using ≈ 9 kg (20 lb) traction force, although up to 14 kg (30 lb) may be necessary.[26,57]

The advantage of the rigid cups, in addition to their lower risk of pop-off, is that the vacuum port is placed laterally or recessed – which allows placement of the cup over the flexion point in cases of deflexed occipito-transverse and occipito-posterior positions. The problem with the soft cups that have a central stem is that it is not possible, due to this stem, to place the cup over the flexion point in many of these deflexed positions. Another disadvantage of the soft cup is that it is not possible to use the finger and thumb placement as easily as with the hard cup. However, using the fingers and thumb spread around the periphery of the soft cup the same principles can be applied.

No attempt should be made to encourage rotation of the fetal head by applying shearing tangential pressure to the cup. Provided the cup has been placed with a correct flexing median application the head will undergo autorotation during traction at the level in the pelvis most suitable for that particular head in that pelvis. In some cases of occipito-posterior position the head does not rotate but is delivered OP.

If the head has descended to the perineum with traction but further progress is slow check posteriorly between the fetal head and the sacrum. Vacca has described entrapment of the fetal hand between the sacrum and the fetal head – which he calls the 'sacral hand wedge' and which can delay final delivery of the head over the perineum.[59] Thus, if there is delay in descent check posteriorly and, if present, grasp the fetal wrist with the fingers and deliver the posterior arm.

If the vacuum cup detaches during traction the situation should be carefully reappraised. If everything still seems suitable for vacuum assisted delivery the cup can be reapplied and traction carried out. If the cup detaches for a second time then further reappraisal will have to be undertaken to determine whether vaginal delivery is safe or whether one should move to caesarean section – which would be necessary if there is inadequate descent and rotation. If the head has rotated and descended to the perineum delivery can be assisted with forceps. This needs especially careful evaluation as it is associated with a higher risk of fetal trauma. At times the chignon can prevent accurate re-application of the vacuum cup.

It is useful to regard vacuum assisted delivery as having two phases. The *descent phase* is from the time of cup application until the head is at the pelvic outlet, at which level the vacuum cup will be completely visible at the introitus. The *outlet phase* is the time from when the cup is completely visible until delivery of the head.[59]

Traction during one uterine contraction is regarded as one 'pull'. One should expect that during three pulls delivery will occur or the head will have progressively descended to the perineum (with the cup completely visible) so that vaginal delivery is clearly safe and feasible. Sometimes it takes two to five more pulls to gently assist delivery of the fetal head over the perineum. When there is progressive descent with traction the pull on the scalp is less compared with no descent. Hence the three pulls during three contractions should have produced enough descent and rotation to signify that additional pulls will achieve safe delivery without trauma to the fetus. Thus, the vast majority of vacuum assisted deliveries should be carried out within 20 minutes from the initial application of the cup. Just as with forceps delivery certain vacuum assisted deliveries should be carried out as a trial of vacuum with the obstetrician prepared to back off in the face of any difficulty and move straight to caesarean section.

Once delivered, the vacuum is released and the cup removed. The chignon should be explained to the parents and that the majority of this swelling will disappear within hours and usually completely within 48 hours. Although subgaleal haemorrhage is rare, its potential should be considered in all infants delivered by vacuum and the appropriate nursing observation in the postnatal ward instituted.

In the postpartum period the events leading to assisted vaginal delivery, either by forceps or vacuum, and its implications should be explained to the woman. She can be reassured that in the vast majority of cases (>80%) spontaneous delivery will occur in a subsequent delivery.[60,61]

SEQUENTIAL INSTRUMENTAL DELIVERY

The most common type of sequential instrumental use is forceps delivery following a failed attempt at vacuum extraction. National guidelines urge caution in the use of sequential instrumental attempts at delivery,[38,39,41] and some large population-based studies show a worse neonatal outcome.[62,63] However, smaller, and more detailed hospital-based reports do not show any

increased neonatal morbidity with the use of forceps after failed vacuum extraction.[57,64–67]

The reported failure-to-deliver rate for vacuum extraction varies from 2%[68] to 35%,[69] with most studies reporting a 10–20% failure rate – higher for nullipara than multipara.[57] In practical terms this means that the obstetrician is faced with this clinical dilemma every 1 in 5 to 1 in 10 attempted vacuum assisted deliveries. In most of these cases the head is low in the pelvis (≥3 cm), presenting the most technically difficult type of caesarean section; with increased maternal morbidity from extension of the uterine incision, bleeding and sepsis and fetal trauma from traumatic attempts to elevate the deeply impacted fetal head (see Chapter 13). The clinically relevant point is to distinguish between those cases that fail to descend below station +2 cm after traction, and those that progressively descend to station ≥3 cm. In most cases the former are best delivered by caesarean section while the latter group can be safely delivered by forceps.[37,67,70,71] The much higher failure-to-deliver rate with the vacuum, compared to forceps (<5%), brings into clinical focus the need for careful appraisal in the selection of instrument with which to assist delivery.

COMPLICATIONS OF ASSISTED VAGINAL DELIVERY

Maternal

Instrumental vaginal delivery is associated with a higher incidence of maternal injuries compared with spontaneous vaginal delivery. These include perineal, vaginal, labial, periurethral and cervical lacerations. There is often significant haemorrhage of an insidious nature associated with these lacerations. Assisted delivery of the head with an emphasis on posteriorly directed traction risks trauma to the perineum and anal sphincter complex, while traction that is directed more anteriorly will result in anterior labial and periurethral lacerations.

In general, vaginal and perineal trauma is less with vacuum assisted delivery than with forceps delivery. The management of lower genital tract trauma is covered in Chapter 23.

Fetal

In general there are more fetal complications with assisted vaginal delivery, although in many instances these may be due to the complication of the labour that led to the necessity for the use of forceps or vacuum assisted delivery.[72–74]

Scalp and Facial Skin Trauma

Superficial bruising, blistering and even minor lacerations can occur at the site of the vacuum cup on the fetal scalp. These are usually trivial and of no lasting significance. Similarly, with forceps assisted delivery, bruising can occur over the fetal cheeks, which is equally benign. These features should be explained to the parents immediately after delivery along with appropriate reassurance.

Caput Succedaneum

Caput succedaneum is a serosanguinous, subcutaneous and extraperiosteal fluid collection with poorly defined margins. It extends across suture lines – in contrast to cephalhaematoma (Fig 10-26a). Caput succedaneum is found normally in spontaneous vaginal delivery and is associated with pressure on the presenting part by the dilating cervix and pelvis. It is often more marked in assisted vaginal deliveries, due to the dystocia present in many of these cases. The vacuum cup produces a well-defined caput succedaneum which is known as a 'chignon'. Both the chignon

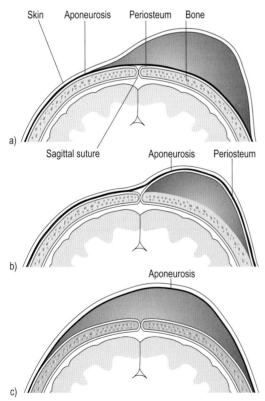

a)

b)

c)

FIGURE 10-26 ■ Fetal scalp trauma. (a) Caput succedaneum. (b) Cephalhaematoma. (c) Subgaleal haemorrhage.

and the physiological caput succedaneum usually resolve within 24–48 hours and have no long-term significance.

Cephalhaematoma

Cephalhaematoma is a subperiosteal collection of serosanguinous fluid secondary to rupture of small blood vessels between the bony skull and the periosteum. The swelling does not cross the suture line, in contrast to both caput succedaneum and subgaleal haemorrhage (Fig 10-26b). Cephalhaematoma is more common following vacuum delivery compared with forceps delivery. Other than the disfigurement, which should be explained to the parents, most cephalhaematomas are benign and resolve within a few weeks. Occasionally there may be residual calcification leading to a hard swelling for several months.

Subgaleal Haemorrhage

Subgaleal haemorrhage is one of the most serious and potentially life-threatening complications of vaginal delivery. It is also known as subaponeurotic haemorrhage, as the bleeding develops in the space between the periosteum and the galea aponeurotica (Fig 10-26c). This aponeurosis is a sheet of fibrous tissue that extends from the orbital margins anteriorly, the temporal fascia laterally and the nuchal ridges posteriorly. In the loose subaponeurotic area lie emissary veins connecting the dural sinuses and the scalp veins. In term infants the subaponeurotic space has a capacity of about 250 ml and this therefore can lead to life-threatening hypovolaemia in the newborn.

A recent review reported the incidence of subgaleal haemorrhage as approximately 1 in 2000–3000 spontaneous deliveries and 1 in 150–200 vacuum assisted deliveries.[75] The rate with forceps assisted delivery is higher than spontaneous vaginal delivery, but about one-third that of vacuum assisted delivery. The occurrence is the same for vacuum assisted delivery with both rigid and soft cups and is likely to be increased with improper placement of the cup and with failed vacuum delivery.

Subgaleal haemorrhage presents as a diffuse, firm but fluctuant mass that crosses suture lines and will shift as the infant's head is repositioned. It is usually observed within the first 12 hours of delivery but may progress insidiously over the next 48–72 hours. Anaemia and hypovolaemic shock are the presenting signs. The treatment is early detection and correction with transfusion of blood products if necessary.

Eye Injuries

Minor injuries such as periorbital oedema, subconjunctival haemorrhages and retinal haemorrhages can occur after spontaneous and assisted vaginal delivery. These are usually trivial and of no long-term significance. Retinal haemorrhage is more common with vacuum assisted delivery compared with spontaneous and forceps delivery.

Facial Palsy

The facial nerve is vulnerable to compression as it exits the stylomastoid foramen or as it passes over the ramus of the mandible. The nerve may be compressed by forceps or by pressure against the bony pelvis, usually the sacral promontory. Facial nerve palsy occurs in about 1 in 2000 spontaneous deliveries, 1 in 1000 vacuum assisted deliveries and 1 in 200 forceps deliveries. The injury is virtually always a neuropraxia and recovery is complete.

Brachial Plexus Injury

Brachial plexus injury is increased with assisted vaginal delivery, probably due to the fact that the indication for assistance is dystocia and often associated with fetal macrosomnia. In most reviews there is a slightly increased risk of shoulder dystocia with vacuum assisted delivery rather than forceps, although this association is by no means consistent.[76]

Skull Fracture

Skull fracture can occur with spontaneous and assisted vaginal delivery. Most fractures are linear, of no clinical significance and require no treatment. Depressed skull fractures are rare and, if greater than 2 cm in width and accompanied by neurological symptoms, require neurosurgical elevation. The fracture may be associated with forceps or vacuum delivery or due to pressure of the skull against the maternal bony pelvis.

Intracranial Haemorrhage

Symptomatic intracranial haemorrhage occurs in about 1 in 2000 deliveries. The risk for assisted vaginal delivery is approximately twice that of spontaneous delivery. The risk seems about equal between vacuum (both rigid and soft cups) and forceps delivery. The highest risk is with failed vacuum followed by forceps assisted delivery.

Spinal Cord Injury

Cervical spine cord injury is very rare, about 1 in 80 000 deliveries. It is more likely to be associated with delivery by rotation, particularly with forceps. The possible pathogenesis and safeguards against this injury have been outlined in the section on forceps rotation earlier in this chapter.

Perhaps the evolution of assisted vaginal delivery is best shown by the attitude expressed by Sir Anthony Carlisle in 1834, when he addressed the select committee on medical education in the British Parliament.[77]

'I consider it derogatory to any liberal man to assume the office of a nurse, of an old woman: it is an imposture to pretend that a medical man is required at labour. The craft therefore involves imposture, mischievous interference and gross indecency. Not only is it beneath our dignity, but it is not within our province. I do not consider the delivery of a woman as a surgical operation: it is a natural operation. The man-midwives have recourse to surgical operations, to make themselves in request, and to make it believed that parturition is a surgical act, which it ought not to be. All interference in my opinion is injurious, particularly premature interference, or a meddling with the process of nature'.

REFERENCES

1. Aveling JH. The Chamberlens and the midwifery forceps. London: J & A Churchill; 1882.
2. Spencer HR. The history of British midwifery from 1650 to 1800. London: John Bale, Sons and Danielsson; 1927.
3. Radcliffe W. A secret instrument. London: William Heinemann; 1947.
4. Radcliffe W. Milestones in midwifery. Bristol: John Wright & Sons; 1967.
5. Chapman E. A treatise on the improvement of midwifery; chiefly with regard to the operation. 3rd ed. London: L. Davis and C. Reymers; 1759.
6. Pugh B. A treatise of midwifery, chiefly with regards to the operation. London: J. Buckland; 1754.
7. Smellie W. A treatise on the theory and practice of midwifery. London: E. Wilson; 1752.
8. Tarnier ES. Descriptions des deux nouveaux forceps. Paris: Martinet; 1877.
9. Saxtorph M. Theoria de diverso partu. Copenhagen: A. H. Godiche; 1772.
10. Ferguson JH. A simple and improved modification of the midwifery forceps. Trans Edinb Obstet Soc 1925–26; 46:78–92.
11. Das K. Obstetric forceps: its history and evolution. Calcutta: The Art Press; 1929.
12. Murray RM. The axis-traction forceps: their mechanical principles, construction and scope. Trans Edinb Obstet Soc 1891;16:58–89.
13. Kielland C. Eine neue form und einfuhrungsweise der geburtszange, stets biparietal an den kindlichen schadel gelegt. Munchen Med Wscher 1915;62:923.

14. Baskett TF. On the shoulders of giants: eponyms and names in obstetrics and gynaecology. 2nd ed. London: RCOG Press; 2008. p. 188–9, 222–3.
15. Jones EP. Kielland's forceps. London: Butterworth and Co.; 1952.
16. Barton LG, Caldwell WE, Studdiford WE. A new obstetric forceps. Am J Obstet Gynecol 1928;1516–26.
17. Moolgaoker A. A new design of obstetric forceps. J Obstet Gynaecol Br Commonw 1962;69:450–7.
18. Baskett TF. The history of vacuum extraction. In: Vacca A. Handbook of vacuum delivery in obstetric practice. 2nd ed. Brisbane: Vacca Research; 2003. p. 11–23.
19. Yonge J. An account of balls of hair taken from the uterus and ovaria of several women. Phil Trans R Soc Lond 1706;725–6:2387–92.
20. Arnott N. Elements of physics or natural philosophy. vol. 1. 4th ed. London: T&G Underwood; 1829. p. 650–2.
21. Simpson JY. On a suction-tractor; or new mechanical power as a substitute for the forceps in tedious labours. Monthly J Med 1849;9:556–9.
22. Malmström T. The vacuum extractor: an obstetrical instrument and the parturiometer: a tokographic device. Acta Obstet Gynecol Scand 1957;36(Suppl. 3): 7–50.
23. Chalmers JA. The ventouse. The obstetric vacuum extractor. Chicago: Yearbook Medical Publisher; 1971.
24. Bird GC. Modification of Malmström's vacuum extractor. BMJ 1969;2:52–6.
25. Bird GC. The importance of flexion in vacuum delivery. Br J Obstet Gynaecol 1976;83:194–200.
26. Vacca A. Operative vaginal delivery: clinical appraisal of a new vacuum extraction device. Aust NZ J Obstet Gynaecol 2001;41:156–60.
27. Drife JO. Choice and instrumental delivery. Br J Obstet Gynaecol 1996;103:608–11.
28. O'Grady JP, Pope CS, Hoffman DE. Forceps delivery. Best Pract Res Clin Obstet Gynaecol 2002;16:1–16.
29. Johanson RB, Mennon V. Vacuum extraction versus forceps for assisted vaginal delivery. Cochrane Database Syst Rev 2004;(2).
30. Johanson RB, Heycook E, Carteer J, Sultan AH, Walklate K, Jones PW. Maternal and child health after assisted vaginal delivery: five-year follow-up of a randomised controlled study comparing forceps and ventouse. Br J Obstet Gynaecol 1999;106:544–9.
31. Baskett TF. Non-progressive labour: dystocia. In: Essential management of obstetric emergencies. 4th ed. Bristol: Clinical Press Ltd; 2004. p. 119–33.
32. Goodfellow CF, Howell MGR, Swaab DF. Oxytocin deficiency at delivery with epidural analgesia. Br J Obstet Gynaecol 1983;90:214–19.
33. Saunders NJ, Spiby H, Gilbert L. Oxytocin infusion during second stage of labour in primiparous women using epidural analgesia: a randomised double-blind placebo-controlled trial. BMJ 1989; 299:1423–6.
34. Tuuli MG, Frey HA, Odibo AO, Macones GA, Cahill AG. Immediate compared with delayed pushing in the second stage of labor: a systematic review and metaanalysis. Obstet Gynecol 2012;120:660–8.
35. Sherer DM, Onyje CI, Bernstein PS. Utilization of real-time ultrasound on labor and delivery in an active academic teaching hospital. Am J Perinatol 1989;16: 303–7.
36. Crichton D. A reliable method of establishing the level of the fetal head in obstetrics. South Afr Med J 1974;48: 784–7.
37. Baskett TF, Arulkumaran S. Assisted vaginal delivery. In: Intrapartum care. 2nd ed. London: RCOG Press; 2011. p. 99–115.
38. Royal College of Obstetricians and Gynaecologists. Operative vaginal delivery. Guideline No. 26. London: RCOG; 2011.
39. Society of Obstetricians and Gynaecologists of Canada. Guidelines for operative vaginal birth. Clinical practice guideline No. 148. J Obstet Gynaecol Can 2004;26: 747–53.
40. Cheung YW, Hopkins LM, Caughey AB. How long is too long? Does a prolonged second stage of labor in nulliparous women affect maternal and neonatal morbidity? Am J Obstet Gynecol 2004;191:933–8.
41. American College of Obstetricians and Gynecologists. Practice Bulletin No. 17. Operative vaginal delivery. Washington, DC: ACOG; 2009.
42. Allen VM, Baskett TF, O'Connell CM, McKeen D, Allen AC. Maternal and perinatal outcomes with increasing duration of the second stage of labour. Obstet Gynecol 2009;113:1248–58.
43. Bleich AT, Alexander JM, McIntire DD, Leveno KJ. An analysis of second-stage labor beyond 3 hours in nulliparous women. Am J Perinatol 2012;29:717–22.
44. Cheong YC, Abdullahi H, Lashen H, Fairlie FM. Can formal education and training improve the outcome of instrumental delivery? Eur J Obstet Gynecol Reprod Biol 2004;113:139–44.
45. Dupuis O, Decullier E, Clerc J, Moreau R, Pham MT, Bin SD, et al. Does forceps training on a birth simulator allow obstetricians to improve forceps blade placement? Eur J Obstet Reprod Biol 2011;159: 305–9.
46. Douglass LH, Kaltreider DF. Trial forceps. Am J Obstet Gynecol 1953;65:889–96.
47. Jeffcoate TNA. The place of forceps in present-day obstetrics. BMJ 1953;2:951–7.
48. Langeran A, Mercier G, Chauleur C, Varlet MN, Patural H, Lima S, et al. Failed forceps extraction: risk factors and maternal and neonatal morbidity. J Gynecol Obstet Reprod Biol (Paris) 2012;41:333–8.
49. Leslie KK, Lehnerz PD, Smith M. Obstetric forceps training using visual feedback and the isometric strength testing unit. Obstet Gynecol 2005;105:377–82.
50. Menticoglu SM, Perlman M, Manning FA. High cervical spinal cord injury in neonates delivered with forceps: report of 15 cases. Obstet Gynecol 1995;86: 589–94.
51. Pomeroy RH. The treatment of occipito-posterior positions. Am J Obstet Dis Wom 1914;69:354–6.
52. Royal Australian New Zealand College of Obstetricians and Gynaecologists. Rotational forceps. College Statement C-Obs13. RANZCOG: Melbourne; 2012.
53. Burke N, Field K, Mujahid F, Morrison JJ. Use and safety of Kielland's forceps in current obstetric practice. Obstet Gynecol 2012;120:766–70.
54. Maryniak GM, Frank JB. Clinical assessment of the Kobayashi vacuum extractor. Obstet Gynecol 1984;64: 431–5.
55. O'Mahoney F, Hofmeyr GJ, Menon V. Choice of instruments for assisted vaginal delivery. Cochrane Database Syst Rev 2010;11:CD005455.
56. Royal Australian New Zealand College of Obstetricians and Gynaecologists. Instrumental vaginal delivery. College Statement C-Obs16. RANZCOG: Melbourne; 2012.
57. Baskett TF, Fanning CA, Young DC. A prospective observational study of 1000 vacuum-assisted deliveries with the OmniCup device. J Obstet Gynaecol Can 2008; 30:573–80.
58. Whitlow BJ, Tamizian O, Ashworth J, Kerry S, Penna LK, Arulkumaran S. Validation of traction force indicator in ventouse devices. Int J Gynecol Obstet 2005;90: 35–8.

59. Vacca A. The 'sacral hand wedge': a cause of arrest of descent of the fetal head during vacuum assisted delivery. Br J Obstet Gynaecol 2002;109:1063–5.

60. Mawdsley SD, Baskett TF. Outcome of the next labour in women who had a vaginal delivery in their first pregnancy. Br J Obstet Gynaecol 2000;107:932–4.

61. Bahl R, Strachan BK. Mode of delivery in the next pregnancy in women who had a vaginal delivery in their first pregnancy. J Obstet Gynaecol 2004;24:272–3.

62. Towner D, Castro MA, Eby-Wilkins E, Gilbert WM. Effect of mode of delivery in nulliparous women on neonatal intracranial injury. N Engl J Med 1999;341:1709–14.

63. Gardella C, Taylor M, Benedetti T, Hitti J, Critchlow C. The effect of sequential use of vacuum and forceps for assisted vaginal delivery on neonatal and maternal outcomes. Am J Obstet Gynecol 2001;185:896–902.

64. Edozien LC, Williams JL, Chatterjee IC, Hirsch PJ. Failed instrumental delivery: how safe is the use of a second instrument? J Obstet Gynaecol 1999;19:460–2.

65. Ezenagu LC, Kakaria R, Bofill JA. Sequential use of instruments at operative vaginal delivery: is it safe? Am J Obstet Gynecol 1999;180:1446–9.

66. Melamed N, Yogev Y, Stainmetz S, Ben-Haroush A. What happens when vacuum extraction fails? Arch Gynecol Obstet 2009;280:243–8.

67. Edgar DC, Baskett TF, Young DC, O'Connell CM, Fanning CA. Neonatal outcome following failed Kiwi Omnicup vacuum extraction. J Obstet Gynaecol Can 2012;34:620–5.

68. Mola GD, Kuk JM. A randomised controlled trial of two instruments for vacuum assisted delivery (Vacca reusable Omnicup and the Bird anterior and posterior cups) to compare failure rates, safety and use effectiveness. Aust NZ J Obstet Gynaecol 2010;50:246–52.

69. Attilakas G, Sibanda T, Winter C, Johnson N, Draycott T. A randomised controlled trial of a new handheld vacuum extraction device. BJOG 2005;112:1510–15.

70. Edozien LC, Williams JL, Chatterjee IC, Hirsch PJ. Failed instrumental delivery: how safe is the use of a second instrument? J Obstet Gynaecol 1999;19:460–2.

71. Vacca A. Trials and tribulations of operative vaginal delivery. BJOG 2007;114:519–21.

72. Baskett TF, Allen VM, O'Connell CM, Allen AC. Fetal trauma in term pregnancy. Am J Obstet Gynecol 2007;197:499–503.

73. Contag SA, Clifton RG, Bloom SL, Song CY, Varner MW, Rouse DJ, et al. Neonatal outcomes and operative vaginal delivery versus caesarean delivery. Am J Perinatal 2010;27:493–6.

74. Werner EF, Janevic TM, Illuzzi J, Fumai EF, Savitz DA, Lipkind HS. Mode of delivery in nulliparous women and neonatal intracranial injury. Obstet Gynecol 2011;118:1239–46.

75. Uchil D, Arulkumaran S. Neonatal subgaleal hemorrhage and its relationship to delivery by vacuum extraction. Obstet Gynecol Surv 2003;58:687–93.

76. Caughey AB, Sandberg PL, Zlatnik MG, Thiet MP, Parer JT, Laros RK. Forceps compared with vacuum: rates of neonatal and maternal morbidity. Obstet Gynecol 2005;106:908–12.

77. Arulkumaran S, Gibb DMF, Tamby Raja RL, Heng SH, Ratnam SS. Rising caesarean section rates in Singapore. Singapore J Obstet Gynaecol 1985;16:5–14.

BIBLIOGRAPHY

Chalmers JA. The ventouse – the obstetric vacuum extractor. London: Lloyd-Luke; 1971.

Dennen PC. Dennen's forceps deliveries. 4th ed. Washington, DC: American College of Obstetricians and Gynecologists; 2001.

Dill LV. The obstetrical forceps. Springfield, Illinois: Charles C. Thomas; 1953.

Laufe LE, Berkus MD. Assisted vaginal delivery: obstetric forceps and vacuum extraction techniques. New York: McGraw-Hill; 1992.

O'Grady JP. Modern instrumental delivery. Baltimore: Williams and Wilkins; 1988.

O'Grady JP, Gimovsky ML, McIlhargie CJ. Vacuum extraction in modern obstetric practice. New York: Parthenon Publishing Group; 1995.

O'Mahony F, Settatree R, Platt C, Johanson R. Review of singleton fetal and neonatal deaths associated with cranial trauma and cephalic delivery during a national intrapartum-related confidential enquiry. Br J Obstet Gynaecol 2005;112:619–26.

Patel RP, Murphy DJ. Forceps review in modern obstetric practice. BMJ 2004;328:1302–5.

Vacca A. Handbook of vacuum delivery in obstetric practice. 3rd ed. Brisbane: Vacca Research; 2009.

Vacca A. Vacuum assisted delivery. Best Pract Res Clin Obstet Gynecol 2002;16:17–30.

Vacca A, Grant A, Wyatt G, Chalmers I. Portsmouth operative delivery trial. A comparison of vacuum extraction and forceps delivery. Br J Obstet Gynaecol 1983;90:1107–12.

Whitby EH, Griffiths PD, Rutter S, et al. Frequency and natural history of subdural haemorrhages in babies and relation to obstetric factors. Lancet 2004;363:846–51.

CHAPTER 11

MALPRESENTATIONS

TF Baskett • AA Calder

Fetal malpresentation exists when the presenting part is other than the normal vertex of the fetal head. This includes two malpresentations that are covered in other chapters: breech (Chapter 16) and cord presentation (Chapter 18). The remaining malpresentations that will be covered in this chapter are face, brow, transverse lie with shoulder or arm presentation, and compound presentations. In modern obstetrics, particularly in the developed world, the incidence of malpresentations has fallen. This is due to the association of many malpresentations with high parity and the fact that women are having fewer children.

The various anteroposterior diameters (Fig 11-1) of the term fetal head vary depending upon the position: normal flexed vertex (9.5 cm), deflexed occipito-posterior position (11–12 cm) and malpresentation: face presentation, submento-bregmatic (9.5 cm) and brow, mento-vertical (13.5 cm). These are illustrated in Figure 11-2.

FACE PRESENTATION

In face presentation the attitude of the fetal head is one of complete extension with the chin as the denominator and leading pole. The presenting diameter is the submento-bregmatic, which in the term fetus is about 9.5 cm. This is the same as the favourable flexed vertex presentation, but the facial bones do not mould to the same extent as the cranial vault does in vertex presentation. The incidence of face presentation is about 1 in 500 births.

Causes

- Fetal anomalies are found in about 15% of face presentations. The commonest are major CNS anomalies such as anencephaly and meningomyelocoele. Tumours of the neck may also cause extension and face presentation.
- Prematurity.

- Mild cephalopelvic disproportion has been incriminated. It is probable that in some cases of deflexed occipito-posterior position with relative disproportion the fetal head may extend completely to a face presentation.
- It has been postulated that excessive tone in the extensor muscles may predispose to face presentation. This theory has been used to explain cases of primary face presentation which occur before the onset of labour. The development of face presentation during labour is called secondary face presentation.
- High parity is associated in the majority of cases.
- In most cases, other than parity, no obvious cause is found.

Diagnosis

The presenting part of the face is between the chin and supraorbital ridges. Usually the characteristic landmarks of the eyes, nose, mouth and chin can be felt with the examining finger during labour. Considerable oedema often develops which may, to a degree, obscure these landmarks. Although the distinction is usually obvious there may be confusion in distinguishing between the mouth and the anus. If this is so, the finger is inserted into the orifice and the gum ridges can easily be felt as a distinguishing landmark.

Diagnosis before labour is rare but may be suspected if on abdominal examination the fetus is easily palpated and its back is lying dorsoanterior. In cases with a normally flexed vertex, palpation of the back and head will reveal only a slight depression at the neck between the back and occiput. In face presentations on the other hand, with the head extended, there is a marked depression between the back and occiput. If there is clinical suspicion, ultrasound will establish or refute the diagnosis.

The position of a face presentation is defined with the chin as the denominator and is therefore recorded as mento-anterior, mento-posterior

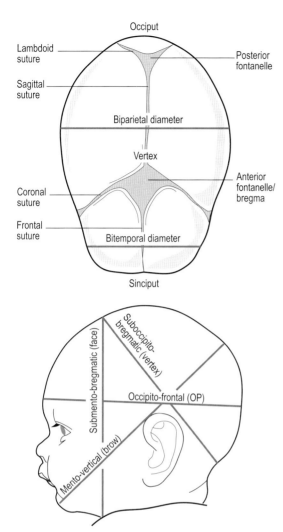

FIGURE 11-1 ■ Diameters and landmarks of the fetal skull.

or mento-transverse, left or right accordingly. The majority of cases are mento-anterior.

Management

On the rare occasions that face presentation is diagnosed before labour a careful ultrasound examination should be made to exclude structural fetal anomalies. One can make the case for observation until the onset of labour or full term, on the grounds that a number of these cases will revert spontaneously to a normal flexed vertex position. However, if face presentation persists and the fetus is normal, it should be delivered by elective caesarean section.

When the diagnosis is made in labour a gross fetal anomaly should be excluded and clinical pelvimetry should rule out obvious pelvic contraction or deformity. The position of the face presentation is then assessed. Depending upon the estimated fetal weight, the position, station, clinical assessment of pelvic capacity and the progress of labour the following guidelines may be used:

If the fetus has an anomaly incompatible with life then progress to vaginal delivery should be followed.

If the position is mento-anterior, which presents the same diameters as a flexed vertex, if the fetus is normal or small in size and the pelvis is of good capacity, progress can be followed with the expectation of spontaneous vaginal delivery. The majority of cases with mento-transverse position will rotate to the more favourable anterior position.

Fifty years ago, when the morbidity and mortality associated with caesarean section was high, vaginal manipulation was used to try and convert face presentations to a vertex presentation. This was carried out at advanced or full cervical dilatation and usually done under deep general anaesthesia with uterine relaxation. In a previous edition of this book Chassar Moir (1964) described his technique:

> 'In cases discovered early in labour (mentolateral) positions, I succeeded in five consecutive cases in correcting the position to a vertex position by the simple intrauterine manipulation of hooking down the occiput with the fingers and simultaneously pressing up the chin and brow with the thumb, labour then proceeded normally in each case.'

Nowadays, we would not advise such manipulation, except perhaps a tentative attempt which is most likely to succeed with a small fetus and a large pelvis. One would only continue with such a manoeuvre if it proved easy and atraumatic.

> 'When the chin is turned towards the pubis, at the lower part of that bone, the woman must be laid on her back, the forceps introduced … and when the chin is brought out from under the pubis, the head must be pulled half round upwards; by which means, the fore and hind head will be raised from the perineum.'
> William Smellie
> A Treatise on the Theory and Practice of Midwifery. London: D. Wilson, 1752, p281

Provided labour continues normally and there is good progress in the second stage with mento-anterior positions, spontaneous delivery is likely.

If progress is inadequate with mento-anterior positions consideration of forceps delivery is appropriate. One has to be very careful that

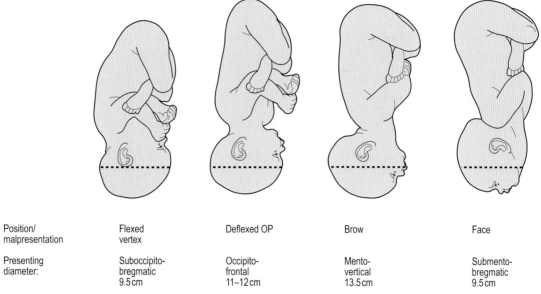

Position/ malpresentation	Flexed vertex	Deflexed OP	Brow	Face
Presenting diameter:	Suboccipito- bregmatic 9.5 cm	Occipito- frontal 11–12 cm	Mento- vertical 13.5 cm	Submento- bregmatic 9.5 cm

FIGURE 11-2 ■ Positions and malpresentations of the fetal head.

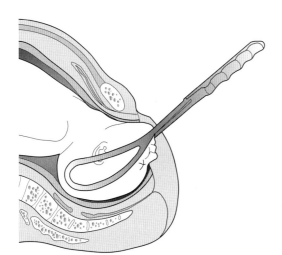

FIGURE 11-3 ■ Face presentation, mento-anterior. Delivery with classical forceps.

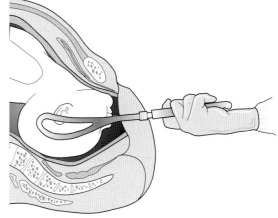

FIGURE 11-4 ■ Face presentation, mento-anterior. Delivery with Kielland's forceps.

there is adequate descent for safe forceps assisted delivery. Even when the face is visible at the vulva the cranium may not be fully through the pelvic brim. The guiding dictum is 'the head is higher than you think'. If forceps delivery is to be considered there should be no head palpable at the pelvic brim and the sacral hollow should be filled with the cranium. Either classical or Kielland's forceps can be used and in face presentations the chin replaces the occiput for orientation. If Kielland's forceps are used the directional buttons on the shanks should point toward the chin. With both types of forceps the blades are applied as for classical forceps to the occiput anterior positions (see Chapter 10). The orientation is along the mento-occipital

diameter of the head. With the pelvic curve of the classical forceps the chin is between the heels of the blades and the face is beneath the level of the shanks (Fig 11-3). With Kielland's forceps the upper part of the blades is at the level of the supraorbital ridges with the face above the level of the shanks (Fig 11-4).

Once locked in position the handles of both types of forceps should be slightly lowered to give maximum extension of the head, which presents the narrowest diameter. With both types of forceps a slight downward traction is applied during a uterine contraction and with maternal effort until the chin is delivered beneath the symphysis. With the classical forceps the handles are gradually elevated up to about 45° to

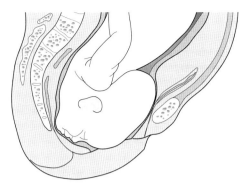

FIGURE 11-5 ■ Face presentation, impacted mento-posterior position.

allow flexion of the occiput over the perineum. Using Kielland's forceps, with their lack of pelvic curve, the handles should only be elevated up to the horizontal level to achieve flexion and delivery of the occiput.

In cases of mento-posterior position which do not rotate to anterior during labour, vaginal delivery is impossible (Fig 11-5). In the past Kielland's forceps were sometimes used to rotate mento-posterior and mento-transverse cases to mento-anterior. However, the risks associated with this are considered excessive in modern obstetrics. Thus, these cases should be delivered by caesarean section.

BROW PRESENTATION

In brow presentation the attitude of the fetal head is midway between the flexed vertex and face presentation. It is the most unfavourable of all cephalic presentations with its mento-vertical diameter of 13 cm in the term fetus. The incidence is approximately 1 in 1000–2000 births.

The potential causes are the same as those for face presentation, although the prevalence of lethal fetal anomalies is less with brow presentation than with face presentation. In a number of cases the cause is cephalopelvic disproportion, in which the fetal head deflexes progressively from vertex, to occipito-posterior, to brow.

Diagnosis

It is rare to diagnose brow presentation before the onset of labour. During labour the landmarks for the examining fingers are the root of the nose, the supraorbital ridges and the anterior fontanelle. Over this presenting area, in neglected cases, considerable moulding and caput can occur, making the identification of these landmarks difficult. Usually, however, the supraorbital ridges and root of the nose can be identified.

Management

In a small number of cases brow presentation is associated with a small fetus in a capacious pelvis. In such cases labour may progress normally to spontaneous delivery. In the normally grown term fetus the wide presenting diameter, unless there is an exceptionally capacious pelvis, is incompatible with vaginal delivery. Attempts have been described with digital manipulation to try and flex the head to a vertex presentation – these are usually fruitless. The other alternative is to manually encourage deflexion to a face presentation. In modern obstetrics neither of these options is usually feasible or desirable. Thus, in the vast majority of cases with brow presentation, caesarean section should be performed.

> 'The child appearing in a very unnatural posture ... with the arm and the shoulder foremost. I then endeavoured with all the strength I had to bring back the arm and shoulder, but to no purpose, this being one of the most troublesome cases that can happen to a man-midwife ... I got my hand into the womb as well as I could ... At last I got hold of one foot, which whilst I was pulling toward me the arm that was before in the passage drew back within the womb of course, and the other foot following the first to the orifice of the womb, I joined them close together, and delivered the child, which proved a daughter and alive ...'
>   Paul Portal
>   The Compleat Practice of Men and Women Midwives. London: J. Johnson, 1763, p178–179

TRANSVERSE LIE

Transverse lie is the most unfavourable lie which the fetus can assume. At term the incidence is about 1 in 500 births. The fetus may be either dorso-anterior or dorso-posterior. In many cases the lie is oblique rather than transverse, with either the head or breech occupying one iliac fossa. With a transverse or oblique lie in labour the most common presentation is the shoulder and sometimes the arm prolapses through the cervix (Fig 11-6).

Causes

- Placenta praevia, which should be considered in all cases.
- Uterine anomaly – most often a septate or subseptate uterus. When this is the cause the fetus is usually relatively fixed in its position and not amenable to version.
- Polyhydramnios.

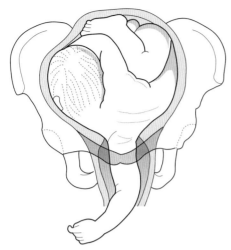

FIGURE 11-6 ■ Shoulder presentation with prolapsed arm.

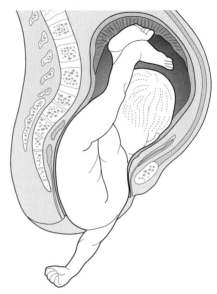

FIGURE 11-7 ■ Spontaneous evolution.

- Fetal anomaly – abnormal babies do abnormal things, including lying abnormally within the uterus. A dead, toneless fetus may also lie transversely.
- Fibroid in the lower uterine segment. On rare occasions an ovarian tumour may have the same effect by preventing the presenting part from entering the lower uterine segment.
- Gross prematurity.
- High parity. Both the uterine and abdominal musculature will lack tone, which may facilitate transverse or oblique lie of the fetus.
- Full bladder can on rare occasions prevent descent of either fetal pole into the lower uterine segment.

Diagnosis

Diagnosis may be suspected by simply inspecting the abdomen, where the uterus is enlarged transversely and shortened vertically. With palpation the emptiness of the lower pole of the uterus is obvious and the head and breech can usually be felt at each side connected by the transverse or obliquely lying fetal back. Only in cases of considerable maternal obesity should it be necessary to resort to ultrasound to confirm the diagnosis. However, ultrasound is usually advisable to rule out placenta praevia or structural fetal anomaly.

In labour the presentation can be confirmed by vaginal examination and it is usually the shoulder that comes to present. This is felt as a small rounded body and the palpable landmarks are the clavicle and the ribs. In a neglected labour after the membranes have ruptured one or more limbs may prolapse through the cervix. The most common is for an arm to prolapse but both a foot and an arm can prolapse together. The prolapsed hand, which may be quite oedematous, can be distinguished from a foot by the absence of the projecting heel (see Chapter 16).

Course of Labour

There are four possible outcomes for a transverse/oblique lie in labour:
- As uterine tone increases in early labour while the membranes remain intact the fetus may convert to a longitudinal lie. This is most likely to happen when the aetiology is lax uterine musculature associated with high parity.
- The shoulder presents and is pushed down into the pelvis. This results in total obstruction and the uterus may become exhausted or rupture.
- Spontaneous delivery of the fetus with the body doubled-up (*partus conduplicato corpore*). This only occurs when the fetus is unusually small or macerated. The head and thorax or pelvis are pressed together and deliver doubled-up.
- Spontaneous evolution, in which the shoulder becomes impacted behind the symphysis and the trunk, the breech and limbs are driven past, followed by the shoulders and head (Fig 11-7). This is exceptionally rare and only occurs with a small premature or macerated fetus with a capacious maternal pelvis.

Management

There are three circumstances to consider in the management of transverse lie and shoulder presentation: late pregnancy before the onset of labour, during labour with the fetus alive and during labour with the fetus dead.

Late Pregnancy Before the Onset of Labour

When transverse or oblique lie is diagnosed ≥36 weeks' gestation, the common associated causes should be sought. This involves the use of ultrasound to rule out placenta praevia, fetal anomaly and multiple pregnancy. It is also essential to ensure that the gestational age is correct. If these causes are ruled out then external cephalic version should be carried out as outlined in Chapter 28. If this is successful and the fetus remains stable as a cephalic presentation, the rest of the antenatal care can be normal. The problem arises, and this is most often in cases of higher parity, when the lie remains unstable, changing from day to day, or even hour to hour between transverse, oblique, cephalic and breech. In such cases, close to term the risk of labour or spontaneous rupture of membranes occurring with the fetus transverse or oblique could result in umbilical cord prolapse or obstructed labour. In these cases it is best to admit the woman to the antenatal ward so that at the earliest signs of labour external cephalic version can be performed, or immediate caesarean section be carried out should there be spontaneous rupture of the membranes and prolapse of the umbilical cord or of an arm.

In many of these cases uterine tone increases in the days before labour and either spontaneous version or external cephalic version successfully stabilizes the fetus to a favourable presentation. In these cases, provided gestational age is a secure ≥38 weeks, a stabilizing induction can be considered. For a stabilizing induction the patient is taken to the labour ward, the lie is corrected to vertex presentation if necessary, and intravenous oxytocin is started as per the normal induction protocol (see Chapter 8). Once uterine contractions have become established a pelvic examination is performed and amniotomy carried out, after excluding cord presentation. The fetal head is carefully controlled with the other abdominal hand during this procedure and amniotic fluid slowly drained off until the head is well settled in the lower uterine segment on to the cervix.

If the transverse lie is not amenable to version then elective caesarean section should be carried out at 39 weeks' gestation.

SPONTANEOUS EVOLUTION

'In the year 1772, I was called to a poor woman in Oxford Street ... I found the arm much swelled and pushed through the external parts in such a manner, that the shoulder nearly reached the perineum. The woman struggled vehemently with her pains, and during her continuance, I received the shoulder of the child to descend ... I remained at the bed-side til the child was expelled and I was very much surprised to find, that the breech and inferior extremities were expelled before the head, as if the case had originally been a presentation of the inferior extremities'.

Thomas Denman
Observations to prove that in cases where the upper extremities present, at the time of birth, the delivery may be affected by the spontaneous evolution of the child. Lond Med J 1784; 564–570

During Labour with the Fetus Alive

In early spontaneous labour it is sometimes possible to carry out external cephalic version in between the uterine contractions. The mother's bladder should be emptied before version. This is most likely to be successful in patients with high parity as the cause of the transverse lie. Unless this is simple and in cases where labour is well established, caesarean section should be performed immediately.

Caesarean section for transverse and oblique lie requires careful appraisal of the lower uterine segment once the abdomen has been entered. Unless the membranes are intact and a broad well-developed lower uterine segment is present, which is not likely in these circumstances, a vertical incision should be made, starting in the lower uterine segment. This incision will usually have to be extended into the upper uterine segment to allow adequate room to manoeuvre the fetus into position for delivery. If accessible it is usually better to deliver the feet first, unless the head is much lower.

During Labour with the Fetus Dead

This is a situation which should rarely, if ever, be encountered in well-developed health services. However, it still has to be confronted in areas of developing countries with limited hospital resources. In these circumstances decapitation with the Blond–Heidler saw is the most appropriate treatment if the skill exists to carry this out. The rationale and technique of this procedure is covered in Chapter 28. In regions where there is less experience with such procedures, or where the mother may not accept this management, caesarean section may be preferable.

COMPOUND PRESENTATION

By definition, compound presentation is prolapse of part or all of one or more limbs in association with cephalic presentation and of prolapse of a hand or arm in association with breech presentation. In practical clinical terms, compound presentation is usually confined to cephalic presentations.

Any condition which interferes with the engagement of the fetal head may predispose to the prolapse of a limb or limbs along with the head. These include contracted pelvis, pelvic tumours and polyhydramnios. Prematurity and a dead macerated fetus are additional causes. It is very unusual for a foot to be alongside or below the fetal head, and if it is the fetus is usually so premature as to be pre-viable or it is macerated.

The commonest situation is a small fetus with a roomy pelvis and a hand and forearm beside and just below the head. Having ruled out any of the other serious causes it is usually a simple matter to push the hand and forearm back beside and above the fetal head. Retaining one's fingers in this position, subsequent uterine contractions

will usually cause the fetal head to descend and the hand and arm to remain above. If the arm prolapses beside and in front of the head it obstructs labour and if it cannot be replaced delivery will have to be by caesarean section.

BIBLIOGRAPHY

Breen JL, Weismeier E. Compound presentation: a survey of 131 patients. Obstet Gynecol 1968;32:419–22.

Cruikshank DP, Cruikshank JE. Face and brow presentation: a review. Clin Obstet Gynecol 1981;24:333–50.

Edwards RL, Nicholson HO. The management of the unstable lie in late pregnancy. J Obstet Gynaecol Br Commonw 1969;76:713–15.

Kawatheker P, Kasturilal MS, Srinivis P, Sudda G. Etiology and trends in the management of transverse lie. Am J Obstet Gynecol 1973;117:39–44.

Kovacs SG. Brow presentation. Med J 1972;280–4.

Laufe LE, Berkus MD. Assisted vaginal delivery: obstetric forceps and vacuum extraction techniques. New York: McGraw-Hill; 1992.

Moore EJT, Dennen EH. Management of persistent brow presentation. Obstet Gynecol 1955;6:186–9.

O'Grady JP. Modern instrumental delivery. Baltimore: Williams and Wilkins; 1988. p. 150–2.

Posner AC, Friedman S, Posner LB. Modern trends in the management of the face and brow presentations. Surg Gynecol Obstet 1957;104:485–90.

Posner LB, Ruben EJ, Posner AC. Face and brow presentations: a continuing study. Obstet Gynecol 1963;21:745–9.

Vacca A. The 'sacral hand wedge', a cause of arrest of descent of the fetal head during vacuum assisted delivery. Br J Obstet Gynaecol 2002;109:1063–5.

Weissberg SM, O'Leary JA. Compound presentation of the fetus. Obstet Gynecol 1973;41:60–2.

CHAPTER 12

SHOULDER DYSTOCIA

JF Crofts

'The delivery of the head with or without forceps may have been quite easy … time passes. The child's face becomes suffused. It endeavours unsuccessfully to breathe. Abdominal efforts by the mother or by her attendants produce no advance, gentle head traction is equally unavailing. Usually equanimity forsakes the attendants. They push, they pull. Alarm increases. Eventually "by greater strength of muscles or by some infernal juggle" the difficulty appears to be overcome, and the shoulders and trunk of a goodly child are delivered. The pallor of its body contrasts with the plum coloured cyanosis of the face and the small quantity of freshly expelled meconium about the buttocks. It dawns upon the attendants that their anxiety was not ill-founded. The baby lies limp and voiceless, and only too often remains so despite all efforts and resuscitation'.
W Morris
J Obstet Gynaecol Br Emp 1955;62:302

DEFINITION

Shoulder dystocia simply means difficult delivery of the fetal shoulders, and is defined as a vaginal cephalic delivery that requires additional obstetric manoeuvres to deliver the fetal body after routine axial traction on the fetal head has been unsuccessful at completing the birth.[1] Shoulder dystocia occurs when the anterior fetal shoulder impacts on the maternal symphysis pubis, or, less commonly, the posterior fetal shoulder impacts on the maternal sacral promontory.

PATHOPHYSIOLOGY OF SHOULDER DYSTOCIA

In the majority of women the antero-posterior (AP) diameter of the pelvic inlet is narrower than the oblique or transverse diameter. The fetal shoulders usually enter the pelvis in the oblique diameter. However, if the fetal bisacromial diameter is large and the fetal shoulders attempt to enter the pelvis in the narrower AP diameter, the anterior fetal shoulder will become impacted on the maternal symphysis pubis – this is shoulder dystocia (Fig 12-1). On extremely rare occasions both shoulders may remain above the pelvic brim – bilateral shoulder dystocia; this requires considerable extension of the fetal neck and is usually associated with instrumental delivery.

INCIDENCE

The incidence of shoulder dystocia in the largest series is reported to be between 0.58% and 0.70% of vaginal births.[2]

RISK FACTORS FOR SHOULDER DYSTOCIA

There are a number of antenatal factors that increase the risk of shoulder dystocia, and in most of these the common denominator is fetal macrosomia:

Macrosomia

The greater the fetal birth weight the higher the risk of shoulder dystocia.[2] A review[3] of 175 886 vaginal births of infants born to non-diabetic mothers reported rates of shoulder dystocia of:
- 5.2% in infants weighing 4001–4250 g
- 9.1% in infants weighing 4251–4500 g
- 14.3% in infants weighing 4501–4750 g
- 29.0% in infants weighing 4751–5000 g.

Infants weighing over 4000 g are significantly more likely to suffer shoulder dystocia compared to those weighing less than 4000 g (11.1% and 0.6% respectively).[4] However, macrosomia remains a weak predictor of shoulder dystocia. The large majority of infants with a birth weight of greater than 4500 g do not develop shoulder dystocia and up to 50% of cases of shoulder dystocia occur in infants with a birth weight less than 4000 g.

Maternal Diabetes Mellitus

Maternal diabetes mellitus increases the risk of shoulder dystocia.[2] Infants of diabetic mothers have a three- to fourfold increased risk

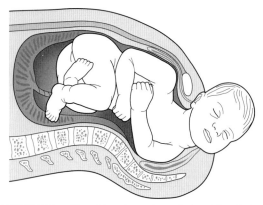

FIGURE 12-1 ■ Shoulder dystocia: relationship of the anterior and posterior shoulder to the pelvic brim.

of shoulder dystocia compared to infants of non-diabetic mothers for the same birth weight. These infants tend to have a higher shoulder-to-head circumference ratio, because the tissues that contribute to shoulder girth are insulin-sensitive and respond to hyperglycaemia and hyperinsulinism.

Instrumental Delivery

Compared to a spontaneous delivery shoulder dystocia is approximately twice as likely to occur with instrumental delivery.[3]

Maternal Obesity

Shoulder dystocia is associated with obesity; however, obese women tend to have larger babies and the association may be due to fetal macrosomia, rather than maternal obesity *per se*.[5]

Previous Shoulder Dystocia

Previous shoulder dystocia is a risk factor for recurrent shoulder dystocia. The rate of repeat shoulder dystocia in a subsequent vaginal delivery has been reported to be between 1.1% and 16.7%.[1] The average recurrence rate is 10%, approximately 10 times the incidence in the general population. However, due to selection bias these recurrence rates may be under-estimated; elective caesarean section may be performed in some pregnancies following a previous birth complicated by shoulder dystocia.

A woman who has had a previous shoulder dystocia should be referred to a consultant-led antenatal clinic in subsequent pregnancies to discuss antenatal care and mode of delivery.

Intrapartum Risks

The risk of shoulder dystocia is increased in any labour in which progress is slow (prolonged first stage, prolonged second stage, use of oxytocin for augmentation of labour, instrumental delivery).[1]

PREDICTION OF SHOULDER DYSTOCIA

Antenatal detection of macrosomia is poor. Clinical fetal weight estimation is unreliable; third trimester ultrasound scans have at least a 10% margin for error for actual birth weight and sensitivity of just 60% for macrosomia (>4.5 kg).[1]

A retrospective review of 267 228 vaginal births reported that even the most powerful predictors for shoulder dystocia have a sensitivity of just 12% and positive predictive value of under 5%.[6] The majority of cases of shoulder dystocia occur in women with no risk factors. Shoulder dystocia is, therefore, an unpredictable and largely unpreventable event. Maternity staff must always be alert to the possibility of shoulder dystocia with any vaginal delivery.[1]

PREVENTION

Induction of Labour

In women with gestational diabetes the incidence of shoulder dystocia is reduced with early induction of labour.[7] The NICE diabetes in pregnancy guideline recommends that pregnant women with diabetes should be offered delivery through induction of labour, or by elective caesarean section if indicated, after 38 completed weeks.[8] This recommendation was made due to the increased risk of late stillbirth associated with diabetes; however, the intervention may also reduce this risk of shoulder dystocia in this cohort.

Induction of labour, however, does not prevent shoulder dystocia in non-diabetic women with a suspected macrosomic fetus and therefore should not be offered to non-diabetic women to reduce the risk of shoulder dystocia.[1]

Caesarean Section

Infants of diabetic mothers have a two- to four-fold increased risk of shoulder dystocia compared with infants of the same birth weight born to non-diabetic mothers.[3,9] A decision-analysis model estimated that in diabetic women with an estimated fetal weight (EFW) of greater than 4.5 kg, 443 caesarean sections would need to be performed to prevent one permanent brachial plexus injury (BPI).[10] Therefore, National Guidelines in the UK[1] and USA[11] recommend the consideration of an elective caesarean section in pregnancies complicated by pre-existing or gestational diabetes if the EFW is greater than 4.5 kg.

It has been estimated that 3695 caesarean sections would be required to prevent one permanent BPI in the non-diabetic population. Therefore National Guidelines suggest that an elective caesarean section should only be considered if the EFW is above 5.0 kg, or there has been a previous severe shoulder dystocia, especially if it was associated with neonatal injury.[1]

MANAGEMENT

Shoulder dystocia is unpredictable and therefore all maternity staff should have the skills required to manage the emergency. There are numerous techniques described that can be used to relieve shoulder dystocia. The Royal College of Obstetricians and Gynaecologists (RCOG) have published an evidence based algorithm for the management of shoulder dystocia (Fig 12-2).[1] No one manoeuvre is superior to another. The algorithm begins with simple measures, which are often effective, and leads progressively to more invasive manoeuvres.

Recognition of Shoulder Dystocia

Shoulder dystocia can occur following spontaneous or assisted delivery of the fetal head. The face and chin may be difficult to deliver and when the head does deliver it remains tightly applied to the vulva, retracts and depresses the perineum – the 'turtle-neck' sign. Restitution may not occur because the fetal head is so tightly applied to the perineum. When routine axial traction is applied to the fetal head the anterior shoulder fails to deliver.

Assistance Is Required

When shoulder dystocia is suspected or diagnosed help must be immediately summoned. This should include senior midwifery staff, the most experienced obstetrician available and a neonatologist. If shoulder dystocia is not resolved quickly then an anaesthetist should also be called.

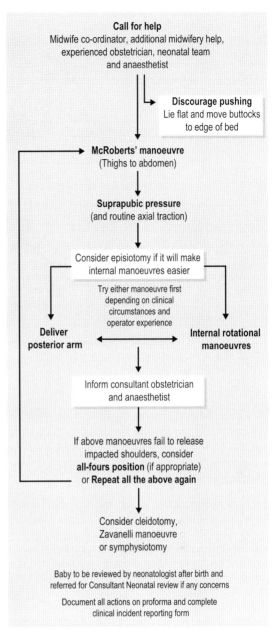

FIGURE 12-2 ■ Algorithm for the management of shoulder dystocia. (Reproduced from reference 1 with the permission of the Royal College of Obstetricians and Gynaecologists).

State the Problem and Stop the Woman Pushing

The mother and her partner should be told that the baby's shoulders are difficult to deliver, that additional help is required, and that someone will explain what is happening and what she needs to do. When help arrives, 'shoulder dystocia' should be clearly stated so that attendants immediately understand the problem to be

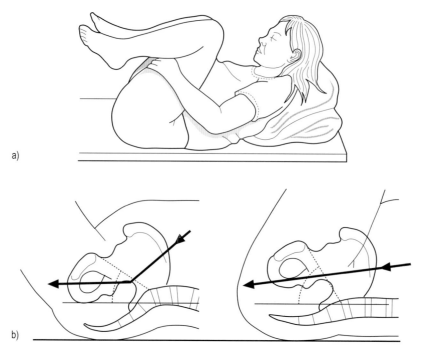

a)

b)

FIGURE 12-3 ■ (a) McRoberts' manoeuvre. (b) Effect is to reduce both the lumbo-sacral angle and the angle of pelvic inclination.

managed. Maternal pushing should be discouraged as it will not resolve shoulder dystocia, and may increase the impaction of the shoulders.

McRoberts' Position

McRoberts' position is the most widely advocated first-line manoeuvre.[12] This involves hyper-flexion of the maternal legs, which increases the relative AP diameter of the pelvis by straightening the sacrum relative to the lumbar spine and rotating the maternal pelvis cephalad. The success rate is reported to be between 40% and 90%.[2]

To assume McRoberts' position the mother should be laid supine with all pillows removed. An assistant on each side should then hyperflex her legs against her abdomen (Fig 12-3). Apply routine traction to the fetal head (i.e. the same degree of traction as applied during a normal delivery) that is axial (i.e. in the axis of the fetal spine). If the shoulders are not released in McRoberts' position by the application of routine, axial traction to the fetal head, traction should be stopped and an additional resolution manoeuvre attempted.

There is no evidence that using McRoberts' position in anticipation of shoulder dystocia is helpful, therefore prophylactic McRoberts' positioning is not recommended.[1]

Suprapubic Pressure

Suprapubic pressure has two aims: (1) to reduce the bisacromial diameter of the fetal shoulders by adduction and (2) to rotate the shoulders into the wider oblique or transverse diameter of the maternal pelvis.[13]

Whilst two assistants hold the woman in the McRoberts' position, the third assistant should apply pressure superior to the maternal symphysis pubis. Pressure should be applied in a downward direction from the side of the fetal back (if this is known). The application of pressure from behind the fetal back will adduct the shoulders and rotate them into the wider oblique diameter of the pelvis (Fig 12-4). If the side of the fetal back is unknown, suprapubic pressure should be applied from the side thought most likely to be the side of the fetal back, and if this pressure is not effective, pressure should be applied from the opposite side. If the shoulders are not released with a combination of McRoberts' position, suprapubic pressure and routine axial traction, traction should be stopped and a different manoeuvre attempted.

Evaluate the Need for Episiotomy

An episiotomy will not relieve the bony obstruction that causes shoulder dystocia and therefore

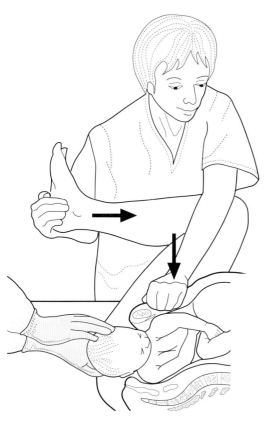

FIGURE 12-4 ■ Assistant applies directed suprapubic pressure and facilitates McRoberts' manoeuvre.

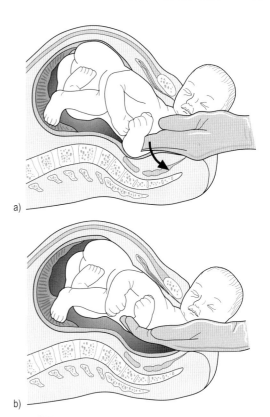

a)

b)

FIGURE 12-5 ■ Delivery of the posterior arm.

by itself will not resolve the dystocia.[1] In some cases an episiotomy may be required to improve access to the pelvis to facilitate internal vaginal manoeuvres.

Internal Manoeuvres

There are two different internal manoeuvres that can be performed – delivery of the posterior arm or internal rotation. There is no evidence that one is superior to the other.[1] All internal manoeuvres start with the same action – gaining access to the pelvis; this is best achieved posteriorly as the sacral hollow is the most spacious part of the pelvis. The whole hand is inserted into the vagina (sacral hollow) posteriorly and, if the fetal arms are flexed across the fetal chest, delivery of the posterior arm should be attempted first. If the posterior fetal arm is extended behind the fetal back, internal rotation is the best option, followed by delivery of the posterior arm.

Delivery of the Posterior Arm

Delivery of the shoulders may be facilitated by delivery of the posterior arm, described by Barnum in 1945.[14] The rationale is that by

delivering the posterior arm the diameter of the fetal shoulders is narrowed by the width of the arm, providing enough room to resolve the shoulder dystocia.

If the fetal arms are flexed the posterior fetal hand and forearm will be encountered on entry into the sacral hollow. The fetal wrist can be grasped by the accoucheur's fingers and thumb. The posterior arm can then be removed from the maternal pelvis through gentle traction in a straight line (Fig 12-5). Once the posterior arm has been delivered, gentle traction can be applied to the fetal head; if the shoulder dystocia has resolved the fetus should be easily delivered. However, if despite delivering the posterior arm, the shoulder dystocia has not resolved the fetus can be rotated through 180° with traction across the fetal chest. The posterior shoulder will become the new anterior shoulder and will be below the symphysis pubis, resolving the dystocia.

The posterior arm is much more difficult to deliver if it is extended. An extended posterior arm needs to be flexed before it can be delivered. Flexion can be achieved by the application of pressure to the antecubital fossa. Once the posterior arm has flexed the wrist can be grasped. Direct traction on the upper arm should be avoided as it may result in humeral fracture.

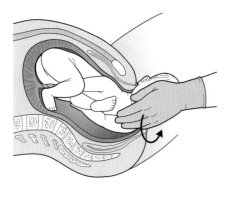

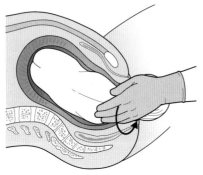

FIGURE 12-6 ■ Internal rotation (a) pressure on anterior aspect of posterior shoulder and (b) pressure on the posterior aspect of posterior shoulder.

Internal Rotational Manoeuvres

The aims of internal rotation are to:

1. move the fetal shoulders out of the narrowest diameter of the pelvis (the anterior-posterior) and into a wider diameter (the oblique or transverse)
2. reduce the fetal bisacromial diameter by adducting the shoulders
3. utilize the pelvic anatomy: as the shoulders rotate they descend through the pelvis due to the pelvic bony architecture.

Rotation can be most easily achieved by pressing on the anterior or posterior aspect of the posterior fetal shoulder[13,15] (Fig 12-6). Pressure on the posterior aspect of the posterior shoulder has the additional benefit of reducing the shoulder diameter through adduction.[13] Rotation moves the shoulders into the wider oblique diameter of the pelvis, which should resolve the dystocia. The shoulders should deliver with routine axial traction. If delivery does not occur, the pressure can be continued and the shoulders rotated through 180° to achieve delivery.

If pressure in one direction is not effective, efforts should be made to rotate the shoulders in the opposite direction by pressure on the opposite aspect of the fetal posterior shoulder.

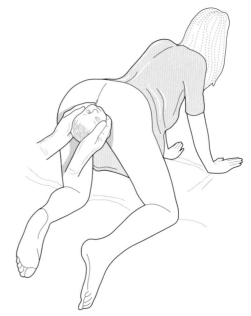

FIGURE 12-7 ■ All-fours position.

An assistant providing suprapubic pressure may help during attempted internal rotation. The person performing internal rotation needs to ensure suprapubic pressure is applied in the correct direction and rotation is with, not against, each other.

Internal rotational manoeuvres were described by Woods[15] and Rubin[13] in 1943 and 1964 respectively. However, both Woods and Rubin included the application of fundal pressure in their descriptions. Fundal pressure is no longer recommended as it can be associated with uterine rupture and BPI.[1] Therefore, internal rotational manoeuvres should no longer be described as a 'Woods' screw' or 'Rubin'. A simple description of what was done is sufficient, for example: 'Rotation and subsequent delivery of the fetal shoulders was achieved by applying pressure on the posterior aspect of the fetal posterior shoulder in an anti-clockwise direction'.

All-Fours Position

The all-fours manoeuvre may dislodge the anterior shoulder and facilitate access to the posterior shoulder to enable internal manoeuvres to be performed.[16] The mother should be asked to transfer onto her hands and knees and gentle traction should be applied to the fetal head to determine if the shoulders have been released (Fig 12-7).

The individual circumstances should guide the accoucheur when to attempt the 'all-fours' technique. For a slim mobile woman without epidural anaesthesia and with a single midwifery attendant, the 'all-fours' position is probably more appropriate, and should be used early in a community setting. For a woman with regional anaesthesia in situ other manoeuvres may be more appropriate.

Manoeuvres of Last Resort

Surgical manoeuvres such as cephalic replacement followed by caesarean section and symphysiotomy are rarely used and have serious potential maternal morbidity. They are considered to be last resort measures and should only be performed if the fetal heartbeat is still present.[1]

Zavanelli Manoeuvre

Cephalic replacement of the head and subsequent delivery by caesarean section was first performed by Zavanelli. In a series of 59 cases, cephalic replacement was unsuccessful in six (10%), and two mothers (3%) suffered a ruptured uterus. It is important to note that the uterus retracts after delivery of the fetal head, so tocolysis is required prior to unrestituting, flexing and replacing the fetal head into the uterine cavity to reduce the risk of uterine rupture[17] (see Chapter 28).

Symphysiotomy

Symphysiotomy is the surgical division of the symphyseal ligament to increase pelvic dimensions. It is associated with high incidence of serious maternal morbidity, including urethral and bladder injury, infection, pain and long-term walking difficulty, and poor neonatal outcome (see Chapter 28).

What Not to Do

Do not pull hard, do not pull down and do not pull quickly. It is instinctive to want to apply traction to the fetal head in an attempt to deliver the baby. However, strong downward traction on the fetal head is associated with neonatal trauma, including permanent BPI. Traction will not resolve the dystocia and traction above that used during a normal delivery should be avoided. Evidence suggests that traction applied quickly with a 'jerk', rather than applied slowly, may be more damaging to the nerves of the brachial plexus;[18] therefore, traction should be applied slowly. Downward traction increases the stretch on the brachial plexus; gentle traction should be carefully applied in the axis of the fetal spine to reduce stretching of the brachial plexus.

Fundal pressure, in the absence of other manoeuvres, is associated with a 77% complication rate, including uterine rupture[19] and BPI in the neonate. Therefore, fundal pressure is no longer a recommended manoeuvre in the management of shoulder dystocia and should not be used.

MANAGEMENT AFTER A SHOULDER DYSTOCIA

Immediate Neonatal Assessment

Following shoulder dystocia the neonate is at risk of stillbirth, hypoxia and birth trauma, which includes BPI, and fractures of the humerus and clavicle. A neonatologist (or equivalent) should be called to attend the birth as soon as shoulder dystocia is diagnosed.

Maternal Assessment and Treatment

There is significant maternal morbidity associated with shoulder dystocia; particularly postpartum haemorrhage (11%) and fourth degree perineal tears (3.8%).

The Baby Should be Examined for Injury by a Neonatal Clinician

BPI is one of the most important complications of shoulder dystocia, complicating 2.3% to 16% of such deliveries.[20–22] Other reported fetal injuries associated with shoulder dystocia include fractures of the humerus and clavicle, pneumothoraces and hypoxic brain damage.[1,4]

BRACHIAL PLEXUS INJURY

The brachial plexus is the most complex structure in the peripheral nervous system conveying motor, sensory and sympathetic nerve fibres to the arm and shoulder. The brachial plexus contains five roots (C5–C8, T1) that terminate in five main peripheral nerves. Sympathetic nerve fibres from the first thoracic root provide the autonomic nerve supply to the head, neck and upper limbs, and control sweat glands, pupil dilatation and eyelid movement.

The brachial plexus is vulnerable to trauma due to its position between two highly mobile structures, the neck and arm. The incidence of BPI in the United Kingdom and Republic of Ireland in 1998–9 was 1 in 2300 live births.[23]

The proportion of BPIs reported to be permanent, an injury lasting more than 12 months, ranges between 8 and 12%.

Classification of Brachial Plexus Injury

Erb's Palsy

Erb's palsy, or upper BPI, is the most common form of BPI with a frequency of 73–86%.[24] The affected cervical nerve roots are the fifth (C5) and sixth (C6), with the seventh cervical root (C7) sometimes also involved. The classic Erb's palsy posture is a result of paralysis or weakness in the shoulder muscles, the elbow flexors and the forearm supinators. The affected arm hangs down and is internally rotated, extended and pronated. If C7 is involved, the wrist and finger extensors are also paralyzed. The loss of extension causes the wrist to flex and the fingers to curl up in the 'waiter's tip position'. Full functional recovery is reported to occur in 65–90% of cases; the prognosis is worse with C7 involvement.[24]

Total Brachial Plexus Injury

Complete involvement of the brachial plexus occurs in approximately 20% of BPIs.[24] The entire plexus from C5–T1 is involved, with total sensory and motor deficits of the entire arm, resulting in a paralyzed arm with no sensation. The phrenic nerve may also be damaged, resulting in a hemi-paralysis of the diaphragm, manifesting in respiratory distress and feeding difficulties in the neonate. Horner's syndrome, caused by sympathetic nerve injury, resulting in contraction of the pupil and ptosis on the affected side may also be present with a total BPI and is associated with a worse prognosis. Full functional recovery is very rare without surgical intervention.

Any baby with a suspected injury following shoulder dystocia should be reviewed by a neonatologist. In the UK the Erb's Palsy Group is an excellent source of information and supports families and healthcare practitioners caring for children with brachial plexus injuries (http://www.erbspalsygroup.co.uk).

DOCUMENTATION

The RCOG shoulder dystocia guideline suggests that a proforma may be helpful in documenting key events after delivery[1] and there is some evidence that this is effective.[25]

Documentation should include the times of delivery of the head and the body, the anterior shoulder at the time of the dystocia, the resolution manoeuvres performed, their timing and sequence, the staff in attendance and the time they arrived, and the neonatal assessment of the baby for injury.

RECOMMENDATIONS AND REQUIREMENTS FOR SHOULDER DYSTOCIA TRAINING

Poor outcomes following shoulder dystocia can be a result of inappropriate clinical management. The 5th Confidential Enquiries into Stillbirths and Deaths in Infancy (CESDI) in England and Wales found grade three suboptimal care in 66% of neonatal deaths following shoulder dystocia.[26] In 2003 the NHS Litigation Authority produced a report on the 264 claims for obstetric brachial plexus injury (OBPI) in England.[27] Medico-legal experts judged 46% (72/158) of the reviewed cases to involve substandard care. The most common criticism related to failure to carry out standard shoulder dystocia resolution manoeuvres.

Staff may lack confidence[28] and competence[29] managing this unpredictable and largely unpreventable condition. Therefore, training for the management of shoulder dystocia might be the most effective means of reducing the associated morbidity and mortality. The 5th CESDI Report recommended a 'high level of awareness and training for all birth attendants' as 'professionals will be exposed to it (*shoulder dystocia*) relatively infrequently, but urgent action is needed when it does occur'.[26] Annual 'skill drills', including shoulder dystocia, are recommended jointly by both the Royal College of Midwives and the RCOG and are one of the requirements in the Clinical Negligence Scheme for Trusts (CNST) maternity standards.

Where training has been associated with improvements in clinical outcomes following shoulder dystocia, all staff have attended on an annual basis. Practical shoulder dystocia training has been shown to improve knowledge,[30] confidence and management of simulated shoulder dystocia.[29,31]

Training staff in the management of shoulder dystocia can improve neonatal outcomes. An 8-year retrospective review of shoulder dystocia management before and after the introduction of annual shoulder dystocia training for all staff in one UK hospital demonstrated a significant reduction in neonatal injury at birth following shoulder dystocia (9.3% pre-training, 2.3% post-training).[22]

REFERENCES

1. Royal College of Obstetricians and Gynaecologists. Shoulder dystocia. Green-top guideline No. 42. London: RCOG; 2012.
2. Gherman RB. Shoulder dystocia: an evidence-based evaluation of the obstetric nightmare. Clin Obstet Gynecol 2002;45:345–62.
3. Nesbitt TS, Gilbert WM, Herrchen B. Shoulder dystocia and associated risk factors with macrosomic infants born in California. Am J Obstet Gynecol 1998;179:476–80.
4. Nocon JJ, McKenzie DK, Thomas LJ, Hansell RS. Shoulder dystocia: an analysis of risks and obstetric maneuvers. Am J Obstet Gynecol 1993;168:1732–7.
5. Robinson H, Tkatch S, Mayes DC, Bott N, Okun N. Is maternal obesity a predictor of shoulder dystocia? Obstet Gynecol 2003;101:24–7.
6. Ouzounian JG, Gherman RB. Shoulder dystocia: Are historic risk factors reliable predictors? Am J Obstet Gynecol 2005;192:1933–5.
7. Horvath K, Koch K, Jeitler K, Matyas E, Bender R, Bastian H, et al. Effects of treatment in women with gestational diabetes mellitus: systematic review and meta-analysis. BMJ 2010;340:c1395.
8. National Institute of Health and Clinical Excellence. Diabetes in pregnancy: management of diabetes and its complications from pre-conception to the postnatal period. London: NICE; 2008.
9. Acker DB, Sachs BP, Friedman EA. Risk factors for shoulder dystocia. Obstet Gynecol 1985;66:762–8.
10. Rouse DJ, Owen J, Goldenberg RL, Cliver SP. The effectiveness and costs of elective cesarean delivery for fetal macrosomia diagnosed by ultrasound. JAMA 1996;276:1480–6.
11. Chauhan SP, Berghella V, Sanderson M, Magann EF, Morrison JC. American College of Obstetricians and Gynecologists practice bulletins: an overview. Am J Obstet Gynecol 2006;194:1564–72.
12. Gonik B, Stringer CA, Held B. An alternate maneuver for management of shoulder dystocia. Am J Obstet Gynecol 1983;145:882–4.
13. Rubin A. Management of shoulder dystocia. JAMA 1964;189:835–7.
14. Barnum CG. Dystocia due to the shoulders. Am J Obstet Gynecol 1945;50:439–42.
15. Woods CE. A principle of physics as applicable to shoulder delivery. Am J Obstet Gynecol 1943;45:796–804.
16. Bruner JP, Drummond SB, Meenan AL, Gaskin IM. All-fours maneuver for reducing shoulder dystocia during labor. J Reprod Med 1998;43:439–43.
17. O'Leary JA. Cephalic replacement for shoulder dystocia: present status and future role of the Zavanelli maneuver. Obstet Gynecol 1993;82:847–50.
18. Allen R, Sorab J, Gonik B. Risk factors for shoulder dystocia: an engineering study of clinician-applied forces. Obstet Gynecol 1991;77:352–5.
19. Gross TL, Sokol RJ, Williams T, Thompson K. Shoulder dystocia: a fetal-physician risk. Am J Obstet Gynecol 1987;156:1408–18.
20. Gherman RB, Ouzounian JG, Goodwin TM. Obstetric maneuvers for shoulder dystocia and associated fetal morbidity. Am J Obstet Gynecol 1998;178:1126–30.
21. Acker DB, Gregory KD, Sachs BP, Friedman EA. Risk factors for Erb-Duchenne palsy. Obstet Gynecol 1988;71:389–92.
22. Draycott TJ, Crofts JF, Ash JP, Wilson LV, Yard E, Sibanda T, et al. Improving neonatal outcome through practical shoulder dystocia training. Obstet Gynecol 2008;112:14–20.
23. Evans-Jones G, Kay SP, Weindling AM, Cranny G, Ward A, Bradshaw A, et al. Congenital brachial palsy: incidence, causes, and outcome in the United Kingdom and Republic of Ireland. Arch Dis Child Fetal Neonatal Ed 2003;88:F185–7.
24. Benjamin K. Distinguishing physical characteristics and management of brachial plexus injuries. Advances in Neonatal Care 2005;5:240–51.
25. Crofts JF, Bartlett C, Ellis D, Fox R, Draycott TJ. Documentation of simulated shoulder dystocia: accurate and complete? BJOG 2008;115:1303–8.
26. Maternal and Child Health Research Consortium. Confidential enquiry into stillbirths and deaths in infancy: 5th Annual Report. London; 1996.
27. NHS Litigation Authority. Summary of substandard care in cases of brachial plexus injury. NHSLA Journal 2003;2:ix–xi.
28. Neill AM, Sriemevan A. Shoulder dystocia: room for improvement? J Obstet Gynaecol 1999;19:132–4.
29. Crofts JF, Bartlett C, Ellis D, Hunt LP, Fox R, Draycott TJ. Training for shoulder dystocia: a trial of simulation using low-fidelity and high-fidelity mannequins. Obstet Gynecol 2006;108:1477–85.
30. Crofts J, Ellis D, Draycott T, Winter C, Hunt L, Akande V. Change in knowledge of midwives and obstetricians following obstetric emergency training: a randomised controlled trial of local hospital, simulation centre and teamwork training. BJOG 2007;114:1534–41.
31. Deering S, Poggi S, Macedonia C, Gherman R, Satin AJ. Improving resident competency in the management of shoulder dystocia with simulation training. Obstet Gynecol 2004;103:1224–8.

CHAPTER 13

CAESAREAN SECTION

TF Baskett · AA Calder

Caesarean section represents the most significant operative intervention in all of obstetrics. Its development and application has saved the lives of countless mothers and infants. On the other hand, its inappropriate use can be a direct and avoidable cause of maternal mortality and morbidity. For these reasons, caesarean section probably represents the largest source of controversy and debate in modern obstetrics. The frequency with which it is carried out continues to rise and has in many hospitals and health regions, reached rates in excess of 30%. The detailed reasons for the rise in caesarean delivery rates are covered later in this chapter. One of the more controversial indications is caesarean delivery on maternal request and it is worth reflecting that in only 150 years caesarean section has evolved from an operation of last resort, usually leading to maternal death, to a method of delivery by maternal choice.

HISTORICAL BACKGROUND

Caesarean section is almost certainly one of the oldest operations in surgery with its origins lost in the mists of antiquity and mythology – as historians are wont to say when they don't know. It has probably been performed by traumatic accident or post-mortem for several millennia. Ancient myth and legend has it that Aesculapius and Bacchus, the Gods of Medicine and Wine respectively, were born by caesarean section.[1] Thus, at least in legend, those born by caesarean section are in good company.

The origin of the word 'caesarean' is unclear. The weak myth that Julius Caesar was born by this route is contradicted by the fact that his mother survived his birth by many years. It is likely that the term comes from the lex regia or royal law legislated by one of the early kings of Rome, Numa Pompilius in 715 BC.[2] This law proclaimed that women who died before delivering their infant had to have the infant removed through the abdomen before burial. This law continued under the ruling Caesars when it was called lex caesarea.

Traumatic caesarean sections have probably occurred throughout the course of history during war, acts of violence and accidents. Among the more well documented are those in which the horns of cattle have torn open the woman's abdomen and uterus.[3] One of the best known cases was reported from Zaandam, Holland, in 1647, in which a bull attacked a farmer and his wife, tearing open her abdomen and uterus with its horn.[4] The woman and her husband later died but the infant survived. Self-performed caesarean section has probably been carried out for many centuries as some women, alone and in desperation, sought to relieve the unrelenting pain of non-progressive labour. Authentic cases are reported from the 18th century.[1,5,6] Caesarean section performed by lay persons also has a long history. One of the earliest reported cases in 1500 was by Jacob Nufer, a swine gelder, who delivered his wife after several days of apparent labour.[1] There was some doubt whether this was an abdominal pregnancy or a caesarean section. Apparently both the mother and infant survived.[7] In Northern Ireland in 1738 Mary Donnally, an illiterate but experienced lay midwife, carried out the first caesarean with survival of the mother in the British Isles.[8]

During the 15th and 16th century caesarean section was carried out after the mother's death, primarily to fulfil religious edicts that were proclaimed in order to save the soul of the infant by baptism. The first medical text advocating caesarean section before the mother was in extremis was published in 1581 by the French physician Francois Rousset (c1530–1603).[9] Rousset advised caesarean section in the living woman, when it was obvious that she could not deliver vaginally, and before she became so moribund that her death and that of her baby was inevitable. For his temerity he was widely criticised, and with considerable vitriol, by the medical establishment of the day. His book has recently been published in English and with a commentary of caesarean delivery in that era.[10]

The first witnessed and documented caesarean section by a physician was performed by Jeremias Trautmann in Wittenberg, Germany in 1610.[1] However, a number of obstetric texts in the 16th and 17th centuries described the rare performance of caesarean section in cases of contracted pelvis. From the 16th to the 18th centuries the prevailing medical wisdom was strongly against caesarean section, with its almost inevitable fatal outcome for the mother. This viewpoint is summed up in the quote by the prominent Dublin obstetrician Fielding Ould (1710–1789) in 1742: 'Repugnant, not only to all rules of theory or practice, but even of humanity'.[11]

The reason for the high mortality in the pre-anaesthetic era was that caesarean sections were usually performed after prolonged labour on women who were dehydrated, exhausted and infected. In

HISTORICAL BACKGROUND (Continued)

addition, after removal of the fetus the uterus was not sutured, adding haemorrhage to the morbidity equation. Jean Lebas first advocated suturing the uterus in 1769 but his advice was not followed for a century.[2] In addition to haemorrhage, sepsis was the commonest cause of death. Eduardo Porro (1842–1902) of Pavia, Italy, carefully studied this problem and, after experiments with animals, he performed a caesarean section followed by subtotal hysterectomy in 1876.[12] He sutured the cervical stump to the lower end of the abdominal wound to control the haemorrhage and to exteriorize any septic drainage. By controlling the haemorrhage and sepsis Porro dramatically reduced the maternal mortality by about half from its usual rate of 80–90%.[13]

Throughout the 19th century obstetricians devised techniques to try and reduce the risk of sepsis and to preserve the uterus; including a lateral extraperitoneal approach by Ferdinand Ritgen (1787–1867) of Giessen in 1821.[14] Fritz Frank (1856–1923) modified the transperitoneal operation by suturing the edges of the incised lower uterine segment visceral peritoneum to the margins of the abdominal wall incision to contain any sepsis and promote its drainage.[14]

Ferdinand Kehrer (1837–1914) of Hiedelberg is one of the under-appreciated contributors to the development of the modern caesarean section.[4,14] In 1881 he performed a transverse lower segment caesarean section, virtually as it is done today.[15] He emphasized the need for careful suturing of the uterine muscle and a separate suture of the peritoneum over the lower uterine segment – the Doppelnaht or 'double layer' technique. About a year later Max Sänger (1853–1903), working in Leipzig, emphasized the need for careful suturing of the uterine incision which he performed longitudinally in the uterus and called the classical caesarean incision.[13,16] It was Sänger's classical caesarean section that held sway while Kehrer's transverse lower segment technique was forgotten. The classical caesarean section was adopted in Britain, most notably by Murdoch Cameron in Glasgow. Cameron was confronted by a great demand for the procedure because his city had seen an enormous growth of population, especially of poor migrant workers. Many of his patients lived in conditions guaranteed to produce skeletal rickets. Poor housing, poor diet, atmospheric pollution and consequent lack of exposure to sunlight meant that vitamin D deficiency was rife. In 1888 he began a series of elective classical caesarean sections on rachitic dwarfs which was immediately and dramatically successful. In the first 2 years, all but one of the 23 mothers and all the infants survived[17] (Fig 13-1).

In addition to careful suturing of the classical uterine incision, Cameron owed his success to two factors. The first was his recognition that the procedure should be carried out before the mother's condition was compromised by exhaustion and the associated infection of a long obstructed labour. This required that the diagnosis of a hopelessly contracted pelvis should be made before, or at least early in labour. This required the refinement of the clinical science of pelvimetry in the era before x-rays, and depended on the digital assessment of the shape and capacity of the pelvis. The first case

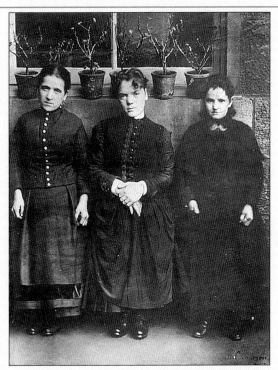

FIGURE 13-1 ■ The first three cases in Murdoch Cameron's historic series of elective classical caesarean section performed on rachitic women with gross pelvic deformities. The photograph was taken outside Glasgow Royal Maternity Hospital and the windowsill on which the flowerpots stand is approximately one metre from the ground.

was the subject of fierce argument among Cameron and his colleagues, the pelvis being considered 'borderline' with an obstetric conjugate of 4 cm! Cameron's second advantage derived from his use of a vulcanized rubber ring which he effectively applied as a tourniquet around the lower part of the uterus after delivery of the infant, constricting the blood flow to the uterus while the wound was repaired. The success of this series of cases resounded across and beyond Europe and was a milestone in the operation's journey from a desperate and usually futile gesture to an acceptable clinical option.

Munro Kerr was a 20-year-old medical student when Murdoch Cameron began his celebrated series and would have undoubtedly attended the Glasgow Royal Maternity Hospital at around that time. He cannot possibly have been unaware of this dramatic development and seems likely to have been attracted to obstetrics by the work of Cameron, whom he would succeed 39 years later as Regius Professor of Midwifery in that city. Indeed, it was Munro Kerr who would be largely responsible for the change from the classical incision to the low transverse incision. When Kehrer performed his low transverse procedure it was to reduce and contain the risk of sepsis. Kerr's main argument was that the healed incision was stronger and less liable to rupture in a subsequent pregnancy. As he wrote:

Continued on following page

The role of caesarean section has been transformed in little more than a century from a procedure of desperation, performed only in the rarest and most terrible circumstances, to one that is commonplace and frequently applied, especially in affluent society, for what some would regard as trivial indications. During that time the operation has changed from one carrying terrifying risks in which the prospect of maternal survival was slim to one in which maternal death is an extreme rarity. During the last quarter of the 20th century in particular, caesarean section rates increased worldwide. A variety of reasons have improved the safety of caesarean section and increased the indications for its performance:

- The introduction of anaesthesia a century and a half ago – itself driven by the search for pain relief in labour, as well as to facilitate surgery.
- Continued improvement in anaesthetic techniques along with the emergence of specialists in obstetric anaesthesia has greatly increased the effectiveness and safety of this component of caesarean delivery.
- Improvements in blood transfusion, antibiotics and thromboprophylaxis have increased the perioperative safety.
- Improved surgical techniques have reduced not only the immediate perioperative complications of caesarean section, but also lessened the risks in subsequent pregnancy.
- There is less experience with certain types of operative vaginal delivery and an unwillingness to accept even small increased risks associated with these techniques. Vaginal breech delivery is the most obvious but by no means only example of this.
- There are now social and medico-legal expectations of a perfect perinatal outcome, which has undoubtedly influenced obstetric care. It is almost unheard of for anyone to be sued for performing a caesarean section, but liability for not performing a caesarean section is not uncommon.
- Advanced maternal age, infertility and assisted reproductive technologies have led to a rise in the number of so-called 'premium' pregnancies. These women also tend to have more complications in pregnancy and labour.
- Although not common there is an increasing demand on the part of some women for elective delivery by caesarean section for what many regard as trivial clinical or social reasons. These may include a fear of labour and vaginal delivery, and the perceived benefits of reducing or eliminating rare fetal risks in labour and long-term sequelae of pelvic floor damage.
- Dramatic advances in neonatal care and outcome have lowered the gestational age at which intervention for fetal indications is appropriate.

As the risks to the woman have progressively diminished, the operation has been found to be justifiable for ever widening clinical and social indications. As more and more women enter second and subsequent pregnancies with a uterine scar it is important to emphasize the long-term potential for serious consequences of caesarean section, which are not often perceived by a short-sighted focus on the immediate decision concerning mode of delivery. It is worth reiterating the view of Myerscough in the 10th edition of this text (1982, p 296), written at a time when the tide of caesareans was at an early point in its inexorable rise:

'I do not doubt that this extension of caesarean section is in the main justified. The remarkable reduction in both maternal and fetal mortality

rates bears this out. Nevertheless, I fear that today, more than ever before, there is a danger of abdominal delivery being regarded as the legitimate method of dealing with each and every obstetric abnormality. Although low, the maternal death rate is not negligible … Nor should it be forgotten that a woman's obstetric future is prejudiced by the uterine scar … The problem today is to select the cases best suited for delivery by caesarean section, having regard not only to the immediate needs of the mother and her unborn child, but also to her more remote obstetric future'.

INDICATIONS

The justification for caesarean section arises from clinical judgement that the interests of the mother, fetus or both are better served by resorting to caesarean delivery in order to avoid the continuation of pregnancy or the onset or the continuation of labour. The conditions that inform this judgement vary widely depending on the population served and the clinical skills and facilities available. As with a number of aspects which make obstetrics such a challenging discipline, the interests of the mother and those of the fetus can at times pull in opposite directions, so that careful assessment is demanded to reach the optimum solution. Recent trends have resulted in a radical change from the need to justify every caesarean against the stern criticism of the obstetric hierarchy to the orthodoxy of today which seems to preach 'if in doubt do a caesarean'. This attitude still needs to be challenged, however, if we are to avoid 'the easy way out', in more than one sense, becoming the norm. Obstetricians in training should be encouraged to develop clinical judgment which they can defend in the courts of the 'obstetric gods' as well as those of the legal system. Defensive obstetrics can be pernicious and must be resisted if we are to do the best for our patients rather than for ourselves. A degree of courage is required if we are not to find that trends in obstetric practice are to be led by external influences rather than clinical ideals.

The indications and proportions of caesarean delivery will vary from country to country and from hospital to hospital. Nonetheless, there are four main indications that account for 60–90% of all caesarean sections. These include: repeat caesarean section (35–40%), dystocia (20–35%), breech (10–15%) and fetal distress (10–15%).[19] Each hospital and health region can analyse its own caesarean delivery indications using the universally applicable Robson 10-group method.[20,21]

In many cases it is not one discrete indication but a combination of relative indications that necessitate caesarean delivery. For example, prolonged non-progressive labour in association with a non-reassuring fetal heart rate pattern may not represent absolute dystocia or definite fetal hypoxia, but relative degrees of each.

Most of the indications for caesarean section are discussed in the individual chapters of this book. However, it may be useful to consider them under three main categories:

Indisputable Indications

- Placenta praevia, except possibly in the most minor degrees of this condition.
- Demonstrable fetal hypoxia or imminent fetal demise. Except in the second stage of labour when vaginal delivery may be a safer and quicker option, clear evidence of fetal hypoxia or its inevitability mandates immediate caesarean delivery. This includes antepartum or intrapartum asphyxia confirmed by fetal blood gas measurement or unequivocal cardiotographic evidence; umbilical cord prolapse; vasa praevia; uterine rupture; and severe abruptio placentae where the fetus is still viable.
- Unequivocal cephalopelvic disproportion, soft tissue obstruction or fetal malpresentation, not caused by gross fetal malformations incompatible with life.

Generally Accepted Indications

This includes many conditions which, depending on their severity, may present ranging from an absolute to a relative need for caesarean section.

- Previous caesarean section is one of the commonest indications. As outlined in the next chapter a variety of additional circumstances will dictate whether or not this is an absolute indication for repeat caesarean section or a trial for vaginal delivery. Within this category most would regard the woman with a previous classical caesarean scar as representing an absolute indication for repeat caesarean section.
- Breech presentation at term is now accepted as an indication for delivery by caesarean section when safe facilities for this exist. This is discussed in Chapter 16.
- Dystocia, manifest by non-progressive labour, makes up an increasing proportion of all caesarean deliveries. Aspects of this diagnosis are discussed in Chapters 5 and 10.

- Fetal distress has been the indication for many caesarean sections for perceived fetal compromise, which was in fact quite misleading. This is discussed in detail in Chapter 6.
- Maternal indications are not common but there are a number of maternal disorders in which, depending upon the severity, it might be advisable to avoid labour. These include severe pre-eclampsia/eclampsia, cardiovascular disease and diabetes. In a number of these cases conditions may be favourable for vaginal delivery but in others caesarean delivery is warranted.

Marginal Indications

This is a small category but has the potential to increase. Included here are those women who have a morbid fear of labour, possibly based on a previous bad experience. Another example is the woman who wants elective caesarean delivery to obviate the perceived risks of fetal injury or asphyxia during labour, or to minimize the risks of damage to her pelvic floor. Others may have worries about their body image or sexuality after vaginal delivery. Each of these women deserves a rational discussion and the provision of full information about the pros and cons of both routes of delivery. Often their concerns can be alleviated by the provision of balanced information, but if not, their wishes should be accommodated within the context of fully informed consent. There is an urgent need to gather data on the short- and long-term sequelae of elective caesarean versus planned vaginal birth so that women can be provided with accurate information for their own clinical and demographic context.[22,23]

CLASSIFICATION OF URGENCY

In recent years a number of organizations have tried to establish guidelines for time limits within which caesarean section should be performed for urgent indications.[24] This debate has taken place within the context of clinical care, hospital accreditation and the spectre of litigation. A recent guideline[25] based on reasonable rationale and some validation has been proposed:[26]

- *Category 1* Immediate threat to the life of the woman or fetus. This will include caesarean sections for severe prolonged fetal bradycardia, fetal scalp blood pH <7.2, cord prolapse, abruptio placentae and uterine rupture. These caesareans should occur as quickly as possible and certainly within 30 minutes.

- *Category 2* Maternal or fetal compromise which is not immediately life-threatening. These include conditions such as antepartum haemorrhage and non-progressive labour with maternal or fetal compromise, but not to the degree of category 1. These cases should also be delivered within 30 minutes if possible but one has to take into account the potential risks in meeting this deadline. For example, the use of general anaesthesia with its increased risks to the mother compared to the slightly more time consuming institution of spinal anaesthesia.

- *Category 3* No maternal or fetal compromise but early delivery required. This will include non-progressive labour without maternal or fetal compromise, and women booked for elective caesarean section who are admitted with ruptured membranes or in early labour. It is recommended that these women be delivered within 75 minutes. There are other cases with slowly worsening conditions such as pre-eclampsia and intrauterine growth restriction (IUGR) in which delivery is indicated. If they are preterm and induction of labour is deemed likely to fail an early caesarean delivery may be necessary.

- *Category 4* Elective planned caesarean section timed to suit the woman and staff. Unless there is urgency for maternal or fetal reasons, elective caesarean section should be planned after 39 completed weeks' gestation to reduce the risk of neonatal respiratory morbidity.

ANAESTHESIA

Regional anaesthesia (epidural or spinal) should be chosen when possible as it has the least associated maternal and neonatal morbidity. General anaesthesia may be given if there is a need for extreme speed, such as in acute fetal distress; patient preference; and for women in whom regional anaesthesia fails (usually less than 5%).

PREOPERATIVE CONSIDERATIONS

- Consent – it has to be admitted that informed consent for caesarean section can vary from the very brief statement of need in acute fetal distress to a much more considered and prolonged discussion in women requesting elective caesarean section for personal reasons. In general the indications for recommending caesarean delivery should be outlined along with the alternatives. The procedure and its complications should be reviewed in the context of the alternatives, which usually include allowing labour to continue or assisted vaginal delivery. The effect of caesarean delivery on future pregnancies should also be reviewed in relevant cases.

- Unless indicated by other medical complications, a complete blood count, blood group and antibody screen comprise adequate preoperative blood testing.
- A urinary (Foley) catheter is placed in the bladder once regional anaesthesia has been established.
- Antacid prophylaxis should be administered in the form of a histamine H_2 receptor blocker (ranitidine or cimetidine).
- The woman should be placed in a 15° left lateral tilt to avoid aorto-caval compression.
- Preoperative shaving of the incision site is not required. If the pubic hair over the proposed incision site is thick it can be clipped short, rather than shaved.

PERIOPERATIVE CARE

- Antibiotic prophylaxis should be given in the form of a single dose of a first-generation cephalosporin or ampicillin. This is given for both elective and emergency caesarean sections and should be administered intravenously either 30 minutes before incision or after the baby is delivered and the umbilical cord is clamped. In women with more prolonged labour and evidence of chorioamnionitis repeat doses of the same antibiotic can be given for the first 48 hours postoperatively.
- Thromboprophylaxis in the form of adequate hydration and early mobilization should apply to all postpartum women. Most women delivered by caesarean section should also receive subcutaneous heparin prophylaxis unless there is a contraindication. This can be administered after discussion with the anaesthetist and usually after removal of the epidural catheter or institution of spinal anaesthesia.
- The Foley catheter can be removed once regional anaesthesia has worn off and the woman is ambulant – usually about 12 hours post-caesarean.
- Postoperative analgesia is best achieved by intrathecal administration of diamorphine or morphine. Non-steroidal anti-inflammatory drugs can also be given, by suppository if necessary.
- Oral fluid and food intake should be administered when the woman feels thirsty or hungry, after confirming bowel peristalsis. In complicated cases, when the possibility of return to the operating theatre exists, oral intake should be withheld until her condition is stable.

TYPES OF CAESAREAN SECTION

Low Transverse Caesarean Section

In about 98% of cases a low transverse segment caesarean section can be performed. The uterine incision is confined to the lower uterine segment so that healing in this relatively non-contractile portion of the uterus in the puerperium is optimal. In addition, the risk of rupture in a subsequent pregnancy is lower than with the other types of caesarean section.

Low Vertical Caesarean Section

This technique is rarely used. Its potential role is in those cases in advanced labour with a well-developed lower uterine segment but at an earlier gestational age, when the overall width of the uterine segment is reduced. In such cases an attempt at a transverse lower segment incision may extend into the major uterine vessels laterally and still not provide a large enough incision for atraumatic delivery of the infant. By making a vertical incision in the lower uterine segment it can be enlarged directly into the upper uterine segment should the size of the incision be inadequate for delivery of the infant. Those who advocate this technique feel that in these circumstances the advantages of the lower segment incision will be gained in most cases. However, most obstetricians feel that in many of these cases the upper uterine segment is entered, providing the same drawbacks as the classical incision in subsequent pregnancies.

Classical Caesarean Section

Classical caesarean section is undertaken when access to the lower segment is prohibited by extensive adhesions, uterine fibroids or, rarely, huge vascularity associated with placenta praevia with or without accreta. On rare occasions when extreme speed is deemed necessary to deliver the fetus, a classical rather than a low transverse caesarean may be undertaken. With an experienced operator, the time saved in performing a classical over a low transverse caesarean is very little, so this indication is extremely rare. It would, however, have application in the very rare case of postmortem caesarean section (see later).

In most units classical caesarean section makes up <2% of all caesarean deliveries. However, this figure is increasing modestly because of the falling gestational age at which caesarean section is performed.[27] This is particularly so in cases performed below 34 weeks' gestation without labour. In such cases the lower segment may not be adequately formed to allow a transverse incision of sufficient size to accommodate atraumatic delivery of the fragile premature infant. It is best to take this decision after the abdomen has been opened and the lower uterine segment carefully inspected. In many cases it is possible to perform a low transverse caesarean section with adequate room to deliver the fetus. The advantages of this to the woman's future obstetric career are obvious. If after making the transverse incision one finds that it is of inadequate size then one has to add a vertical incision in the middle into the upper uterine segment. This will produce an inverted 'T' incision which in subsequent pregnancies will have to be treated as a classical caesarean scar. The advantage of this approach, however, is that in the majority of cases a low transverse incision will be achieved and in those cases in which the inverted 'T' has to be performed the morbidity to the mother and infant is no greater than for a classical caesarean section.[28]

> 'The abdominal incision should possess two qualities – it should be high and it should be sufficiently long … My rule is to make the incision 8 to 10 inches [20 to 25 cm] in length … two-thirds of this incision is made above and one-third below the level of the umbilicus'.
> Munro Kerr
> Operative Midwifery, 1908, p409

SURGICAL TECHNIQUES

For the majority of types of caesarean section the transverse Pfannenstiel incision or Joel–Cohen incision is appropriate. The main reason for using a lower midline incision instead is when speed of entry is paramount. This may be necessary with acute fetal compromise, massive haemorrhage, uterine rupture (in which speed is required for fetal reasons as well as the extra room that may be needed for additional surgical manoeuvres) and the very rare case of perimortem caesarean delivery.[29]

During labour the bladder becomes an abdominal organ and therefore the peritoneal cavity should be opened as high as possible and then extended down under transillumination. After opening the peritoneal cavity the uterus is checked for dextro- or laevo-rotation – the former is more common due to the sigmoid colon. This appraisal of the orientation of the uterus is very important in placing the uterine incision, otherwise it may be eccentric and extend into the uterine vessels on one side.[19] The loose utero-vesical peritoneum is identified. The attachment of this peritoneum, where it adheres to the surface of the uterus, is the upper margin of the lower uterine segment. This peritoneum should be divided about 2–3 cm below the level of this attachment in the midline and then extended laterally towards each side. The loose areolar tissue between the lower uterine segment and the bladder is gently separated with the forefinger and a Doyen or similar retractor placed to move the bladder down and keep it from the line of uterine incision.

In prolonged labour with disproportion the lower uterine segment is stretched and drawn up, forming a considerable portion of the lower uterus. It is important to identify the upper margin of the lower uterine segment where the utero-vesical peritoneum reflects from the uterus. The uterine incision is usually made about 2–3 cm below this point. If one does not use this landmark it is possible to place the uterine incision so low as to be in the vagina rather than the uterus. In making the uterine incision one should be constantly aware of the risk of laceration to the fetal presenting part. The risk is greatest in obstructed labour with a thin lower uterine segment stretched over the fetal head and face. Identify the midline and gently palpate with the fingers at the site of the proposed incision, which will give some idea of the thickness involved. Using a scalpel and with very gentle strokes make a 2 cm horizontal incision. After the first stroke and with each succeeding stroke sweep the index finger of the opposite hand across the incision so that the layers can be clearly seen. When the incision is partially through the muscle, press and release the centre of the incision with the forefinger – if the remaining layer is very thin this will usually raise a 'bleb' of membranes which can then be incised, almost like a blister, without risk to the underlying fetus. Alternatively, one can use the forefinger or the scalpel handle to 'burrow' through the final thin layer. Either way, obsessional attention to this point should virtually eliminate the risk of fetal laceration.

Once the uterus is entered, the forefinger is placed between the fetus and the uterine muscle towards one side and the incision is continued with either curved Mayo or bandage scissors for about 2 cm on each side from the initial entry point with a slight curve upwards. Both fingers are then hooked into this incision and pulled laterally for the final blunt extension of the incision. Once again, care should be taken to balance the pull on each side to avoid extension into the uterine blood vessels. In earlier gestation, when the width of the lower uterine segment may be marginal, the angles of the uterine incision can be directed upwards, which will produce an enlarged 'trap-door' effect.

If the fetus is in cephalic presentation manual delivery of the head is, in most cases, straightforward. Insert the flat of the lower hand downwards between the head and the lower uterine segment. Using the lightly flexed fingers it should be possible to elevate the fetal head into the uterine incision. At the same time an assistant applies firm fundal pressure on the breech of the infant which facilitates delivery of the head (Fig 13-2). In elevating the head the occiput should be identified and the head flexed so that the narrowest diameter passes through the uterine incision. If there is difficulty in delivering the head manually, Simpson's or similar forceps can be used to guide the fetal head through the uterine incision, making sure that the orientation of the head is appropriately identified so that the forceps can be placed correctly.

Once the head is delivered the oropharynx and nasal passages are cleared, if necessary with gentle suction. At this point the anaesthetist should give 5 units of oxytocin intravenously, followed by an oxytocin infusion. Once the infant is completely delivered it should be rapidly dried and the cord double-clamped and a specimen kept for cord blood pH analysis. The placenta should be removed by controlled cord traction once signs of separation have occurred. Routine manual removal of the placenta is discouraged as it increases blood loss and postoperative sepsis[29,30] and even occasionally acute uterine inversion.[31] Once the placenta has been delivered the uterine cavity should be checked to ensure there are no retained portions of placenta or membranes.

Exteriorization of the uterus should not routinely be carried out. In some women under regional anaesthesia this will cause nausea, vomiting and pain. With appropriate assistance and reasonable surgical skill it is quite possible to suture the uterine incision without this manoeuvre. On the other hand, if there is an extension of the uterine incision, or exposure is limited by heavy bleeding, then one should not hesitate to bring the uterus out of the abdominal incision to facilitate haemostasis and repair.

If there is more than slight bleeding from the cut edges of the uterine incision Green–Armytage or ring forceps can be used to compress the bleeding edges. Even if these are not required for bleeding it is useful to place at least one such forcep on the lower edge of the uterine incision for identification. The lower edge of the uterine incision often recedes inferiorly and may be obscured by blood. The posterior wall of the lower uterine segment may protrude forward and even mimic, to the unwary, the lower edge of the uterine incision.

Traditionally, closure of the uterine incision has been in two layers – although in the past 15 years an increasing number of obstetricians have moved to single-layer closure. This is usually with a continuous suture, either running or locked. In general this saves about 7 minutes operating time and results in slightly less blood loss.[32] There are as yet conflicting and inadequate data on the outcome of single- versus double-layer closure upon the integrity of the scar in subsequent labour.[24,32] One large cohort study showed a fourfold increase of uterine rupture in subsequent pregnancy for single- versus double-layer closure.[33] Until firm evidence is available the authors recommend two-layer closure. The first layer should include the cut edges of the muscle only and not the decidua. It should be a running suture, which avoids the bunching and elevation of tissues seen with a continuous locking suture, and facilitates the placement of the second layer which can be either running or locking (Fig 13-3). The second layer of sutures should raise a fold of muscle on the upper and lower side to cover the first layer of sutures. The most commonly used sutures are

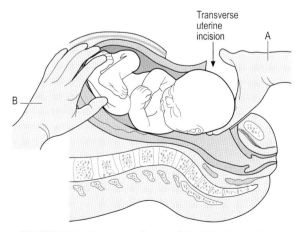

FIGURE 13-2 ■ Manual delivery of the fetal head. Identify the occiput and flex the head (A) through the uterine incision with concomitant fundal pressure by an assistant (B).

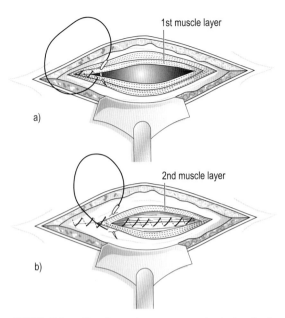

a)

1st muscle layer

b)

2nd muscle layer

FIGURE 13-3 ■ Two-layer lower segment uterine incision closure. The first running layer includes muscle but excludes the decidua. The second layer folds muscle over the first layer of sutures and can be a running or locking suture.

0 or No. 1 polyglactin (Vicryl) or polyglycolic acid (Dexon).

Another change in surgical technique in recent years has been to omit closure of both the visceral peritoneum over the uterine segment and the parietal peritoneum. Reviews of the trials suggest that closure of neither of these layers is necessary and omission of this step is associated with a marginally shorter operating time and less postoperative pain.[24,29,34] However, a recent study has shown that closure of both these peritoneal layers significantly reduces adhesions found at subsequent caesarean section.[35]

For closure of the abdominal wall some will approximate the medial edges of the rectus muscles loosely with two or three interrupted and lightly tied sutures but many omit this step. The rectus sheath is closed with a running suture. It is unnecessary to place sutures in the subcutaneous fat as this does not improve healing and only serves to provide more foreign material for potential infection. The skin can be closed with staples, interrupted percutaneous sutures or a subcuticular suture. Recent data suggests that subcuticular skin closure may reduce the risk of delayed infection.[36]

A simplified variation of the above technique has been developed by Michael Stark at the Misgav Ladach Hospital in Jerusalem and named after that hospital. In the Misgav Ladach method the Joel–Cohen transverse skin incision is used,

which is about 2–3 cm higher than the Pfannenstiel incision. The rectus sheath is incised, again higher than the traditional Pfannenstiel approach. At this level the rectus muscles move more freely beneath the fascia. The rectus muscles are pulled apart with the fingers. The parietal peritoneum is then stretched and entered bluntly as high as possible with the index finger. The lower uterine segment is identified and the utero-vesical peritoneum divided as for the normal technique of transverse lower segment caesarean. A Doyen retractor is used to retract the bladder. The uterus is entered with a scalpel in the normal manner and the incision then enlarged with the fingers. After delivery of the fetus and placenta the uterus is closed in one layer. Neither the visceral or parietal peritoneum is closed, nor are the rectus muscles. The rectus sheath is closed with a running suture. This operative technique has been described in detail.[37] Experience with this method of caesarean section suggests that it results in a shorter operating time, less blood loss and less postoperative analgesic requirement.[38,39]

COMPLICATED CAESAREAN SECTION

Classical Caesarean Section

The abdominal incision is the same as for a low transverse caesarean section. With appropriate retraction a classical caesarean section can be performed through a low transverse abdominal wall incision. Using the scalpel, a 2–3 cm incision is made in the upper part of the lower uterine segment, with care taken to avoid the underlying fetus. Once the uterine cavity is entered two fingers are placed inside to protect the fetal parts and using either the scalpel or scissors the incision is extended 10–12 cm upwards in the longitudinal plane. Once the fetus and placenta have been delivered it is helpful to exteriorize the uterus as the classical incision is much more vascular and access to it is limited with the transverse abdominal wall incision. This allows the assistant's hands to encircle the incision with the fingers on one side and the thumbs on the other to compress the uterine incision and assist its closure (Fig 13-4). This manoeuvre of the assistant's hands is key in reducing blood loss and, by providing progressive compression, reduces the tension on the sutures as they are placed, facilitating closure of the thick gaping muscle. Depending on the thickness of the incised muscle, one or two running sutures may be required to bring

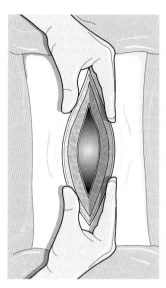

FIGURE 13-4 ■ Classical caesarean section. The assistant's hands encircle the incision to reduce blood loss and facilitate its closure.

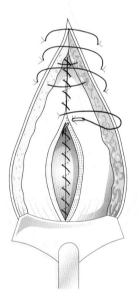

FIGURE 13-5 ■ Suture closure of the classical caesarean incision. The deep layers are closed by 2–3 running sutures, with a final wide locking suture of the seromuscular layer.

together the deeper layers of the uterine muscle. This should aim to leave about 1 cm of the outer layer of uterine muscle gaping, which is closed by a final locking seromuscular suture (Fig 13-5).

Low Vertical Caesarean Section

In low vertical caesarean section the uterine incision requires careful dissection of the bladder

from the lower uterine segment. This dissection should not extend too far lateral or much bleeding will ensue from the vascular pillars of the bladder. An initial 2 cm vertical incision is made in the lower uterine segment in the midline, with the same precautions for fetal protection as the low transverse incision. With the finger through the incision protecting the fetus, scissors are used to extend the incision downwards and upwards. One has to strike a balance between extending too far down and getting into the very vascular area of the vagina at the base of the bladder and too far upwards and extending into the upper uterine segment. In fact, in many cases extension to the upward uterine segment is necessary to provide a large enough incision for delivery of the fetus. The lower end of the incision should be captured with a stay suture in order to delineate the lower edge and, using traction on this stay suture, facilitate haemostatic closure of the lower part of the incision. Otherwise the incision is closed using the same principles as for the transverse lower segment incision.

Deeply Engaged Fetal Head

Caesarean section at full cervical dilatation with the head deeply impacted in the pelvis can be associated with increased maternal and perinatal morbidity.[29,40] The deep impaction of the fetal head is compounded by the fact that the amniotic fluid has drained away and the uterine muscle tightly 'hugs' the fetus, reducing the room for elevation of the fetal body and for intrauterine manipulation. The following options are available to deal with this situation:[41]

1. Push the flat of the lower hand between the uterine incision and the fetal head deep into the vagina. Using the upper hand to grasp the wrist of the lower hand may aid in elevation of the lower hand and head without excessive levering movements of the lower hand, which risk extension of the uterine incision. This is the standard technique of delivering the fetal head which may be unsuccessful with a deeply engaged head.

2. An assistant cups the fetal head vaginally in one hand and elevates it to meet the operator's hand (Fig 13-6). Some obstetricians will do this just before they scrub for such caesarean sections.

3. Deliver the fetal head through the uterine incision using forceps. This is particularly suitable for the head in occipito-posterior position. With gentle pressure on the fetal

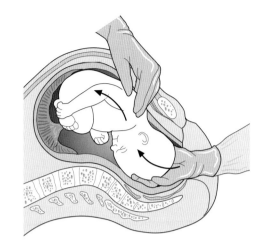

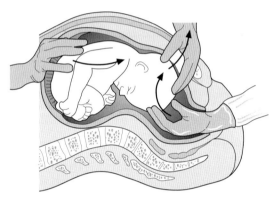

FIGURE 13-6 ■ Vaginal elevation of the deeply engaged fetal head into the lower uterine segment.

chin rotate the head towards the direct occipito-posterior position and apply the forceps alongside the fetal head with the pelvic curve towards the pubic symphysis. The fetal head is then elevated from the pelvis with the forceps and up through the uterine incision.

4. Reverse breech extraction. The operator reaches up and grasps the fetal feet and pulls them down through the uterine incision, which elevates the fetal trunk and head. Continued traction on the fetal legs, in essence, carries out an internal podalic version and the breech is delivered through the uterine incision first.[42,43]

5. It is helpful, and is in some cases essential, to provide uterine relaxation as an aid to all the above manoeuvres. This is best achieved by pre-caesarean co-ordination with the anaesthetist in order to have intravenous nitroglycerine ready for administration (see Chapter 28).

6. Extend the uterine 'T' incision. Because of the implications for future pregnancies

this is the last resort, but it may be necessary to achieve delivery without fetal trauma.

Breech Presentation

For breech presentation all of the manoeuvres are the same up until delivery of the fetus. In the preterm fetus, however, in which the body of the breech is significantly smaller than the head, there is the risk of entrapment of the fetal head by the narrower isthmic portion of the uterus and by the uterine incision and contracted uterus after delivery of the body. This is particularly so with regional anaesthesia which does not provide any uterine relaxation. Thus, the anaesthetist should be forewarned and have intravenous nitroglycerine drawn up and ready to administer should this be necessary (see Chapter 16).

Transverse Lie

With caesarean section for transverse lie the lower uterine segment may not be well developed due to the absence of a presenting part in the pelvic brim. Once the abdomen has been opened a careful assessment of the development and capacity of the lower uterine segment should be made. In some cases it is possible to turn the fetus to a longitudinal lie and find that the lower uterine segment is sufficiently developed to carry out a transverse lower segment incision. Alternatively, internal podalic version followed by breech extraction through a lower segment incision may be feasible, if necessary aided by tocolysis with nitroglycerine. If the lower segment is inadequately developed, a vertical incision will have to be made, starting low and extending into the upper uterine segment.

Placenta Praevia

There are a number of potential complications of caesarean section specific to placenta praevia and placenta praevia accreta. These are covered in Chapter 19.

Obesity

Caesarean section, which is more commonly indicated in the morbidly or super-obese (body mass index >50), presents a major surgical challenge.[44]

One of the main surgical decisions in these women is the choice of abdominal incision. It may be possible to perform a Pfannenstiel incision in the healthy skin 3–4 cm above the natural skin crease. In many, however, the pannus is too large or unhealthy (oedematous and/or ulcerated) to carry out the standard Pfannenstiel incision. In women with a large pannus the umbilicus will be dragged down to the level of the symphysis pubis in the standing position. Thus, a transverse incision made above the umbilicus may, paradoxically, allow access through the thinner part of the abdominal wall above the main pannus.[45] Other surgical aspects include adequate retraction and full antibiotic and thromboprophylaxis.[46]

There is much to be said for providing obstetric services to this very high risk group of women in specialized clinics.[46]

DOCUMENTATION

After every caesarean delivery a detailed note should be recorded in the chart. This should include a summary of events in labour, the indication and surgical details of the operation. This is necessary for audit purposes and so that the information is available to those who may look after the woman in a subsequent pregnancy. The perioperative decisions and procedures should also be reviewed with the woman during her postpartum stay in hospital.

POSTMORTEM AND PERIMORTEM CAESAREAN SECTION

As outlined in the historical background of this chapter, postmortem caesarean section has a long history and associated rich mythology, and almost invariably the infant did not survive.[4] Within 6 minutes of cessation of cerebral blood flow in the mother there is neurological injury.[47] Thus, if the mother dies the fetus ideally should be delivered within 5 minutes. If delivery cannot be achieved within 10–15 minutes then it should not be attempted, as the chance of a normally surviving infant is remote.

The term perimortem caesarean section has been used to describe the situation in which the mother has had cardiac arrest but is being actively resuscitated. Cardiopulmonary resuscitation is most effectively carried out with the woman in the supine position. Up to 26 weeks' gestation the uterus does not reach above the bifurcation of the aorta so that aorto-caval compression does not occur. Thus, up to 26 weeks' gestation resuscitation of the woman in the supine position can occur, and at this gestation caesarean section will not help the mother and is unlikely to result in a surviving infant. This is particularly so when the circumstances arise, as they most commonly do at this gestation, far from the immediate availability of a neonatal intensive care unit.[48] It bears emphasis that at this gestation no personnel or resources should be diverted from maternal resuscitation.

In the third trimester of pregnancy the uterus will cause aorta-caval compression so that CPR should be performed in the head down lateral tilt position, which is more difficult. If adequate CPR cannot be achieved in this position then classical caesarean section through a lower midline incision, preferably within 5 minutes of starting CPR, is advantageous – both to the mother and the infant.[47,49] A recent review of perimortem caesarean sections has shown this principle to be appropriate, with half of the cases showing a marked improvement in haemodynamic status immediately after the uterus was emptied by caesarean section.[47] Thus, this approach benefits both the mother and the infant.

POSTMORTEM CAESAREAN

'It is, indeed, possible to save a child by the caesarian operation, or cutting it out of the womb of its mother just expired; but what man in his senses would put his character upon this footing'.'
　　Edmund Chapman
　　A Treatise on the Improvement of Midwifery. London: L. David and C. Reymers, 1759:xiv

REFERENCES

1. Young JH. Caesarean section. The history and development of the operation from earliest times. London: H. K. Lewis; 1944.
2. Fasbender H. Geschichte der geburtshulle. Jena: Gustav Fisher; 1906. p. 979–1010.
3. Harris RP. Cattle-horn lacerations of the abdomen and uterus in pregnant women. Am J Obstet Dis Women Child 1887;20:673–85.
4. Trolle D. The history of caesarean section. Copenhagen: C. A. Rietzel; 1982.
5. Cawley T. Case of a self performed caesarean section. London Med J 1785;6:372.
6. Mosley B. Self performed caesarean section. London: 1795.
7. Pickrell KL. An inquiry into the history of cesarean section. Bull Soc Med Hist Chicago 1935;4:414–53.
8. Stewart D. The caesarean operation done with success by a midwife. Edin Med Essays and Observ 1771;5:37.
9. Rousset F. Traitte Nouveau de L'Hysterotomotokie ou Enfantement Caesarien. Paris: Denys du Val; 1581.
10. Cyr RM, Baskett TF. Caesarean birth: the work of Francois Rousset in Renaissance France. London: RCOG Press; 2010.
11. Ould F. A treatise of midwifry. Dublin: O. Nelson; 1742. p. xxiii.
12. Porro E. Della amputazione utero-ovarica come complemeno di talio cesareo. Ann Univ Med Chir (Milan) 1876;237:289–350.

13. Baskett TF. On the shoulders of giants: eponyms and names in obstetrics and gynaecology. 2nd ed. London: RCOG Press; 2008. p. 282–3, 306–7.

14. Marshall CM. Caesarean section lower segment operation. Bristol: John Wright; 1939.

15. Kehrer FA. Ueber ein modificintes verfahren biem kaiserschnitte. Arch Gynakol 1882;19:177–209.

16. Sänger M. Zur rehabilitirung des classischen kaiserschnitte. Arch Gynakol 1882;19:370–99.

17. Dow DA. The Rottenrow, the history of the Glasgow Royal Maternity Hospital 1834–984. Lancaster: Parthenon Press; 1984.

18. Kerr JM. The lower uterine segment incision in conservative caesarean section. J Obstet Gynaecol Br Emp 1932;28:475–87.

19. Baskett TF, Arulkumaran S. Intrapartum care. 2nd ed. London: RCOG Press; 2011. p. 155–68.

20. Robson MS. Classification of caesarean sections. Fetal Mat Med Rev 2001;12:23–39.

21. Allen VM, Baskett TF, O'Connell CM. Contribution of select maternal groups to temporal trends in caesarean delivery rates. J Obstet Gynaecol Can 2010;32:633–41.

22. Royal Australian and New Zealand College of Obstetricians and Gynaecologists. Caesarean delivery on maternal request. College Statement, C-Obs 39. Melbourne: RANZCOG; 2010.

23. Lavender T, Hofmeyr GT, Neilson JP, Kingdom C, Gyte GM. Caesarean section for non-medical reasons at term. Cochrane Database Syst Rev 2012;3: CD004660.

24. National Institute for Clinical Excellence. Clinical guideline: caesarean section. London: RCOG Press; 2004.

25. Royal College of Obstetricians and Gynaecologists and Royal College of Anaesthetists. Classification of urgency of caesarean section – a continuum of risk. Good Practice Guidance No.11. London: RCOG Press; 2010.

26. Lukas DN, Yentis SM, Kinsella SM, Holdcroft A, May AE, Wee M, et al. Urgency of caesarean section: a new classification. J R Soc Med 2000;93:346–50.

27. Bethune M, Pemezel M. The relationship between gestational age and the incidence of classical caesarean section. Aust NZ J Obstet Gynaecol 1997;37:153–5.

28. Patterson LS, O'Connell CM, Baskett TF. Maternal and perinatal morbidity associated with classical and inverted 'T' caesarean sections. Obstet Gynecol 2002;100:633–7.

29. Hema KR, Johanson R. Techniques for performing caesarean section. Best Pract Res Clin Obstet Gynaecol 2001;15:17–47.

30. Baska A, Kalan A, Ozkan A, Baksu B, Tekelicoglu M, Goker N. The effect of placental removal method and site of uterine repair on postcesarean endometritis and operative blood loss. Acta Obstet Gynecol Scand 2005;84:266–9.

31. Baskett TF. Acute uterine inversion: a review of 40 cases. J Obstet Gynaecol Can 2002;24:953–6.

32. Dodd JM, Anderson ER, Gates S. Surgical techniques for uterine incision and uterine closure at the time of caesarean section. Cochrane Database Syst Rev 2008;3: CD004732.

33. Bujold E, Bujold C, Hamilton EF, Harel F, Gauthier RJ. The impact of single-layer or double-layer closure on uterine rupture. Am J Obstet Gynecol 2002;186: 1326–30.

34. CAESAR Study Collaborative Group. Caesarean section surgical techniques; a randomised factorial trial (CAESAR). BJOG 2010;117;1366–76.

35. Lyell DJ, Caughey AB, Hu E, Daniels K. Perinatal closure at primary cesarean delivery and adhesions. Obstet Gynecol 2005;106:275–80.

36. Clay FS, Walsh CA, Walsh SR. Staples Vs subcuticular sutures for skin closure at caesarean delivery: a meta-analysis of randomized controlled trials. Am J Obstet Gynecol 2011;204:378–83.

37. Holmgren G, Sjoholm L, Stark M. The Misgav Ladach method for cesarean section: method description. Acta Obstet Gynecol Scand 1999;78:615–21.

38. Darj E, Nortstrom ML. Misgav Ladach method for cesarean section compared to the Pfannenstiel method. Acta Obstet Gynecol Scand 1999;78:37–41.

39. Hofmeyr GJ, Mathai M, Shah A, Novikova N. Techniques for caesarean section. Cochrane Database Syst Rev 2008;(1):CD004662.

40. Allen VM, O'Connell CM, Baskett TF. Maternal and perinatal morbidity of caesarean section at full cervical dilatation compared with caesarean delivery in the first stage of labour. Br J Obstet Gynaecol 2005;112: 986–90.

41. Royal Australian and New Zealand College of Obstetricians and Gynaecologists. Delivery of the fetus at caesarean section. College Statement: C-Obs 3. Melbourne: 7RANZCOG; 2010.

42. Levy R, Chernomoretz T, Appelman Z, Levin D, Or Y, Haggy ZJ. Head pushing versus reverse breech extraction in cases of impacted fetal head during caesarean section. Eur J Obstet Gynecol Reprod Biol 2005;121: 24–6.

43. Chopra S, Bagga R, Keepanasseril A, Jain V, Suri V. Disengagement of the deeply engaged fetal head during caesarean section in advanced labor: conventional method versus reverse breech extraction. Acta Obstet Gynecol Scand 2009;88:1163–6.

44. Alanis MC, Goodnight WH, Hill EG, Robinson CJ, Villers MS, Johnson DD. Maternal super-obesity (body mass index > or =50) and adverse pregnancy outcomes. Acta Obstet Gynecol Scand 2010;89: 924–30.

45. Tixier H, Thouvenot S, Coulange L, Peyronel C, Filipuzzi L, Sagot P et al. Cesarean section in morbid obese women:supra or subumbilical transverse incision? Acta Obstet Gynecol Scand 2009;88:1049–52.

46. Kingdom JC, Baud D, Grabowska K, Thomas J, Windrim RC, Maxwell CV. Delivery by caesarean section in super-obese women: beyond Pfannenstiel. J Obstet Gynaecol Can 2012;34:472–4.

47. Katz V, Balderstan K, DeFreest M. Perimortem cesarean delivery: were our assumptions correct? Am J Obstet Gynecol 2005;192:1916–21.

48. Baskett TF. Trauma in pregnancy. In: Essential management of obstetric emergencies. 4th ed. Bristol: Clinical Press Ltd; 2004. p. 271–2.

49. Whitten M, Irvine LM. Post-mortem and perimortem caesarean section: what are the indications? J R Soc Med 2000;93:6–9.

CHAPTER 14

Vaginal Birth after Caesarean Section

VM Allen • TF Baskett

ONCE A CAESAREAN ALWAYS A CAESAREAN

'One thing must always be borne in mind, viz., that no matter how carefully a uterine incision is sutured, we can never be certain that the cicatrized uterine wall will stand a subsequent pregnancy and labor without rupture. This means that the usual rule is, once a Caesarean always a Caesarean. Many exceptions occur ... The general rule holds, however, that we cannot depend upon a sutured uterine wall, whether it is done in a Caesarean section or a myomectomy, hence I believe the extension of Caesarean section to conditions other than dystocia from contracted pelvis or tumours should be exceptional and infrequent.'

Edwin Craigin
Conservatism in obstetrics. NY Med J 1916; 104:1–3

One of the most common dictums in obstetrics was put forward almost a century ago by Edwin Craigin: 'once a caesarean always a caesarean'. The main purpose of Craigin's presentation was to point out the maternal risks of caesarean section with a plea that it should be used only for the most stringent indications. In the early 20th century the most common indication for caesarean section was disproportion and contracted pelvis, and the type of caesarean section was classical with its associated significant risk of uterine rupture in a subsequent pregnancy. Thus, when Craigin proposed his dictum it was appropriate, as it would be now under the same circumstances. Craigin's main point was that caesarean section was a dangerous operation and that once it was performed the woman would be subject to the dangers of repeat caesarean section in a subsequent pregnancy. He did, however, point out that vaginal delivery after previous caesarean section was feasible and reported one of his own patients who had three vaginal deliveries after one caesarean section.

As the low transverse caesarean section became more common in the 1930s and 40s, and the indications for caesarean section widened to include non-recurrent reasons, the approach to women previously delivered by caesarean section changed in many countries. The risk of subsequent rupture of low transverse caesarean section was small and increasing numbers of women were encouraged to undergo labour and vaginal delivery. By the late 1970s and 1980s there were many reports of large series showing that spontaneous labour and vaginal delivery following a single low transverse caesarean section was a safe and reasonable option with appropriate safeguards. Consensus statements embraced and encouraged labour and vaginal delivery with a previous caesarean section under these circumstances.

However, as is so often the case in obstetrics, the pendulum of opinion swings too far and labour and vaginal delivery was pursued for widening indications – including more than one previous caesarean section, induction of labour and augmentation of non-progressive labour. Not surprisingly, an increasing number of cases of uterine rupture were reported, some of which resulted in fetal death or severe neonatal neurological damage, as well as maternal morbidity, sometimes including hysterectomy. The possibility of complete uterine rupture in labour ranges from 3 to 7 per 1000 pregnancies,[1,2] while the risk of perinatal death or severe morbidity, should rupture occur, is 4.5 per 1000 more with trial of vaginal delivery than with repeat caesarean delivery.[1] These rare but tragic outcomes and the associated medico-legal sequelae caused the pendulum to swing rapidly back in the opposite direction. Revised national guidelines suggested more stringent facility and personnel requirements in order to conduct labour and vaginal delivery following previous caesarean section.[2–5] Some hospitals, fearing institutional liability, forbade labour and vaginal delivery following previous caesarean section. The most sensible, practical and safest clinical course lies in the middle ground.

The term 'trial of labour' has been applied incorrectly to these cases. Trial of labour is a well-established obstetric principle when labour is undertaken in the face of suspected disproportion, which is contraindicated in a woman with a uterine scar. The term 'trial of scar' should also be avoided. The correct term is 'trial for vaginal delivery'.

This chapter will outline the factors that need to be considered in helping women reach a decision whether or not to undertake labour with a view to vaginal delivery after previous caesarean section.

SELECTION CRITERIA FOR VAGINAL BIRTH AFTER CAESAREAN SECTION (VBAC)

The previous obstetrical record should be reviewed so that details of the labour, indications for caesarean section, operative details and postoperative recovery can be appraised. There are several factors that need to be evaluated in assessing the level of medical risk and, indeed, medico-legal risk so that the appropriate informed consent can be obtained.

Type of Uterine Scar

- *Classical caesarean section scars* are about 10 times more likely to rupture during labour than lower segment caesarean incisions and may rupture before the onset of labour. The rupture rate for a previous classical scar is approximately 3–5%. In addition, this type of scar rupture is potentially much more lethal to both fetus and mother as it tends to give way suddenly and this may be before labour or early in labour. As a result the woman is often not in hospital when the rupture occurs. This is in contrast to the lower segment caesarean scar which is most likely to rupture after some hours of labour when the woman is in hospital and appropriate medical intervention can be undertaken without delay.
- *Low vertical caesarean section* is rarely performed. The indication is usually in earlier gestation when the lower uterine segment has formed to a degree but its transverse dimensions are felt to be inadequate for the normal transverse incision. In these cases the low vertical incision has been advocated as an alternative to classical caesarean

section. However, in many instances the lower segment is not sufficiently developed, even vertically, to allow a big enough incision without encroaching on the upper uterine segment. Thus, these scars, while having a slightly smaller risk of rupture than a classical caesarean scar, are probably best treated in the same manner.
- *Extensions of a transverse lower segment caesarean incision* should be appraised by careful scrutiny of the operative report. If there was any marked extension of one or both angles, or a 'T' extension into the upper uterine segment, these scars are best not subjected to labour.
- *Hysterotomy* scars are not commonly seen in modern obstetrics with medical methods for second trimester termination. However, if present they should be treated in the same manner as a classical caesarean scar and repeat elective caesarean section chosen.
- *Myomectomy* incisions require individual consideration. If the incisions are extensive, and particularly if the uterine cavity was entered, they are probably best not subjected to labour. Similarly, hysteroscopic myomectomy incisions, if associated with perforation of the uterus would be best managed by elective caesarean section. Otherwise, hysteroscopic myomectomies not associated with perforation or deep myometrial excision can be allowed to labour.
- *Previous rupture* of any type of uterine scar in a previous pregnancy is obviously a contraindication to subsequent labour.

In some cases it is impossible to obtain the previous operative record. From the history it is often possible to work out the type of the previous uterine incision. For example, if the previous caesarean section was done at term, and particularly if it was for dystocia, one can reasonably assume that it was a transverse lower segment caesarean section. On the other hand, if the caesarean section was done at less than 32 weeks' gestation and not in labour the chances are more likely that a classical caesarean section was done. Augmentation of labour with oxytocin in the latent phase with an unknown uterine scar has been associated with an increased risk of uterine rupture and dehiscence.[6]

Labour with the Previous Caesarean Section

If the previous caesarean section was carried out electively without labour, or in the early latent phase of labour, the pattern of uterine activity in the subsequent labour is likely to be of the nulliparous type, requiring stronger and longer uterine work to efface and dilate the 'nulliparous' cervix.[7] In contrast, those who had previous caesarean section in active labour are more likely to show a multiparous pattern in a subsequent labour, with less uterine work and less strain on the uterine scar.

Previous Vaginal Delivery

If the woman had a previous vaginal delivery, either before or after the caesarean section, her chances of a successful and safe VBAC are enhanced. This is one of the most positive factors in favour of trial for vaginal delivery.[8,9]

Uterine Incision Closure

One large retrospective review showed a significant increase of subsequent scar rupture in those women in whom the initial caesarean had a single-layer versus a double-layer closure.[10] However, this finding has not been noted in other hospitals and there are many who have not shown an increase in scar rupture rates or changes in infectious morbidity since changing to single-layer closure.[11,12]

Postoperative Infection

Postpartum endomyometritis may interfere with adequate healing of the uterine scar and increase the risk of subsequent rupture in labour.[13] The practical clinical point here is that many cases of postpartum fever are not due to endomyometritis. Thus, it is inappropriate to exclude all women who have had a postpartum fever following the previous caesarean delivery. However, if there is good clinical evidence in the record that the sepsis was intrauterine it may be prudent to avoid labour in a subsequent pregnancy.

Recurrent Indications for Caesarean Section

One of the most common reasons for primary caesarean section is dystocia or cephalo-pelvic disproportion, although a true diagnosis of the latter is rare. These diagnoses are not necessarily a recurrent indication and many will labour and deliver successfully after a previous caesarean for these indications. Overall, however, they have a slightly lower success rate than for other 'non-recurrent' indications.

Inter-Pregnancy Interval

Pregnancy and delivery within 12 months of a previous caesarean section may be associated with an increased risk of scar rupture in that pregnancy.[14]

Twins

A large cohort study suggests risks of uterine rupture with trial for vaginal delivery after caesarean are similar between twin and singleton pregnancies.[15] However, to some extent twin pregnancies have potentially double the price to pay for subsequent scar rupture. In addition, over-distension of the uterus associated with multiple pregnancy and the possible need for intrauterine manipulation for delivery of the second twin increase the risk of scar rupture. These are cases in which other selection criteria and individual considerations have to be weighed very carefully and cautious prudence remains the guiding principle.

External Cephalic Version

The influence of manoeuvres required for external cephalic version (ECV) on the uterine scar is unclear. Uterine rupture is a theoretical risk but has not been well studied. Rates of successful ECV are similar between women with a previous caesarean section and women without a previous caesarean section.[16]

More than One Previous Caesarean Delivery

There are a number of series that have shown success in achieving vaginal delivery in women with two previous caesarean sections. However, the risk of uterine rupture is approximately doubled and the woman should be so informed.[14,17]

Measurement of Lower Uterine Segment Thickness

Small studies using ultrasound to measure the thickness of the lower uterine segment in the third trimester of pregnancy have suggested that those women with a very thin lower uterine segment have an increased risk of scar rupture.[18,19] This work is promising and it is possible that there may be a critical measurement below which trial for vaginal delivery carries too great a risk.

Predicting Adverse Outcomes with Trial for Vaginal Delivery

Validated antepartum prediction tools demonstrate an association between increasing maternal age and post-term pregnancies with an increased risk of emergency caesarean section and uterine rupture in women planning vaginal birth after previous caesarean section.[20]

Hospital Facilities and Personnel

Trial for vaginal delivery can only be undertaken in a hospital which has immediately available midwifery, nursing, anaesthesia and obstetric staff along with the appropriate operating theatre, laboratory and blood transfusion services. These criteria have been reviewed in national guidelines.[2–5]

Decision Aids for Mode of Delivery

Randomized controlled trial data using computer-based decision aids, given to women with a previous caesarean section and their health care professional, demonstrate a reduction in decisional conflict and higher rates of vaginal delivery compared to usual care.[21] The decision aids allowed access to standardized and reliable information and empowerment of the user.[22,23]

Cost

Caesarean delivery in labour has been shown to be associated with increased costs compared to spontaneous delivery and to caesarean delivery without labour.[24] Studies modelling cost-effectiveness demonstrate that the average expected cost of failed trial for vaginal delivery is higher than either vaginal delivery or elective repeat caesarean delivery.[25] If the a priori chance of a successful trial for vaginal delivery is at least 74%, then the cost/benefit profile favours a trial for vaginal delivery.[25]

There are a number of so-called 'soft factors' which, in addition to the above, may influence the decision. These include maternal age, maternal obesity, secondary infertility, the desire for more pregnancies and previous maternal morbidity.

It is essential that the woman and her partner understand and accept the principles involved in a trial for vaginal delivery. From a review of the above selection criteria certain increased risks may be identified and these must be discussed with the woman, along with the advantages of a successful trial for vaginal delivery. It is quite inappropriate to apply any coercion, however subtle, towards labour.

MANAGEMENT OF TRIAL FOR VAGINAL DELIVERY

Antenatal Care

This should be routine other than the detailed review of the previous delivery record and of the selection factors noted above.

Induction of Labour

This is one of the more contentious areas in the debate on VBAC. Obviously, spontaneous labour is the most desirable and induction of labour should only be considered when the indication is compelling. If the cervix is favourable, amniotomy is the method of choice and adds no additional risk to spontaneous labour. If amniotomy fails to induce labour, oxytocin may be cautiously used, which only very slightly increases the risk of uterine rupture.[26] If the cervix is unfavourable and prostaglandins are chosen, the level of risk rises.[27] This is greatest with misoprostol but also significantly higher with the prostaglandin E2 gels.[28] The use of these gels to ripen the unfavourable cervix should only be considered in a hospital with on-site anaesthesia, obstetrics and immediate operating theatre facilities. Even then it is doubtful that this level of increased risk is acceptable and perhaps only in very unusual circumstances (such as fetal death). The woman should be advised that this method of induction does carry a small but significantly increased risk of uterine rupture.[29,30] The risk associated with misoprostol, even in a small series, has shown an unacceptably high rate of uterine rupture and this agent should not be used.[31] Mechanical methods for cervical ripening, such as intracervical balloon catheters,[26] may offer an alternative for eligible women with a previous caesarean section who are considering a trial for vaginal delivery with an unfavourable cervix at term.

Labour

The woman who selects trial of vaginal delivery should be advised to come into hospital early after labour starts. On admission, blood should be taken for group and screen. It is reasonable to allow the woman to ambulate in early labour. Once labour is established, however, an intravenous drip should be established and continuous electronic fetal heart rate monitoring instituted. The latter is wise because fetal heart rate abnormalities are the earliest warning sign of uterine rupture.[32] If requested, epidural analgesia is not contraindicated and fears that it would mask the signs and symptoms of uterine rupture have not been substantiated.

The progress of labour should be carefully monitored and, provided this is satisfactory, an optimistic outcome can be expected. Early signs and symptoms of uterine rupture should be sought. These are discussed in Chapter 15. There is increasing experience with oxytocin augmentation of non-progressive labour but this does carry an increased risk of uterine rupture.[27] The use of augmentation or induction is associated with a reduced likelihood of vaginal delivery.[9] This should only be undertaken in hospitals with on-site anaesthesia and obstetric staff and the woman should understand that this does increase the risk. If oxytocin augmentation is chosen one should expect a smooth and progressive response. If this does not occur discretion is the better part of valour and caesarean section should be performed.

The second stage of labour is the time of maximal strain to the lower uterine segment and this may be shortened with assisted vaginal delivery by forceps or vacuum if the second stage is prolonged and the head is low in the pelvis. The conduct of the third stage of labour is normal. There are those who advocate routine exploration of the caesarean scar following delivery. In fact this can be carried out fairly easily with a vaginal examination through the cervix and feeling across the lower uterine segment for the V-shaped gutter of the scar to assess its integrity. However, most large series have shown that if uterine rupture occurs at the time of delivery the mother will have symptoms that draw attention to this diagnosis. If there are no such signs and symptoms scar rupture that would require treatment has not occurred and the manual exploration itself may cause perforation of the scar.

Rising caesarean section rates worldwide mean that in some countries 10–12% of the obstetric population have previously been delivered by caesarean section. This, then, is one of the most common complications of pregnancy. In some hospitals about 70% of women who undertake a trial for vaginal delivery will achieve their desired result. However, even in hospitals with a well-established policy of VBAC only about 30–40% of all women previously delivered by caesarean section choose and achieve vaginal delivery. Malpractice concerns also contribute to rates of planned vaginal delivery after previous caesarean section.[33]

A meta-analysis from the 1990s shows a slightly increased risk of uterine rupture and neonatal mortality and morbidity with trial for vaginal delivery and increased rates of maternal morbidity with elective caesarean section.[34] More recent case-control data suggest that, among women with a previous caesarean section, the estimated incidence of uterine rupture is 0.2 per 1000 pregnancies overall, and 2.1 and 0.3 per 1000 pregnancies in women planning vaginal or elective caesarean delivery, respectively.[14] Available randomized trial data evaluating risks associated with planned vaginal birth compared to elective repeat caesarean section demonstrate that, among women with one prior caesarean section, planned caesarean section was associated with a lower risk of fetal and infant death and serious neonatal morbidity.[35] The essence of the selection for and management of VBAC is to avoid the extremes. The majority of women with one previous transverse low segment caesarean section and spontaneous progressive labour will achieve vaginal delivery with safety for themselves and their infant. Once exceptions are made to this and additional risks undertaken – such as labour after more than one previous caesarean section, induction of labour and augmentation of non-progressive labour – the risk to both mother and infant increases. There comes a time in this equation when discretion is the better part of valour and it is not appropriate to take additional risks when the chances of increasing the rate of safe vaginal delivery are relatively low and the chances of uterine rupture and its sequelae increase.[36]

From a maternal point of view the safest outcome is spontaneous labour and spontaneous vaginal delivery, while the outcome associated with the greatest morbidity (other than uterine rupture) is a failed trial for vaginal delivery resulting in caesarean section. Compared with caesarean section after a failed trial, elective caesarean section carries much less morbidity for both mother and infant. Careful clinical appraisal should delineate the probability of either of these two extremes occurring and, along with the woman's wishes, provide a sensible guide to either trial of vaginal delivery or repeat elective caesarean section. Blind adherence to either one of these clinical options is not appropriate. For the woman who wants to have more than 2–3 children, the cumulative morbidity of repeated elective caesarean sections will make trial for vaginal delivery a more attractive prospect. However, excessive zeal in the pursuit of vaginal delivery after previous caesarean section, most often manifest in those with limited experience, can put the woman and her infant at unreasonable risk.

REFERENCES

1. Smith GCS, Pell JP, Cameron AD, Dobbie R. Risk of perinatal death associated with labor after previous cesarean delivery in uncomplicated term pregnancies. JAMA 2002;287:2684–90.
2. Royal College of Obstetricians and Gynaecologists. Birth after previous Caesarean birth. Green-top Guideline No. 45. London: RCOG; 2007.
3. American College of Obstetricians and Gynecologists. Vaginal birth after previous cesarean delivery. Practice Bulletin No. 115. Washington, DC: ACOG; 2010. Obstet Gynecol 2010;116:450–63.
4. Society of Obstetricians and Gynaecologists of Canada. Guidelines for vaginal birth after previous caesarean birth. Clinical Practice Guideline No. 155. Ottawa: SOGC; 2005.
5. Royal Australian and New Zealand College of Obstetricians and Gynaecologists. Planned vaginal birth after Casesarean section (Trial of labour). C-Obs 38. Victoria: RANZCOG; 2010.
6. Grubb DK, Kjos SL, Paul RH. Latent labor with an unknown uterine scar. Obstet Gynecol 1996;88: 351–5.
7. Arulkumaran S, Gibb DMF, Ingemarson I, Kitchener S, Ratnam SS. Uterine activity during spontaneous labour after previous lower segment caesarean section. Br J Obstet Gynaecol 1989;96:933–8.
8. Zelop CM, Shipp TD, Repke JT, Cohen A, Lieberman E. Effect of previous vaginal delivery on the risk of uterine rupture during a subsequent trial of labour. Obstet Gynecol 2001;183:1184–6.
9. Eden KB, McDonagh M, Denman MA, Marshall N, Emeis C, Fu R, et al. New insights on vaginal birth after cesarean, can it be predicted? Obstet Gynecol 2010;116:967–81.
10. Bujold E, Hamilton EF, Harel R, Gauthier RJ. The impact of single-layer or double-layer closure on uterine rupture. Am J Obstet Gynecol 2002;186:1326–30.
11. Roberge S, Chaillet N, Boutin A, Moore L, Jastrow N, Brassard N, et al. Single- versus double-layer closure of the hysterotomy incision during cesarean delivery and risk of uterine rupture. Int J Gynecol Obstet 2011; 115:5–10.
12. Caesarean section surgical techniques: a randomised factorial trial (CAESAR): CAESAR study collaborative group. Br J Obstet Gynaecol 2012;117:1366–76.
13. Shipp TD, Zelop C, Cohen A, Repke JT, Lieberman E. Post-cesarean delivery fever and uterine rupture in a subsequent trial of labour. Obstet Gynecol 2003; 101:136–9.
14. Fitzpatrick KE, Kurinczuk JJ, Alfirevic Z, Spark P, Brocklehurst P, Knight M. Uterine rupture by intended mode of delivery in the UK: a national case-control study. PLoS Med 2012;9(3):e1001184. doi:10.1371/journal.pmed.1001184.
15. Ford AAD, Bateman BT, Simpson LL. Vaginal birth after cesarean delivery in twin gestations: a large, nationwide sample of deliveries. Am J Obstet Gynecol 2006;195:1138–42.
16. Abenhaim HA, Varin J, Boucher M. External cephalic version among women with a previous cesarean delivery: a report on 36 cases and review of the literature. J Perinat Med 2009;37:156–60.
17. Bretalle F, Cravello L, Shojair R, Roger V, D'Ercole C, Blanc B. Childbirth after two previous caesarean sections. Eur J Obstet Gynecol Reprod Biol 2001;94: 23–6.
18. Rozenberg P, Goffinet F, Phillipe HJ. Thickness of the lower segment: its influence in the management of patients with previous cesarean sections: Eur J Obstet Gynecol Reprod Biol 1999;87:39–45.
19. Martins WP, Barra DA, Gallarreta FMP, Nastri CO, Filho FM. Lower uterine segment thickness measurement in pregnant women with previous Cesarean section: reliability analysis using two- and three-dimentional transabdominal and transvaginal ultrasound. Ultrasound Obstet Gynecol 2009;33:301–6.
20. Smith GCS, White IR, Pell JP, Dobbie R. Predicting cesarean section and uterine rupture among women attempting vaginal birth after prior cesarean section. PLoS Med 2005;2:e252.
21. Montgomery AA, Fahey T, Jones C, Ricketts I, Patel RR, Peters TJ, et al. Two decision aids for mode of delivery among women with previous caesarean section: randomised controlled trial. BMJ 2007;334:1305.
22. Frost J, Shaw A, Montgomery A, Murphy DJ. Women's views on the use of decision aids for decision making about the method of delivery following a previous caesarean section: qualitative interview study. BJOG 2009;116:896–905.
23. Rees KM, Shaw ARG, Bennert K, Emmett CL, Montgomery AA. Healthcare professionals' views on two computer-based decision aids for women choosing mode of delivery after previous caesarean section: a qualitative study. BJOG 2009;116:906–14.
24. Allen VM, O'Connell CM, Baskett TF. Cumulative economic implications of initial method of delivery. Obstet Gynecol 2006;108: 549–55.
25. Macario A, El-Sayed YY, Druzin ML. Cost-effectiveness of a trial of labour after previous cesarean depends on the *a priori* chance of success. Clin Obstet Gynecol 2004;47:378–85.
26. Bujold E, Blackwell SC, Gauthier RJ. Cervical ripening with transcervical foley catheter and the risk of uterine rupture. Obstet Gynecol 2004;103:18–23.
27. Lydon-Rochelle M, Hoet VL, Easterling TR, Martin BP. Risk of uterine rupture during labor among women with a prior cesarean delivery. N Engl J Med 2001; 345:3–8.
28. Ravasi DJ, Wood SL, Pollard JK. Uterine rupture during induced trial of labor among women with previous cesarean delivery. Am J Obstet Gynecol 2000;183:176–9.
29. McDonagh MS, Osterweil P, Guise JM. The benefits and risk of inducing labour in patients with prior caesarean delivery: a systematic review. Br J Obstet Gynaecol 2005;112:1007–15.
30. Kayani SI, Alfirevic Z. Uterine rupture after induction of labour in women with previous caesarean section. Br J Obstet Gynaecol 2005;112:451–5.
31. Wing DA, Lovett K, Paul RH. Disruption of prior uterine incision following misoprostol for labor induction in women with previous cesarean delivery. Obstet Gynecol 1998;91:828–30.
32. Ridgeway JJ, Weyrich DL, Benedetti TJ. Fetal heart rate changes associated with uterine rupture. Obstet Gynecol 2004;103:506–12.
33. Bonanno C, Clausing M, Berkowitz R. VBAC: a medicolegal perspective. Clin Perinatol 2011;38:217–25.
34. Mozurkewich EL, Hutton EK. Elective repeat cesarean delivery versus trial of labor: a meta analysis of the literature from 1989 to 1999. Am J Obstet Gynecol 2000;83: 1187–97.
35. Crowther CA, Dodd JM, Hiller JE, Haslam RR, Robinson JS. Planned vaginal birth or elective repeat caesarean: patient preference restricted cohort with nested randomised trial. PLoS Med 2012;9(3):e1001192. doi:10.1371/journal.pmed.1001192.

36. Guise JM, Berlin M, McDonagh M, Osterweil P, Chan B, Helfand M. Safety of vaginal birth after cesarean: a systematic review. Obstet Gynecol 2004;103:420–9.

BIBLIOGRAPHY

Guise JM, McDonagh MS, Osterweil P, Nygren P, Chan BKS, Helfand M. Systematic review of the incidence and consequences of uterine rupture in women with previous caesarean section. BMJ 2004;329:19–23.

Landon MB, Spong CY, Thom E, Hauth JC, Bloom SL, Varner MW, et al. Risk of uterine rupture with a trial of labor in women with multiple and single prior cesarean delivery. Obstet Gynecol 2006;108:12–20.

Turner MJA, Agnew G, Langan H. Uterine rupture and labour after a previous low transverse caesarean section. Br J Obstet Gynaecol 2006;113:729–32.

CHAPTER 15

UTERINE RUPTURE

MJ Turner

Uterine rupture is an uncommon but serious obstetric emergency associated with an increase in fetal and maternal mortality and morbidity.[1,2] There are, however, wide variations in its incidence, its aetiology and its adverse outcomes which are closely related to variations in the organization and resources of maternity services worldwide.

Differences in the type of uterine rupture (see below), in the prevalence of previous uterine surgery and in the supervision and management of labour explain why there are wide variations reported in the incidence of uterine rupture and in clinical outcomes. In Dublin, for example, the incidence was 1 in 4889 women delivered compared with 1 in 585 deliveries in Benghazi.[3,4] In a recent UK case–control study of 159 women, uterine rupture was associated with only two maternal deaths and a perinatal mortality rate of 124 per 1000.[2] In contrast, in an 8-year Nigerian review, uterine rupture accounted for 17% of all maternal deaths and the perinatal mortality rate was 86%.[5]

CLASSIFICATION

- *Complete uterine rupture* involves the full thickness of the uterine wall, with or without expulsion of the fetus and/or placenta and includes rupture of the membranes at the site of rupture. It usually presents as a dramatic emergency which threatens the life of both the woman and her baby, particularly if there is any delay in performing laparotomy.
- *Incomplete rupture* or uterine dehiscence occurs when the uterine wall ruptures but the visceral peritoneum remains intact. It is usually asymptomatic and the diagnosis is made incidentally at the time of caesarean section. The time interval between incomplete rupture and diagnosis is usually unknown and incomplete rupture is rarely associated with adverse clinical outcomes. It often goes unrecorded and therefore case ascertainment is unreliable. It is recommended that the term 'dehiscence' be reserved for incomplete rupture and that such cases be excluded from clinical studies of uterine rupture because the impact is clinically of little consequence.

CAUSES

Complete uterine rupture may occur with either a previously scarred or an unscarred uterus. In high-income healthcare settings complete rupture occurs most commonly in the presence of a previously scarred uterus, but in low income healthcare settings complete rupture often occurs in an unscarred uterus following unsupervised obstructed labour.

- Despite the frequent use of oxytocics to induce or augment labour, rupture of the uterus in a primigravida is extraordinarily rare, particularly in the absence of a congenital uterine malformation or trauma.[6–8] Rupture in the absence of trauma in a primigravida raises questions about previously undisclosed uterine surgery or perforation.
- Traumatic uterine rupture is uncommon. Antepartum, the trauma is usually the result of an accident or violence. In such circumstances, the threat to life is high because there may be other injuries and the pregnant woman may not be under medical supervision. Peripartum traumatic rupture may occur when a prolonged labour is inadequately supervised or when an obstetric manoeuvre or operative vaginal delivery goes badly wrong. This is more likely to occur and is more likely to end in catastrophe in poorly resourced countries.
- Rupture of a scarred uterus is usually associated with a history of previous caesarean section.[2,9] The type of the previous caesarean matters. The risk of rupture after a low transverse caesarean ranges from 0.2 to 1.5%.[10–13] More recent American reviews quote a rate of 0.5–1.0%, which is higher than the 0.2% cited in European studies.[2,3] The risk of uterine rupture quoted for a

trial of labour after a caesarean delivery varies widely in national guidelines; although the experts presumably reviewed a similar body of scientific evidence.[13,14]

- A 4–9% rupture rate after a previous classical or T-incision caesarean is quoted.[1,10] There is uncertainty about the risk of rupture if the previous vertical incision was confined to the lower uterine segment.[1]
- Rarely, uterine rupture may complicate delivery following a previous myomectomy, or a uterine perforation which may or may not have been diagnosed at the time. It may also complicate previous uterine surgery such as a metroplasty or cornual resection of an ectopic pregnancy.[15] It has been suggested in the past that the risk of rupture is only increased if the previous surgery involved the full thickness of the uterine wall but evidence to support this is lacking.

Prevention and early diagnosis of uterine rupture in clinical practice are more likely to be successful when a detailed obstetric and gynaecological history is taken at the first antenatal visit. Uterine rupture after previous scarring confined to a low transverse uterine incision may present intrapartum or postpartum and thus the commonest presentation of uterine rupture in developed countries occurs under midwifery or obstetric supervision. Uterine rupture after previous scarring involving the uterine body may present antepartum, intrapartum or postpartum. Indeed, antepartum rupture of a vertical scar may occur remote from term and outside hospital. Thus, rupture with a vertical scar on the uterine body may be associated with higher risks of an adverse clinical outcome.

BANDL'S RING

'The upper parts of the uterus were uniformly hard, the lower somewhat softer. A shallow, transverse furrow, an inch below the umbilicus indicated the boundary between the uterine corpus and the cervix (lower uterine segment)... the head and shoulders were partly palpable through the abdominal wall, covered only by a very thin layer. The whole cervix (lower uterine segment) was uniformly paper-thin and enormously stretched out, so that it must surely have contained half the infant while the body of the uterus and fundus sat on the infant like a cap... the conditions in this case were obviously most favourable for rupture of the uterus. It would have taken only one or two additional contractions of the uterus or the increased pressure of the physician's hand or an instrument to bring it about...'

Ludwig Bandl
Über Ruptur der Gebärmutter und ihre Mechanik. Vienna: Czermak.1875

CLINICAL PRESENTATION

- Uterine rupture complicating a previous low transverse caesarean section commonly presents intrapartum with fetal heart rate abnormalities.[16] Thus, it is recommended that women with previous uterine surgery should have continuous electronic fetal heart rate monitoring in labour.[12] If there are heart rate abnormalities, the diagnosis of rupture should be immediately considered and delivery expedited. The time taken to perform a fetal scalp blood pH for evidence of fetal hypoxia may incur a delay which can be catastrophic if the fetal heart abnormalities are due to uterine rupture. Therefore, early recourse to an emergency caesarean is advisable if there is evidence of fetal compromise in women labouring with a previous uterine scar.
- Intrapartum uterine rupture may also present with cessation of uterine contractions and, therefore, any decision to augment labour with oxytocin should only be made with great caution after clinical assessment by an experienced obstetrician.
- There may be a history of constant rather than intermittent abdominal pain. Tenderness over a previous caesarean scar is a non-specific symptom and not particularly helpful in making the diagnosis.
- Uterine rupture may be associated with haemorrhage which can precipitate clinical shock. Abdominal tenderness or shock which appears disproportionate to any blood loss should raise the suspicion of concealed intra-abdominal bleeding. Primary postpartum haemorrhage unresponsive to the normal treatment, including oxytocics, in a woman with a scarred uterus should also raise the suspicion of rupture.
- If the rupture involves the bladder, haematuria may persist before or after delivery.
- Alteration in the shape of the uterine swelling on abdominal examination is described; however, this may not occur until part of the uterine contents have been expelled into the abdominal cavity.
- Antepartum uterine rupture is rare but should be considered in any woman with a uterine scar who presents with abdominal pain or tenderness, particularly in association with clinical shock and a fall in haemoglobin concentration. If a previous caesarean section has been performed preterm the possibility of a vertical uterine incision should be considered. Ideally, the notes

from all previous caesareans should be available and scrutinized by an obstetrician at the first antenatal visit.

- Blunt trauma, unless substantial, is a rare cause of uterine rupture and usually presents before delivery with a history of an accident or violence.[17]
- Uterine rupture associated with obstetric trauma is manifest at the time or shortly after an obstetric manoeuvre or operative delivery when the obstetrician is still present.

MANAGEMENT

The key to a successful outcome following uterine rupture is early diagnosis, prompt intervention and, if the woman is clinically shocked, resuscitation that often entails blood transfusion. However, laparotomy under general anaesthesia is required as a matter of urgency and cannot be delayed until the resuscitation is complete, especially if there is continuing haemorrhage.

At laparotomy, the diagnosis is confirmed, the extent of the rupture quickly determined and the baby delivered. If the baby or placenta have already been expelled from the uterus, the neonatal outcome is usually poor. Once the baby and placenta have been delivered, control of haemorrhage is the priority. The uterus and surrounding structures must be closely inspected because the trauma may have extended beyond what was seen on initial assessment.

In many cases a simple repair of the site of rupture will suffice and recourse to peripartum hysterectomy may be unnecessary (see Chapter 28). A tubal sterilization at the time of repair is inadvisable unless it was already planned; it is unwise to make an important decision about future fertility in the middle of an obstetric emergency.

DELIVERY AFTER UTERINE RUPTURE

There is a paucity of information on delivery after previous uterine rupture, in part because it is more likely to occur in multigravidas who may decide their family is complete after a previous life-threatening experience. In a study of 18 pregnancies in 15 women who had repair of the uterine tear, 17 babies were delivered by elective caesarean and one delivered vaginally preterm; with no case of recurrent rupture.[18] In two other reviews,[19,20] a total of 11 women were delivered of 15 babies by elective caesarean without

recurrent rupture. In a study of six women, 10 babies were successfully delivered by elective caesarean subsequent to repair of the rupture.[19] In a study of five women, all were delivered by caesarean section and no recurrent uterine rupture occurred.[20] Not surprisingly, previous uterine rupture is considered a contraindication to a trial of labour.

PREVENTION OF UTERINE RUPTURE

As caesarean section has become safer for the mother, technically challenging obstetric manoeuvres and instrumental vaginal deliveries have little role in contemporary obstetrics in high-income countries. As a result, traumatic uterine rupture has become less common and, in the rare cases of accident or violence, is highly unpredictable and almost impossible to prevent.

The number of women whose uterus is scarred following previous gynaecological surgery is small and there is usually a history of infertility. Women with a vertical obstetric scar on their uterus are also few in number and there is often a history of poor perinatal outcome associated with preterm delivery. The threshold for performing an elective caesarean in both these groups is low and thus, uterine rupture is exceptional.

In the UK audit, 87% (139/159) of cases of uterine rupture had a history of previous caesarean section.[2] Fear of uterine rupture and its life-threatening complications has led obstetricians in the USA to largely abandon the practice of a trial of labour after caesarean section except in carefully selected cases.[21,22] This may be related, in part, to the fact that many women with a previous caesarean in the USA deliver in smaller maternity units where labour is not supervised by midwives and the obstetrician, anaesthetist and neonatologist are not on call in the hospital.

Reverting back to the policy of a 'once a Caesarean, always a Caesarean' will prevent cases of uterine rupture which are related to labour. Clinically it is important to remember it will not prevent all cases because rupture is reported, albeit rarely, in women who had planned a repeat elective caesarean section but who went into labour earlier than expected. Thus, if a woman scheduled for a repeat caesarean presents with abdominal pain or in labour she should be assessed with a view to advancing the caesarean delivery. She should not be allowed to labour unsupervised in the antenatal ward. In women with a single previous low transverse caesarean section, it is possible to prevent many cases of uterine rupture by careful selection of women for trial of labour, by avoiding the use of oxytocics for induction and by close supervision in labour.[3]

FETAL OUTCOMES

Uterine rupture has been associated with an increase in perinatal deaths.[1,2] In a recent national case–control study of uterine rupture, after excluding the stillbirths that occurred before rupture, the perinatal mortality rate was 124 per 100 000 (95% CI 75–189), which was significantly higher than the national rate of 7.5 per 100 000 (risk ratio 16.5, 95% CI 10.7–25.4).[2] In addition, nine infants were diagnosed with encephalopathy and 41% (56/137) of the infants were admitted to a neonatal unit.[2]

Apart from the careful selection of women allowed a trial of labour after caesarean section, a key issue is determining the fetal outcome is the decision-to-delivery interval. If uterine rupture occurs in a maternity hospital staffed by well-trained midwives and with specialist medical staff always on duty, it is possible to achieve a short diagnosis–delivery interval. Over a decade, 36 cases of uterine rupture occurred in nine hospitals in Utah during 11 195 trials of labour after previous caesarean.[22] The frequency of rupture was 0.3%. All neonates who delivered within 18 minutes after a suspected uterine rupture had normal umbilical pH levels or Apgar scores >7 at 5 minutes. Poor long-term outcome occurred in three neonates with a decision-to-delivery interval longer than 30 minutes.

MATERNAL OUTCOMES

In the UK national audit, two of 159 women with uterine rupture died, a case fatality of 1.3%, 9% (n = 15) had a hysterectomy and 6% (n = 10) had one or more organs damaged at rupture or removed during surgery.[2] Of the 159, 31% (n = 50) were admitted for critical or high dependency care.[2]

An uncommon clinical challenge is the management of a woman with an intrauterine fetal death where the risk of adverse outcome following rupture concerns the woman only. In a secondary analysis of a multicentre American study, 209 women previously delivered by caesarean section were studied with a singleton antepartum intrauterine fetal death ≥20 weeks' gestation.[24] The trial of labour rate was 75.6% (158/209) and the VBAC (vaginal birth after caesarean section) rate of women who laboured was 86.7%. The authors concluded that induction of labour

should be considered an alternative to repeat caesarean section. However, the rupture rate was 3.4% (n = 4) following induction and none of the four women had a previous vaginal delivery. In contrast, there was no uterine rupture identified in the women who laboured spontaneously with a previous low transverse caesarean section.

The recent RCOG (Royal College of Obstetricians and Gynaecologists) Guidelines on late intrauterine fetal death and stillbirth (IUFD) found no studies on the safety and effectiveness of induction of labour after IUFD in women with a single caesarean section scar.[25] Thus, practices in the management of women with an IUFD and a scarred uterus are guided by expert opinions only.[25] However, induction in these circumstances appears to carry a higher risk of uterine rupture than watchful expectancy.[24,25]

RISKS OF UTERINE RUPTURE

Determining the risks of uterine rupture is difficult. They depend, for example, on the definition used, on the population studied, on the healthcare setting and on obstetric practices.[26,27] In a minority of cases, the acute emergency cannot be anticipated and it must be managed when and where it arises. In the majority of cases of uterine rupture, prevention may be possible. In carefully selected cases of women undergoing trial of labour after previous caesarean section, rupture may occur but the risk is lower than often reported.[2,3] When rupture does occur, the threat to the lives and wellbeing of the woman and her offspring is low in absolute terms in developed countries, particularly if a laparotomy is undertaken urgently.[1,3] While the clinical challenge of uterine rupture can never be underestimated, prevention should not be driven by an exaggerated fear of the complications of attempting a vaginal birth after caesarean section (see Chapter 14).

REFERENCES

1. Turner MJ. Uterine rupture. Best Pract Res Clin Obstet Gynaecol 2002;16:69–79.
2. Fitzpatrick KE, Kurinczuk JJ, Alfirevic Z, Spark P, Brocklehurst P, Knight M. Uterine rupture by intended mode of delivery in the UK: a national case-control study. PLoS Med 2012;9:e1001184.
3. Turner MJ, Agnew G, Langan H. Uterine rupture and labour after a previous low transverse caesarean section. BJOG 2006;113:1–4.
4. Rahman J, Al-Sibai MH, Rahman MS. Rupture of the uterus in labor. A review of 96 cases. Acta Obstet Gynecol Scand 1985;64:311–15.
5. Ola ER, Olamijulo JA. Rupture of the uterus at the Lagos University Teaching Hospital, Lagos, Nigeria. West Afr J Med 1998;17:188–93.

6. Sweeten KM, Graves WK, Athanassiou A. Spontaneous rupture of the unscarred uterus. Am J Obstet Gynecol 1995;172:1851–5.

7. Landon MB. Uterine rupture in primigravid women. Obstet Gynecol 2006;108:709–10.

8. Ravasia DJ, Brain PH, Pollard JK. Incidence of uterine rupture among women with Müllerian duct anomalies who attempt vaginal birth after cesarean delivery. Am J Obstet Gynecol 1999;181:877–81.

9. Gardeil F, Daly S, Turner MJ. Uterine rupture in pregnancy reviewed. Eur J Obstet Gynecol Reprod Biol 1994;56:107–10.

10. Vaginal birth after previous cesarean delivery. ACOG Practice Bulletin No. 115. American College of Obstetricians and Gynecologists. Obstet Gynecol 2010;116: 450–63.

11. Scott JR. Vaginal birth after cesarean delivery: a common-sense approach. Obstet Gynecol 2011;118: 342–50.

12. Foureur M, Ryan CL, Nicholl M, Homer C. Inconsistent evidence: analysis of six national guidelines for vaginal birth after cesarean section. Birth 2010;37: 3–10.

13. Turner MJ. Vaginal birth after cesarean delivery: a common sense approach. Obstet Gynecol 2011;118: 1176–7.

14. Dubuisson JB, Fauconnier A, Deffarges JV, Norgaard C, Kreiker G, Chapron C. Pregnancy outcome and deliveries following laparoscopic myomectomy. Hum Reprod 2000;15:869–73.

15. Ridgeway JJ, Weyrich DL, Benedetti TJ. Fetal heart changes associated with uterine rupture. Obstet Gynecol 2004;103:506–12.

16. Ripley DL. Uterine emergencies. Atony, inversion, and rupture. Obstet Gynecol Clin North Am 1999;26: 419–34.

17. O'Connor RA, Gaughan B. Pregnancy following simple repair of the ruptured gravid uterus. BJOG 1989;96: 942–4.

18. Al Sakka M, Dauleh W, Al Hassani S. Case series of uterine rupture and subsequent pregnancy outcome. Int J Fertil Womens Med 1999;44:297–300.

19. Lim AC, Kwee A, Bruinse HW. Pregnancy after uterine rupture: a report of 5 cases and a review of the literature. Obstet Gynecol Surv 2005;60:613–17.

20. Guise JM, Berlin M, McDonagh M, Osterweil P, Chan B, Helfand M. Safety of vaginal birth after cesarean: a systematic review. Obstet Gynecol 2004;103: 420–9.

21. Gregory KD, Fridman M, Korst L. Trends and patterns of vaginal birth after cesarean availability in the United States. Semin Perinatol 2010;34:237–43.

22. Holmgren C, Scott JR, Porter TF, Esplin MS, Bardsley T. Uterine rupture with attempted vaginal birth after cesarean delivery: decision-to-delivery time and neonatal outcome. Obstet Gynecol 2012;119: 725–31.

23. Ramirez MM, Gilbert S, Landon MB, Rouse DJ, Spong CY, Varner MW, et al. Mode of delivery in women with antepartum fetal death and prior cesarean delivery. Am J Perinatol 2010;27:825–30.

24. Green-top guideline no. 55. Late fetal death and stillbirth. Royal College of Obstetricians and Gynaecologists, October 2010.

25. Kieser KE, Baskett TF. A 10-year population-based study of uterine rupture. Obstet Gynecol 2002;100: 749–53.

26. Spong CY. To VBAC or not to VBAC. PLoS Med 2012;9:e1001191.

27. Turner MJ. Delivery after one previous cesarean section. Am J Obstet Gynecol 1997;176:741–4.

CHAPTER 16

BREECH DELIVERY

TF Baskett

> 'If the feet of the child come foremost, you must take care to baptize them immediately ...'
> Paul Portal
> The Compleat Practice of Men and Women Midwives. London: J. Johnson, 1763, p23

The fetus in breech presentation has a higher perinatal mortality and morbidity due mainly to prematurity, congenital anomalies, birth asphyxia and trauma. At 28 weeks' gestation the incidence of breech presentation is approximately one in five. At term, 3–4% of all fetuses are in breech presentation, making this the commonest malpresentation.

Over the past 30 years there has been a worldwide trend to deliver a greater proportion of breech presentations by caesarean section. In 2000 an international multicentre randomized-controlled trial of planned vaginal delivery versus planned elective caesarean section for uncomplicated term breech presentation confirmed that perinatal mortality and serious neonatal morbidity were significantly lower in the planned caesarean group.[1] Further analysis of the Term Breech Trial showed that prelabour caesarean and caesarean during early labour were associated with the lowest adverse perinatal outcome due to labour or delivery and that vaginal delivery had the highest risk of adverse outcome.[2] Furthermore, the widespread adoption of elective caesarean for breech delivery in the Netherlands was associated with an improvement in neonatal outcome.[3] As a result, although the conclusions of this trial were disputed,[4–7] where appropriate facilities existed caesarean section for the term breech become the standard of care in many hospitals and was supported by national guidelines.[8]

Subsequently, secondary analysis by the Term Breech Trial group showed that the mortality and morbidity outcomes of the children at 2 years of age were similar.[9] In addition, compared to vaginal delivery, maternal morbidity was increased in those women delivered by caesarean section in labour, but not higher in those delivered by elective caesarean without labour.[10] With the availability of the secondary analysis, a number of publications appeared advocating selective vaginal breech delivery, supported by some institutional data.[6,11–13] As a result many national guidelines were modified to support those willing to provide selective vaginal breech delivery under strict selection and management criteria.[14–17]

However, even before the Term Breech Trial results were published, most obstetricians had 'voted with their scalpels'. The trial results and an increasingly critical medico-legal climate only served to consolidate this approach. Furthermore, the discussion involved in fully informed consent often hardens the resolve of the woman to choose elective caesarean delivery. Even in the large multi-institutional study from France and Belgium, which promoted breech vaginal delivery with strict selection and intrapartum management criteria, only 22% of all term breech presentations were delivered vaginally.[12] In Dublin, where obstetric leaders wrote in favour of selective vaginal delivery of the term breech,[6,11] the caesarean breech delivery rate rose from 77% to 90% respectively in the 8-year epochs before and after the Term Breech Trial.[18]

For the preterm breech (24–32 weeks' gestation) recent evidence suggests that caesarean delivery reduces perinatal death and morbidity compared to attempted vaginal delivery.[19] Thus, the majority of obstetricians choose caesarean section for the viable preterm breech.

The above notwithstanding, there are still occasions when vaginal breech delivery will have to be undertaken, for the following reasons:

1. Labour may proceed so rapidly that there is inadequate time to perform caesarean section. Even in the Term Breech Trial almost one in 10 of those assigned to delivery by caesarean section were delivered vaginally.[1]
2. Labour and delivery may occur in a setting where caesarean section is unavailable or carries greater risks than are justified by the perceived perinatal benefit.
3. From erroneous observation or lack of opportunity the diagnosis of breech presentation may not be made until late in the second stage of labour, when it is too late to perform caesarean section.

4. The woman, although informed of the increased perinatal risks, may still choose to proceed with labour and vaginal delivery.

In addition, while caesarean section may reduce the risks of fetal trauma, it is still necessary to know and perform the appropriate manoeuvres required to safely deliver the fetus through the uterine incision. This applies particularly to the after-coming head of the fetus, and these manoeuvres are similar to those required for atraumatic vaginal breech delivery. Thus, it remains essential for the accoucheur to acquire and retain the skills necessary to protect the fetus during vaginal delivery. Unfortunately, one of the side effects of an almost universal policy of caesarean section for breech delivery is that it becomes a self-fulfilling prophecy that obstetric trainees will have limited opportunities to acquire the skills necessary for safe vaginal breech delivery.[20] As in other areas of our specialty, simulation and manikin training have to supplement on-the-job acquisition of experience.[21,22] These skills may also be augmented by the routine and systematic rehearsal of all the manoeuvres during delivery of the breech through the uterine incision at every caesarean section for breech presentation.[23]

INTRAPARTUM FETAL RISKS

The main reasons for the poor outcome of the breech presentation, compared with the fetus in cephalic presentation, are prematurity and congenital anomalies. It is also possible that there are subtle neurological abnormalities that cause the fetus to lie in breech presentation and which may contribute to a poorer outcome irrespective of the method of delivery. During labour and delivery the fetus in breech presentation is subjected to the following risks:

- A higher incidence of cord entanglement or cord prolapse, especially in the footling breech, may lead to asphyxia. In addition, when the after-coming head of the breech enters the pelvic brim the associated cord compression can cause asphyxia if there is undue delay in descent and delivery of the head.
- The fetal buttocks and trunk have a smaller diameter than the head. This is particularly exaggerated in the preterm fetus. Thus, there is a danger that the buttocks and trunk will slip through an incompletely dilated cervix causing entrapment of the arms and/or the head, leading to trauma and asphyxia.

- Fracture or dislocation of limbs may occur and this is most likely with extended or nuchal displacement of the arms.
- Damage to intra-abdominal organs may be sustained, especially the liver and spleen, if the hands of the accoucheur are placed above the pelvis and encircle the abdomen during manipulations.
- Cervical spine dislocation or fracture due to excessive traction during delivery of the head, particularly if there is hyperextension of the neck because of undue elevation of the body of the fetus while the head is still in the pelvis.
- Brachial plexus injury due to inappropriate and excessive traction on the shoulders in an attempt to deliver the head.
- Traction on the fetal trunk while the head remains in the pelvis may tend to pull the base of the fetal skull away from the vault.
- As the fetal head descends across the pelvic floor and perineum there is compression and, if delivery of the fetal head is not carefully controlled, sudden decompression as the head delivers. This may cause a tentorial tear and intracranial haemorrhage, risks which are increased when there is concomitant hypoxia.

In essence, the job of the obstetrician is to protect the fetal brain during labour and delivery, and nowhere is this duty more critical than in breech delivery. The key is to apply a well-rehearsed sequence of manoeuvres and achieve the balance between excessive haste leading to traumatic delivery and undue delay with its risk of asphyxia. In most cases a minimal amount of interference is required but there should always be active control and protection of the fetal head at delivery.

ANAESTHESIA

For some women a combination of narcotic, inhalation and pudendal block will provide adequate analgesia and allow the most natural progression of the first and second stages of labour. Epidural block provides the best pain relief and also has the advantage of blunting the maternal bearing-down effort in the late first stage of labour. In the nulliparous woman epidural block may be required for adequate pain relief, but can prevent the desired maternal bearing-down effort in the second stage of labour. This may lead to uncertainty as to whether such failure of descent is due to impaired maternal propulsive effort or due to feto-pelvic disproportion. In carefully selected cases oxytocin augmentation may be used, but with extreme caution. On the other hand, the multiparous woman often receives adequate pain relief with narcotic, inhalation and pudendal block, but epidural analgesia has the benefit of blunting her bearing-down reflex, which may occur prematurely in the late first stage of labour. The ideal, therefore, is a selective epidural block that allows retention of motor activity, while providing a humane degree of sensory block. Ideally, an anaesthetist should be present at all breech deliveries, either to supervise the regional block or to provide rapid general anaesthesia and/or uterine relaxation if necessary.

FIRST STAGE OF LABOUR

In general, the frank and complete types of breech presentation fill the lower uterine segment and are well applied to the cervix. In contrast, the footling breech (Fig 16-1) may not and there is a much higher incidence of cord prolapse. For this reason, and the propensity of the footling breech to slip through the incompletely dilated cervix, labour is best avoided with a footling breech presentation unless there is no alternative. The frank or complete breech at term, of reasonable size (2000–3800 g), is most likely to result in a safe vaginal delivery if the first stage of labour is smooth and progressive.

Oxytocin augmentation is permissible, particularly in the nulliparous breech, for similar indications to cephalic presentation. However, this would only be undertaken in cases where caesarean delivery is not a realistic alternative. In the Term Breech Trial the perinatal outcome was significantly worse in cases in which oxytocin augmentation was used.[2] Amniotomy in labour is acceptable if the breech is well applied to the cervix. In general, however, one tries to leave the membranes intact as long as possible. X-ray pelvimetry is of no proven value for management of the breech in labour.

When the membranes rupture spontaneously during labour an immediate pelvic examination should be done to exclude cord prolapse.

It is essential to be sure that the cervix is fully dilated and not palpable before encouraging maternal bearing-down effort. Because the breech is usually smaller than the after-coming head it is possible, even at term, for the breech to appear at the introitus before the cervix is fully dilated. The early appearance of male external genitalia can also be misleading. It is therefore a cardinal rule that one must check for full cervical dilatation before proceeding with delivery.

CONDUCT OF BREECH DELIVERY

Delivery of the Breech and Legs

With uterine contractions and maternal effort the breech should be allowed to descend to the perineum. The woman can then be placed in the

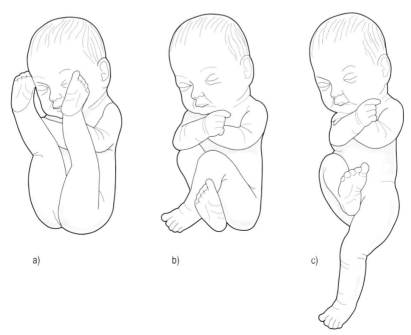

a)

b)

c)

FIGURE 16-1 ■ Types of breech presentation. (a) Frank, (b) complete and (c) footling.

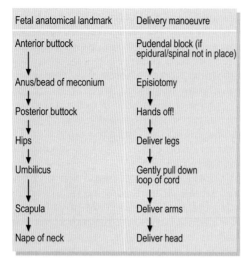

Fetal anatomical landmark	Delivery manoeuvre
Anterior buttock ↓	Pudendal block (if epidural/spinal not in place) ↓
Anus/bead of meconium ↓	Episiotomy ↓
Posterior buttock ↓	Hands off! ↓
Hips ↓	Deliver legs ↓
Umbilicus ↓	Gently pull down loop of cord ↓
Scapula ↓	Deliver arms ↓
Nape of neck	Deliver head

FIGURE 16-2 ■ Breech delivery: fetal anatomical landmarks and sequence of manoeuvres.

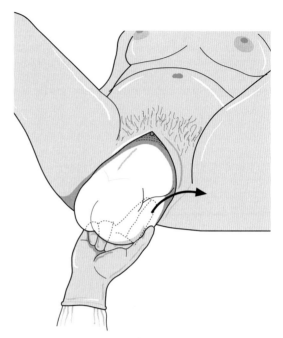

FIGURE 16-3 ■ Assisted delivery of extended legs. The fingers splint the femur, slightly abduct the thigh and then flex the hip and knee.

lithotomy position and, if epidural analgesia has not already been established, a pudendal block is performed along with local anaesthetic infiltration of the perineum. The guiding principle at this time is 'keep your hands off the breech', be patient, and await the appearance of critical anatomical landmarks (Fig 16-2). The most helpful manoeuvres involve flexion and rotation but not traction. The following sequence should be observed:

- As the breech descends it meets the obstruction of the perineum. With further maternal effort the anterior buttock of the fetus 'climbs up' the perineum until the fetal anus is visible over the fourchette – usually manifest by a bead of meconium. The breech does not recede in between contractions. At this point the combination of descent and lateral flexion of the fetus has reached its maximum and further progress will only occur when the obstruction of the perineum is removed. This, therefore, is the point at which episiotomy is performed, with special care to avoid injury to the fetal genitalia. The comparable timing for a footling breech presentation is when the fetal buttocks reach the perineum.

- A combination of the above observations and testing the distension of the perineum with a finger will guide the precise timing of episiotomy, with particular care taken to avoid cutting fetal soft tissues. Wait until the beginning of a contraction and then perform the episiotomy, which ensures maternal effort throughout the entire uterine contraction to help deliver the

buttocks and legs. With a complete breech, maternal effort alone will usually deliver the legs and lower trunk.

- With a frank breech presentation the extended legs often require assistance in the form of slight abduction at the hip and flexion of the knee for delivery. One hip is usually anterolateral and two or three fingers should be placed along the fetal thigh above the knee to slightly abduct and flex the hip, followed by flexion of the knee on the fetal body. The more 'splinting' fingers that can be placed along the thigh to conduct this manoeuvre the greater the distribution of force, which lessens the chance of fracture of the femur. This principle applies to all manoeuvres involving the limbs. Once the anterior leg has been flexed and delivered the breech should be gently rotated so that the other hip is anterolateral and the same procedure repeated on the other side (Fig 16-3).

- The remainder of the abdomen and lower thorax will usually deliver with maternal effort alone. At this point gently bring down a loop of umbilical cord so it is not under tension for the remainder of the delivery.

- Throughout delivery of the legs, abdomen and lower thorax there should be minimal or no traction, which is likely to cause extension of the arms and fetal head – both undesirable. Other than assisting the delivery of extended legs with flexion and ensuring that the fetal back remains anterior, one should rely on maternal effort alone.

Delivery of the Shoulders and Arms

A critical stage of the delivery has now been reached. As the fetal trunk delivers and descends the fetal head will enter the pelvic brim, causing compression of the umbilical cord. Ideally, the rest of the delivery should be accomplished within 2–3 minutes, to avoid asphyxia. On the other hand, one must not panic and employ undue haste, potentially leading to trauma of the arms, brachial plexus, cervical spine and brain. Although it may not seem so, 2–3 minutes is ample time to systematically and carefully go through the manoeuvres to effect safe delivery:

- With maternal effort alone the lower border of the more anterior scapula will become visible under the pubic arch. Provided no undue traction has been applied the arms are usually flexed across the fetal chest. Using two fingers pass them over the fetal shoulder and down along the humerus, splinting and sweeping it across the chest to deliver the elbow and forearm. The fetus is then rotated 90° to bring the other scapula into view and the same procedure is repeated.
- When rotating the fetus for this and other purposes it is important to avoid gripping the fetal abdomen. The obstetrician's hands should grasp the thighs with the thumbs over the sacrum and the index fingers around the iliac crest. In this way the intra-abdominal contents will not be traumatized. The use of a small sterilized towel will assist the correct placement and help maintain the grip (Fig 16-4).

Delivery of the Head

At this point the obstetrician becomes actively involved to protect the fetal head during delivery. The key factors are gentle descent and flexion of the fetal head, protection of the cervical spine from excessive traction or hyperextension, and protection of the fetal brain from the compression and sudden decompression forces during delivery over the perineum. It is this sudden decompression, or 'champagne cork' delivery, that can lead to tentorial tears and intracranial haemorrhage. The following sequence is recommended:

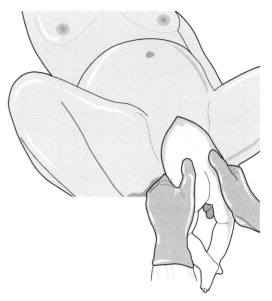

FIGURE 16-4 ■ The manner of grasping the breech for rotation and traction.

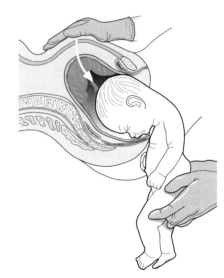

FIGURE 16-5 ■ The fetus suspended vertically, partially supported by the operator's hands. An assistant provides suprapubic pressure. This combination promotes descent and flexion of the fetal head.

- After delivery of the arms, descent and flexion of the fetal head are encouraged by allowing the infant's body, partially supported by the operator's hands, to hang vertically. An assistant applies mild suprapubic pressure to help promote descent and flexion (Fig 16-5). It is important that the infant should not hang by its own weight unsupported as this may promote extension of the head or, in a small infant, allow completely uncontrolled delivery of the head.

- When the hair line on the back of the infant's head (the nape of the neck) is visible under the pubic arch the head has descended adequately and the time has come for its assisted delivery.

In all cases delivery of the head should be carefully controlled. There have been many techniques described for this purpose but the two main ones will be described here.

Forceps to the After-Coming Head

If facilities and assistance are available this is the technique of choice as it provides the greatest degree of control and protection from the compression and sudden decompression forces. The operator kneels while an assistant holds the infant's body at or just above the horizontal plane. It is very important to clearly instruct the assistant not to hold the fetal body higher than this plane as hyperextension of the fetal neck can cause dislocation of the cervical spine, bleeding in the venous plexus around the cervical spinal cord, and even quadriplegia.

Piper's forceps were designed particularly for the after-coming head of the breech, but any of the long handled forceps can be used. The reason the operator kneels is to see under the trunk of the infant and also because the plane of application of the forceps is in a slightly upward manner following the curve of the sacrum. Hold one forcep by the handle with the tips of the fingers of the second hand placed at the end of the blade. The blade is then inserted between four and five o'clock and the tips of the fingers guide the insertion alongside the fetal head. A similar procedure is done with the other forcep blade inserted between 7 and 8 o'clock. Particular care should be exercised in applying the forceps blades. Because the episiotomy has already been performed there is a danger that the tip of the blade can track into the paravaginal tissues under the apex of the episiotomy.

Another advantage of the forceps is that gentle traction promotes flexion of the fetal head, reducing the diameter and aiding descent. During initial descent of the fetal head the body of the fetus must remain in the horizontal plane (Fig 16-6a). Once the chin and mouth are visible over the perineum then the forceps, body and legs of the fetus are raised in unison to complete delivery (Fig 16-6b). The combination of flexion and safe traction on the fetal head, plus the cradling effect of the forceps which provides protection from compression and decompression, make this an ideal method for safe delivery of the head.

> ### FIRST USE OF FORCEPS TO THE AFTER-COMING HEAD OF THE BREECH
>
> 'In the year 1755, I was called to a case ... but after the body was delivered, the head of the child stuck at the brim of the pelvis, on which I made several trials to bring it down into the vagina ... I was afraid of overstraining the neck if I repeated these trials and increased the force. The patient being in a supine position, I introduced a blade of the long forceps, curved to one side, up along each side of the pelvis, while an assistant held up the body of the child to give more room for the application; and having fixed them on the head, and joined the blades of the instrument together, I introduced two fingers of my left hand, and fixed them on each side of the child's nose, while my right hand pulled the head with the instrument and delivered it safely.'
>   William Smellie
>   The Collection of Preternatural Cases and Observations in Midwifery. Vol 3. London: D. Wilson and T. Durham, 1764, p193

Mauriceau–Smellie–Veit Manoeuvre

This technique is invaluable when delivery happens rapidly, there is no assistance, or no time to apply the forceps. The operator's forearm is placed under the fetal body with a fetal leg on

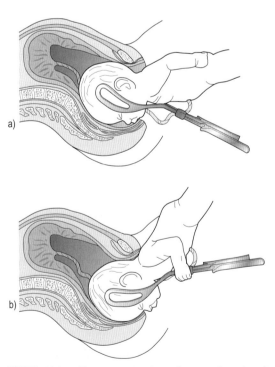

FIGURE 16-6 ■ Forceps to the after-coming head. (a) During initial descent and flexion of the head the fetal trunk is kept horizontal. (b) As the fetal chin is delivered the forceps and body are raised in unison.

either side. The forefinger and middle finger of this hand are placed on the maxilla beside the nose to promote flexion of the fetal head. It is permissible initially to gently flex the lower jaw to bring the maxilla into reach. However, no undue traction should be placed on the lower jaw of the fetus as it risks dislocation and is not as effective in flexing the fetal head as the safer position of the fingers on the maxilla. The other hand is placed on the fetal back with the middle finger pushing up the occiput, to promote flexion, and the other fingers resting on the fetal shoulders. With this grip, the cervical spine is splinted and protected while flexion of the fetal head is promoted (Fig 16-7). Gentle traction in a downward and backward plane should help guide the head over the perineum and control delivery to avoid sudden decompression. Only gentle traction should be used with this technique and its role is usually that of slowing down and controlling the delivery, rather than providing traction. If traction is necessary to cause descent of the fetal head, forceps to the after-coming head is the safer technique.

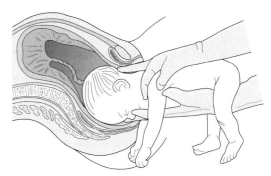

FIGURE 16-7 ■ Mauriceau–Smellie–Veit manoeuvre.

COMPLICATIONS OF BREECH DELIVERY

Extended Arms

Extension of the arms usually occurs when there has been inappropriate traction up to this point in the delivery. It also may occur if the trunk has passed through an incompletely dilated cervix. There are two techniques for dealing with extended arms.

> ### FIRST DESCRIPTION OF WHAT WAS TO BECOME THE MAURICEAU–SMELLIE–VEIT MANOEUVRE
>
> 'I therefore passed my fingers up the child's mouth supporting the breast with my wrist and arm, putting one finger into the mouth, and two others upon the cheeks, I pulled towards me, and at the same time drawing with my other hand above the shoulders, brought out the head'.
> William Giffard
> Cases in Midwifery. London: Motte, 1734

> ### MAURICEAU–SMELLIE–VEIT MANOEUVRE
>
> 'Then I brought the body lower, but finding that the head stopped at the upper part of the pelvis, I insinuated my hand up along the breast, and introduced a finger into the mouth, and by pulling gently brought the forehead into the concave part of the sacrum: being afraid of over-straining the underjaw, I quitted that hold and placed a finger on each side of the nose; then I laid the body of the child on that arm, and by slipping the fingers of my other hand over the shoulders and on each side on the neck, I got the head safely extracted'.
> William Smellie
> The Collection of Preternatural Cases and Observations in Midwifery. Vol 3. London: D. Wilson and T. Durham, 1764, p72

> ### LØVSET'S MANOEUVRE
>
> 'The theoretical basis for this procedure is that the posterior shoulder is always the lower one, owing to the pelvic inclination and the direction of the birth axis in the pelvic outlet … If the body of the foetus is turned 180° with its back to the front, the shoulder will appear under the pubis if the body descends sufficiently during the last 90° to 130° of the manoeuvre. To make this possible the posterior shoulder must be below the promontory when the rotation begins, whether spontaneously or by traction'.
> Jørgen Løvset
> Shoulder delivery by breech presentation. J Obstet Gynaec Br Emp 1937; 44:696–701

Løvset's Manoeuvre

The principle of this elegant manoeuvre is based on the fact that the inclination of the pelvis is such that the posterior shoulder enters the pelvic cavity in advance of the anterior shoulder. Using the pelvic grip on the fetus the trunk is gently drawn downwards with its back in the oblique anterior position. The body is then lifted to cause upward and lateral flexion, which promotes descent of the posterior shoulder below the sacral promontory. Using gentle traction and rotation the posterior shoulder is rotated through 180° to become the anterior shoulder. As it

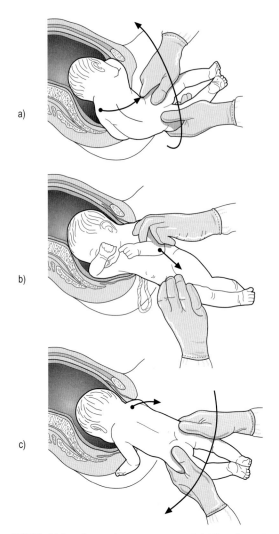

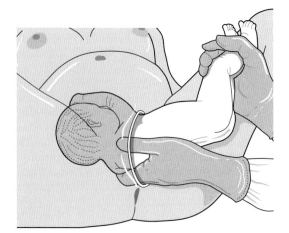

FIGURE 16-9 ■ Bringing down the posterior extended arm.

FIGURE 16-8 ■ Løvset's manoeuvre. (a) The fetus is elevated slightly to facilitate descent of the posterior shoulder below the sacral promontory and then rotated 180°. (b) The posterior shoulder has been rotated to the anterior position and can be delivered. (c) Keeping the back uppermost the body is rotated 180° to allow delivery of the other arm.

started below the pelvic brim it will remain at that level as it rotates to become the anterior shoulder, where it will be easily accessible below the symphysis pubis and the humerus can be swept down across the fetal chest and delivered. Keeping the back uppermost the body is then rotated back 180° bringing the other shoulder into the anterior and accessible position for delivery (Fig 16-8).

Bringing Down the Posterior Arm

This is an alternative to Løvset's manoeuvre, but requires full regional or general anaesthesia.

If the fetal back is toward the mother's right side the operator's right hand grasps the fetal legs and pulls them gently up and over to the mother's left side, which serves to promote descent of the posterior shoulder. The operator's left hand is passed along the spine of the fetus, over its shoulder and laid along the humerus (Fig 16-9). Having reached the fetal shoulder, the index and middle fingers should be placed along the upper arm as far as the bend of the elbow and the arm pushed down across the fetal face. This should bring the humerus and elbow into range to be grasped, splinted and delivered by the whole hand. In the initial manoeuvre it is important not to try and hook the humerus down with one or two fingers or you risk fracture. By pushing it down across the fetal face flexion of the elbow should make the arm more accessible.

Nuchal Arm

On rare occasions, usually because of inappropriate traction and rotational manoeuvres, the shoulder is extended and elbow flexed with the forearm trapped behind the occiput. Attempts to hook down the trapped arm will usually result in fracture of the humerus. Correct treatment is to rotate the fetus in the direction in which the hand is pointing. The occiput slips past the forearm and the friction of the rotation causes the shoulder and elbow to flex and become accessible for delivery (Fig 16-10). In the very rare event of bilateral nuchal arms this type of rotation will assist in releasing one arm but worsen the situation of the other. Thus, gentle rotation is tried in either direction to find which arm can be more easily released first. Rotation

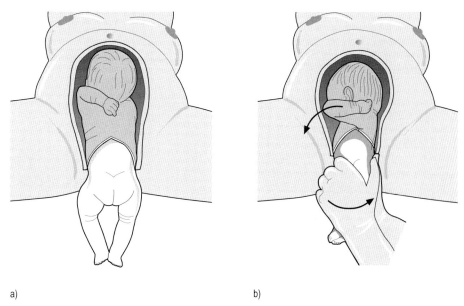

a)   b)

FIGURE 16-10 ■ (a) Nuchal arm. (b) The body is rotated 90° freeing the forearm from the occiput.

in the opposite direction should then allow delivery of the other arm. Bilateral nuchal displacement of the arms is exceptionally rare and can be very difficult to rectify.

Posterior Rotation of the Trunk and Head

This complication should not occur if a competent accoucheur has been in attendance throughout delivery and corrected any tendency of the back to rotate posteriorly. It can happen when the fetal trunk is born before assistance arrives, when of necessity one has to deal with an occipito-posterior position of the head. Even at this stage rotation may often be accomplished using the Mauriceau–Smellie–Veit manoeuvre to elevate and rotate the fetus to the occipito-anterior position. It is very important that the head and trunk are rotated together. If this is accomplished the delivery can be completed either by the Mauriceau–Smellie–Veit manoeuvre or with forceps to the after-coming head.

If rotation is impossible because the head is too firmly fixed low in the pelvis it may be delivered in the occipito-posterior position using the Mauriceau–Smellie–Veit manoeuvre or with forceps. The other alternative is to use the reverse Prague manoeuvre with one hand exerting gentle traction downwards and backwards on the shoulders, while the other lifts the feet to flex the infant and aid delivery of the occiput (Fig 16-11).

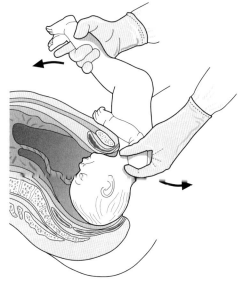

FIGURE 16-11 ■ Reverse Prague manoeuvre to deliver the after-coming head when the occiput is posterior.

Head Entrapment by Incompletely Dilated Cervix

This is one of the most feared complications and, as previously mentioned, all steps should be taken to ensure that the cervix is fully dilated before breech delivery. It is more common in the preterm breech where the small body may easily slip through an incompletely dilated cervix.

Should this occur before the head has descended enough to compress the umbilical cord, every effort should be made to prevent descent of the breech. In a number of these cases, cervical dilatation is occurring quite rapidly and only a few minutes stalling may be required.

If, however, the head has descended so that the cervix encloses the head and chin, the cord will be compressed and delivery must be effected rapidly. If the cervix is sufficiently distensible, forceps may be carefully slipped through the cervix and placed around the head to cradle and protect it while traction guides the head through the cervix to delivery. If the cervix is rigid and unyielding, it will have to be incised at the 4 and 7 o'clock position with long scissors so that the cervix is sufficiently open, but any extension of the incision does not extend upwards and tear the uterine vessels.

BREECH EXTRACTION

Other than in selected cases of the second twin (Chapter 17) this procedure is rarely required in modern obstetrics. It is only justifiable if there is delay in the second stage together with a contraindication to caesarean section, or if the fetus is already dead. Exceptionally, in some geographical circumstances, breech extraction may be performed for cord prolapse at full dilatation in a multiparous patient.

The procedure should be carried out under anaesthesia with uterine relaxation. If the breech has arrested low in the pelvis, groin traction may be all that is required to make the legs accessible and accomplish the rest of the delivery in the manner of an assisted breech delivery. If only the anterior groin is accessible, traction may be provided with the forefinger passed over the thigh and the traction made against the trunk of the fetus. The amount of traction can be increased if the wrist is grasped by the other hand (Fig 16-12). If both the anterior and posterior fetal groins are accessible then a forefinger in each groin is more effective (Fig 16-13). Traction should be applied during a uterine contraction and a generous mediolateral episiotomy performed.

If the breech is higher in the pelvis, such that groin traction will not make the legs accessible, one has to bring down one or both legs. Under anaesthesia and profound uterine relaxation the hand should be passed up along the anterior thigh to beyond the bend of the knee. The lower tibia and foot are then grasped (Fig 16-14). Pinard's manoeuvre, which involves flexing the knee against the fetal abdomen and chest, may

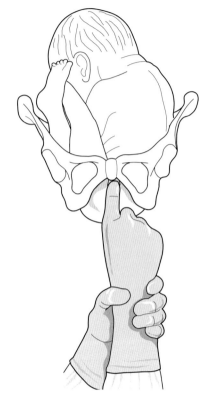

FIGURE 16-12 ■ Breech extraction: traction with forefinger in the anterior groin. The other hand grasps the wrist to allow stronger traction.

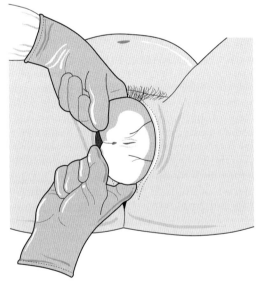

FIGURE 16-13 ■ Traction with a forefinger in each groin.

help make the foot more accessible (Fig 16-15). When reaching up for the ankle the operator should feel for the cord and try and manoeuvre it to the outer side of the hand, so that it lies between the hand and the uterine wall and is less

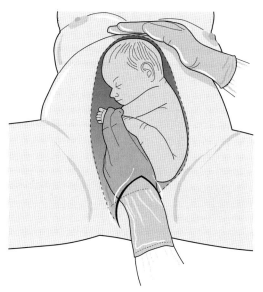

FIGURE 16-14 ■ Breech extraction: bringing down the anterior leg.

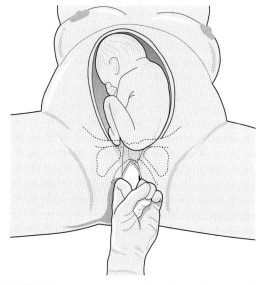

FIGURE 16-16 ■ Breech extraction: if only the posterior leg is brought down, the anterior buttock may be caught up on the pubic symphysis.

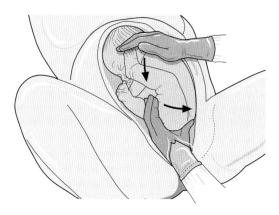

FIGURE 16-15 ■ Breech extraction: Pinard's manoeuvre to make the foot more accessible.

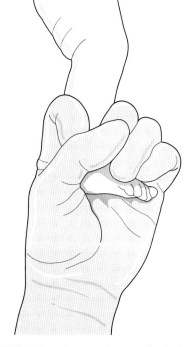

FIGURE 16-17 ■ Breech extraction: method of grasping the foot.

likely to be entangled as the leg is brought down. If possible, the posterior leg should also be brought down. If not, the anterior leg is adequate and if only one leg can be brought down it should always be the anterior one. If only the posterior leg is brought down the anterior buttock may be caught up on the symphysis pubis (Fig 16-16).

Once the anterior or both feet have been brought down the foot or feet are grasped in the manner shown in Figure 16-17. Steady traction should be exerted downwards and backwards in line with the axis of the upper pelvis. If only the anterior leg has been delivered, traction is exerted until the fetal pelvis has been delivered. Rotate the infant so that the posterior hip becomes anterior and the leg is then delivered

with the fingers splinting the femur and flexing the hip and knee upon the fetal abdomen. The remainder of the delivery is performed as for an assisted vaginal delivery. However, because of the traction employed extended arms are more likely to be encountered.

If the posterior leg has been brought down in error, the leg is rotated 180° in a wide arc during downward traction to become the anterior leg.

While this chapter has stressed that the modern standard of care for the term breech is delivery by caesarean section, careful selection and conduct of labour and vaginal breech delivery can bring good perinatal results with less risk to the mother. Depending on circumstances and facilities the obstetrician may be faced with no alternative but to conduct a breech vaginal delivery. Because most breech presentations are now delivered by caesarean section it is important that obstetricians organize a programme of external cephalic version in their practice or hospital in order to reduce the number of infants presenting by the breech. Details of external cephalic version are to be found in Chapter 28.

REFERENCES

1. Hannah ME, Hannah WJ, Hewson SA, Hodnett ED, Saigal S, Willan AR. Planned caesarean section versus planned vaginal birth for breech presentation at term: a randomised multi-centre trial. Term Breech Trial Collaborative Group. Lancet 2000;356:1375–83.
2. Su M, Hannah WJ, Willan A, Ross S, Hannah ME. Planned caesarean section decreases the risk of adverse perinatal outcome due to both labour and delivery complications in the Term Breech Trial. Br J Obstet Gynaecol 2004;111:1065–74.
3. Rietberg CC, Stinkens PME, Visser GHA. The effect of the Term Breech Trial on medical intervention behaviour and neonatal outcome in The Netherlands: an analysis of 35,453 term breech infants. Br J Obstet Gynaecol 2005;112:205–9.
4. Van Roosmalan J, Rosendaal F. There is still room for disagreement about vaginal delivery of breech infants at term. Br J Obstet Gynaecol 2002;109:967–9.
5. Hauth J, Cunningham FG. Vaginal breech delivery is still justified. Obstet Gynecol 2002;99:1115–16.
6. Alarab M, Regan C, O'Connell MP, Keane DP, O'Herlihy C, Foley ME. Singleton vaginal breech delivery at term: still a safe option. Obstet Gynecol 2004;103:407–12.
7. Kotaska A. Inappropriate use of randomized trials to evaluate complex phenomena. BMJ 2004;329:1039–42.
8. Hofmeyer GJ, Hannah ME. Planned caesarean section for term delivery. Cochrane Database Syst Rev 2008;3: CD 000166.
9. Whyte H, Hannah ME, Saigal S, Hannah WJ, Hewson S, Amankwah K, et al. Term Breech Trial Collaborative Group. Outcomes of children at 2 years after planned caesarean birth versus planned vaginal birth for breech presentation at term: The International Randomized Term Breech Trial. Am J Obstet Gynecol 2004;191: 864–71.
10. Su M, Mcleod L, Ross S, Willan A, Hannah WJ, Hutton EK, et al. Factors associated with maternal morbidity in the term breech trial. J Obstet Gynaecol Can 2007;29: 324–30.
11. Turner MJ. The term breech trial: Are the clinical guidelines justified by the evidence? J Obstet Gynaecol 2006; 26:491–4.
12. Goffinet F, Carayol M, Foidart J-M, Alexander S, Uzan S, Subtil D, et al. For the PREMODA Study Group. Is planned vaginal delivery for breech presentation at term still an option? Results of an observational prospective survey in France and Belgium. Am J Obstet Gynecol 2006;194:1002–11.
13. Toivonen E, Palomaki O, Huhtala H, Uotila J. Selective vaginal breech delivery at term –still an option. Acta Obstet Gynaecol Scand 2012;91:1177–83.
14. American College of Obstetricians and Gynecologists. Mode of term singleton breech delivery. Committee Opinion No. 265. Obstet Gynecol 2006;108:235–7.
15. Royal College of Obstetricians and Gynaecologists. The management of breech presentation. Guideline No. 20b. London: RCOG; 2006.
16. Society of Obstetricians and Gynaecologists of Canada. Vaginal delivery of breech presentation. Clinical Practice Guideline No.226. J Obstet Gynaecol Can 2009;31: 557–66.
17. Royal Australian and New Zealand College of Obstetricians and Gynaecologists. Management of the term breech presentation. College Statement C-Obs 11. Melbourne: RANZCOG; 2009.
18. Hehir MP, O'Connor HD, Kent EM, Fitzpatrick C, Boylan PC, Coulter-Smith S, et al. Changes in vaginal breech delivery rates in a single large metropolitan area. Am J Obstet Gynecol 2012;206:498.ei–4.
19. Reddy UM, Zhang J, Sun L, Chen Z, Raju TN, Laughton SK. Neonatal mortality by attempted route of delivery in early preterm birth. Am J Obstet Gynecol 2012;207:e1–8.
20. Chinnock M, Robson S. Obstetric trainees' experience in vaginal breech delivery: implications for future practice. Obstet Gynecol 2007;110:900–3.
21. Queenan JT. Teaching infrequently used skills: vaginal breech delivery. Obstet Gynecol 2004; 103:405–6.
22. Deering S, Brown J, Hodor J, Satin AJ. Simulation training and resident performance of singleton vaginal breech delivery. Obstet Gynecol 2006;107:86–9.
23. Baskett TF. Trends in operative obstetrical delivery: implications for specialist training. Ann R Coll Phys Surg Can 1988;1:119–21.

CHAPTER 17

TWIN AND TRIPLET DELIVERY

JFR Barrett

On Twins: 'It is a constant rule, to keep patients, who have born one child, ignorant of there being another, as long as it can possibly be done'.
  Thomas Denman
    An Introduction to the Practice of Midwifery.
London: J. Johnston, 1795

In recent years the advent of assisted reproductive therapy has resulted in a doubling of the incidence of twins, and a 10-fold increase in triplets.[1] Compared with singleton pregnancies the perinatal mortality, morbidity and long-term neurodevelopmental disability is increased 5–10-fold in twins. Prematurity, low birth weight, congenital anomalies, twin-to-twin transfusion, intrauterine growth restriction, intrapartum asphyxia and trauma are all responsible for these risks.[2]

The second twin is at increased risk during delivery because of malpresentation and placental separation following delivery of the first.[3] A multicentre randomized controlled trial, the Twin Birth Study, has confirmed the safety of vaginal birth in experienced hands.[4] Thus, once again the skills of the obstetric accoucher will be paramount, just as they were when the first edition of this book was published in 1908.

OBSTETRIC FACTORS

Malpresentations

In 60% of twin pregnancies one or both of the twins is non-vertex at the time of delivery; however, the first twin is cephalic in 75–80% of cases. The most common combinations are vertex/vertex (40%), vertex/non-vertex (35–40%) and non-vertex/other (20–25%). The main factor in considering the planned delivery method is the presentation of the first twin. The presentation of the second twin should not be relevant in the decision of the route of delivery, because in about 20% the second twin changes presentation after the first twin has been delivered.[5,6]

Second Twin

The second twin is at increased risk during labour and delivery for two reasons:

1. Placental separation, which reduces oxygen transfer leading to asphyxia. The longer the interval following delivery of the first twin the higher the risk of caesarean delivery for the second twin and the potential for asphyxia (see below).[7,8]

2. Malpresentation and thus vulnerablity to trauma associated with intrauterine manipulations. Some have sought to apply the findings of the Term Breech Trial to the second twin in breech presentation. However, the presentation of the second twin was not related to the risk of adverse outcome in the Twin Birth Study. Furthermore, internal version and breech extraction has been shown to result in a lower incidence of caesarean delivery for the second twin compared to those delivered following external cephalic version.[4]

Individual Considerations

In each case a number of factors will influence the decision for or against labour and vaginal delivery:

- General maternal considerations such as age, parity, infertility and medical complications.
- Potential fetal compromise including fetal growth restriction and abnormal tests of fetal wellbeing are more frequent in twins, and will often lead to delivery by caesarean section.
- Estimated fetal weight. Although there is no evidence to support planned caesarean section for low birth weight twins, many obstetricians will choose this route for those infants less than 32 weeks' gestation or with an estimated fetal weight <1500 g.[9]
- Weight discrepancy. Significant weight discrepancy (>750 g), particularly if twin B is bigger than twin A, is often used as a reason for caesarean delivery. However, the

reproductive history of the mother is relevant; for example, a multiparous woman with previous large babies is unlikely to run into complication at delivery of twin infants, who are usually significantly smaller, even if the second twin is larger than the first.

- Monoamniotic twins are rare but the risk of cord entanglement is high enough to warrant elective caesarean delivery.
- Appropriate facilities and skilled personnel should be available. This involves an obstetrician, anaesthetist and neonatal personnel plus sufficient equipment for two infants.

Maternal Risks

Mothers of twins have a higher risk of maternal morbidity and mortality than singletons.[10–12] The reasons include a higher incidence of anaemia, hypertension and pre-eclampsia, gestational diabetes, postpartum haemorrhage and thromboembolism. In addition, with the high incidence of preterm labour the mother is exposed to the potential risks of tocolytic therapy (see Chapter 9).

ANAESTHETIC FACTORS

Epidural anaesthesia is the analgesic of choice, although for uncomplicated twin delivery inhalation analgesia and pudendal block may be adequate. Less narcotic analgesia is desirable in the preterm fetus and, should intrauterine manipulation or caesarean delivery become necessary, the mother is saved the hazards of rapid induction of general anaesthesia. The anaesthetist should be prepared to provide rapid uterine relaxation with intravenous nitroglycerine (see Chapter 28).

FIRST STAGE OF LABOUR

Currently most authorities recommend induction between 37 and 39 weeks if spontaneous labour does not occur, due to an increase in the stillbirth rate that occurs after this gestation.[13,14] The first stage of labour is managed as a singleton; however, an intravenous infusion should be established. If the presentation of twin A is other than cephalic, caesarean section is usually advisable. Induction of labour and augmentation with oxytocin is used as for a singleton. Both twins should have electronic fetal heart rate monitoring (EFM). Care should be taken that each fetus has a distinct fetal heart rate pattern. The author has seen several cases in which the same twin was

inadvertently monitored, leaving asphyxia undetected. Ideally, a fetal scalp clip should be applied to twin A as soon as possible and twin B monitored externally.[15]

SECOND STAGE OF LABOUR

The necessary anaesthetic, obstetric and neonatal equipment and personnel should be marshalled and the second stage of labour conducted in the operating room. In general the first twin is delivered spontaneously or assisted by forceps or vacuum for the same indications as a singleton. Once delivered, the cord of the first twin should be clamped and 'tagged' and, because there is usually a period of uterine inertia, one should have prepared a solution of oxytocin to 'piggy back' onto the main intravenous line.

> 'Being convinced there is a second child, the membranes must be immediately broke without waiting for pains; and introducing the hand into the womb, to find out the feet, the child must be brought forth by them'.
> Fielding Ould
> A Treatise of Midwifry. Dublin: O. Nelson, 1742, p52

DELIVERY OF THE SECOND TWIN

Once the first twin has been delivered, the lie of the second twin should be established. Ultrasound may help delineate the lie; however, abdominal palpation and vaginal examination will usually confirm the presentation. The following protocol is suggested:

- Continuous EFM should be established.
- If the presentation is cephalic check vaginally to rule out cord presentation, which can also be seen on ultrasound.
- Provided there is no cord, steady the presenting part over the pelvic brim, rupture the membranes and apply the internal scalp electrode. The oxytocin infusion can then be started as needed.
- Provided the fetal heart rate is normal one can wait for spontaneous delivery of the second twin – either cephalic or an assisted breech delivery (see Chapter 16).
- If the second twin is an oblique or transverse lie and the obstetrician is trained in the procedure then a breech extraction with or without internal podalic version should be performed (see Chapters 16 and Chapter 28). If the obstetrician is skilled at this procedure and there is good

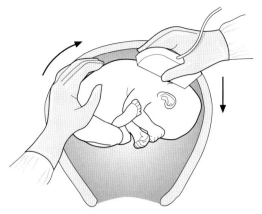

FIGURE 17-1 ■ Use of ultrasound transducer to assist external cephalic version of twin B, while providing continuous observation of the fetal heart rate.

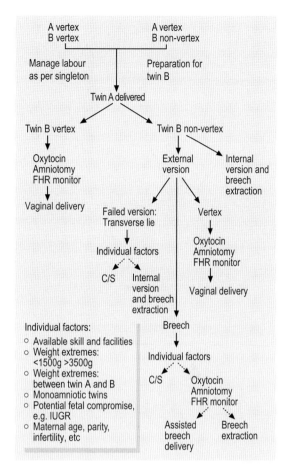

FIGURE 17-2 ■ Intrapartum management of twin pregnancy. (Reproduced with permission from Baskett TF. Essential management of obstetric emergencies. 4th ed. Bristol: Clinical Press, 2004.)

anaesthesia and uterine relaxation this is the method of choice and attended by good results.[5,16,17]

- For those not trained in the above, external cephalic version may be attempted (Fig 17-1) (see Chapter 28).
- If difficulty is encountered with either of these methods, then caesarean section for the second twin may have to be chosen. This may be seen by some as an 'obstetrical defeat'. However, it is better to accept this than risk trauma or asphyxia of the fetus.[18,19]
- If there is a non-reassuring fetal heart rate pattern, intrapartum bleeding or cord prolapse delivery of the second twin will have to be accelerated. If the fetus is in low vertex presentation, forceps or vacuum assisted delivery should be feasible. If the fetal head is at a higher station in the mid-pelvis or at the pelvic brim the vacuum is the better option. It is essential that the vacuum be placed over the flexion point so that the narrowest diameter is presented (see Chapter 10). If the fetus is in breech presentation then breech extraction should be considered. A summary of the intrapartum management is outlined in Figure 17-2.

In the Twin Birth Study, a large international randomized-controlled trial, obstetricians skilled in the conduct of twin vaginal birth used the above protocol. The study showed that planned vaginal birth was not associated with an increased risk of perinatal mortality or morbidity compared to planned caesarean delivery for twins >32 weeks. The result was not affected by parity, chorionicity or presentation of the second twin.[4]

THIRD STAGE OF LABOUR

The over-distended uterus is very prone to uterine atony. Thus, active management of the third stage of labour should be carried out and intravenous oxytocin kept running for 8 hours.

> 'The method of extracting the second immediately after the first child, is never practised by the female adventurers in the art of midwifery; for they leave it all to nature; cutting the funis, tying it to the mother's thigh; they wait for a new labour; and the waters gathering which the poor patient is seldom able to undergo, being much weakened and fatigued by what she has already suffered; yet it sometimes happens, that she has a full week between the bringing forth of two children, and frequently two to three days'.
>   Fielding Ould
>   A Treatise of Midwifry. Dublin: O. Nelson, 1742, p55

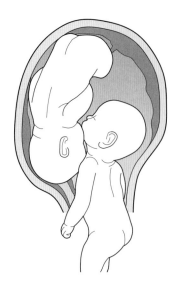

FIGURE 17-3 ■ Locked twins: breech/vertex.

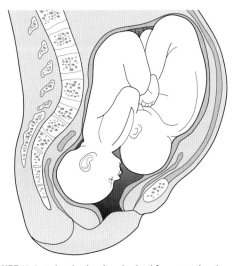

FIGURE 17-4 ■ Locked twins: locked fore-coming heads.

LOCKED TWINS

This is an extremely rare condition occurring in about 1 in 1000 twin gestations; most commonly breech/vertex (Fig 17-3) and vertex/vertex (Fig 17-4). There are two management options:
1. Under anaesthesia and with profound uterine relaxation it may be possible to disimpact the interlocking parts by elevating the first twin and pushing away the second twin.[20]
2. Classical caesarean section.

Historically, decapitation of the first twin using the Blond–Heidler saw may be employed, a manoeuvre associated with risk of rupture of the lower uterine segment (see Chapter 28).

CONJOINED TWINS

Conjoined twins are exceptionally rare and require delivery by caesarean section.[21]

TRIPLETS AND HIGHER-ORDER MULTIPLE PREGNANCY

In many developed countries assisted reproductive techniques have increased the incidence of triplets to 1 in 500–1000 of all deliveries. Maternal morbidity and perinatal morbidity and mortality are higher in triplets compared with both singleton and twin pregnancies.[22] In most hospitals all viable triplet pregnancies are delivered by elective caesarean section because:
- The first presenting fetus of triplets is other than vertex in about one-third of cases.
- The chances of a malpresentation of the second and third of triplets is high.
- There is difficulty in monitoring three fetuses simultaneously.
- There is a need for three neonatal teams at delivery; it is easier to marshal the required personnel for an elective rather than an emergency delivery.

Few centres have enough experience to provide adequate comparison between triplets delivered vaginally as compared to caesarean. Individual hospitals will have to make their own decisions based on local facilities, personnel and experience.[23–26]

REFERENCES

1. Van Voorhis BJ. Outcomes from assisted reproductive technology. Obstet Gynecol 2006;107:183–200.
2. Blondel B, Kogan MD, Alexander GR, Dattani N, Kramer MS, MacFArlane A, et al. The impact of the increasing number of multiple births on the rates of preterm birth and low birthweight: an international study. Am J Public Health 2002;92:1323–30.
3. Hofmeyr GJ, Barrett JF, Crowther CA. Planned caesarean section for women with a twin pregnancy. Cochrane Database Syst Rev 2011;(12):CD006553.
4. Barrett J, Aztaloz E, Willan A, et al. The Twin Birth Study: A multicentre RCT of planned (cs) and planned (VB) for twin Pregnancies. Am J Obstet Gynecol 2013;208(1):S4.
5. Adam C, Allen AC, Baskett TF. Twin delivery: influence of the presentation and method of delivery on the second twin. Am J Obstet Gynecol 1991;165:23–7.
6. Barrett JFR, Ritchie JWK. Twin delivery. Best Prac Res Clin Obstet Gynaecol 2002;16:43–56.
7. Leung TY, Tam WH, Leung TN, Lok IH, Lau TK. Effect of twin-to-twin delivery interval on umbilical cord blood gas in the second twin. Br J Obstet Gynaecol 2002; 109:63–7.
8. Leung TY, Lok IH, Tam WH, Leung TN, Lau TK. Deterioration in cord blood status during the second stage of labour is more rapid in the second twin than

in the first twin. Br J Obstet Gynaecol 2004;111: 546–9.

9. Hutton E, Barrett J, Hannah M. Use of external cephalic version for breech pregnancy and mode of delivery for breech and twin pregnancy: a survey of Canadian practitioners. J Obstet Gynaecol Can 2002;24:804–10.

10. Bouvier-Colle MH, Varnox N, Salanave B. Case-control study of risk factors for obstetric patients admission to intensive care units. Eur J Obstet Gynecol Reprod Biol 1997;74:173–7.

11. Baskett TF, O'Connell CM. Maternal critical care in obstetrics. J Obstet Gynaecol Can 2009;31:218–21.

12. Blickstein I. Maternal mortality in twin gestations. J Reprod Med 1997;42:680–4.

13. Breathnach FM, McAuliffe FM, Geary M, Daly S, Higgins JR, Dornan J, et al for the Perinatal Ireland Research Consortium. Optimum timing for planned delivery of uncomplicated monochorionic and dichorionic twin pregnancies. Obstet Gynecol 2012;119: 50–9.

14. Dodd JM, Crowther CA, Haslam RR, Robinson JS. Elective birth at 37 weeks of gestation versus standard care for women with an uncomplicated twin pregnancy at term: the Twins Timing of Birth Randomised Trial. BMC Pregnancy and Childbirth 2010;10:68–74.

15. Barrett J, Bocking A. The Society of Obstetricians and Gynaecologists of Canada. Consensus statement on management of twin pregnancies (part I). J Obstet Gynaecol Can 2000;22:519–29.

16. Boggess KA, Chisholm CA. Delivery of the nonvertex second twin: a review of the literature. Obstet Gynecol Surv 1997;52:728–35.

17. Pschera H, Jonasson A. Is cesarean section justified for delivery of the second twin? Acta Obstet Gynecol Scand 1988;67:381–2.

18. Persad VL, Baskett TF, O'Connell CM, Scott HM. Combined vaginal-cesarean delivery of twin pregnancies. Obstet Gynecol 2001;98:1032–7.

19. Wen SW, Fung KF, Oppenheimer L, Demissie K, Yang Q, Walker M. Occurrence and predictors of cesarean delivery for the second twin after vaginal delivery of the first twin. Obstet Gynecol 2004;103:413–9.

20. Saad FA, Sharara HA. Locked twins: a successful outcome after applying the Zavanelli manoeuvre. J Obstet Gynaecol 1997;17:366–7.

21. Bianchi A, Maresh M, Rimmer S. Conjoined twins. In: Hillard T, Purdie D, editors. The yearbook of obstetrics and gynaecology. London: RCOG Press; 2004;11: 37–47.

22. Cassell KA, O'Connell CM, Baskett TF. The origins and outcomes of triplet and quadruplet pregnancies: 1980 to 2001. Am J Perinatol 2004;21:439–45.

23. Wildshut HIJ, Van Roosmalen J, Van Leeuwen E, Keirse MJNC. Planned abdominal compared with planned vaginal birth in triplet pregnancies. Br J Obstet Gynaecol 1995;102:292–6.

24. Dommergues M, Mahieu-Caputo D, Mandelbrot L, Huon C, Moriette C, Dumez Y. Delivery of uncomplicated triplet pregnancies: is the vaginal route safer? A case-control study. Am J Obstet Gynecol 1995;172: 513–7.

25. Dommergues M, Mahieu-Caputo D, Dumez Y. Is the route of delivery a meaningful issue in triplets and higher order multiples? Clin Obstet Gyneol 1998;41:25–9.

26. American College of Obstetricians and Gynecologists. Practice Bulletin No. 56. Multiple Gestation: Complicated twin, triplet, and high-order multi-fetal pregnancy. Obstet Gynecol 2004;104:869–83.

CHAPTER 18

CORD PROLAPSE

TF Baskett

'Yet sometimes the navel string falls down and comes before it; for which cause the child is in much danger of death ... As soon as 'tis perceived, you must immediately endeavor to put it back, to prevent the cooling of it, behind the child's head, lest it be bruised ... But sometimes, not withstanding all these cautions, and the putting back of it, it will yet come forth every pain; then without further delay, the chirurgeon must bring the child forth by the feet, which he must search for, tho the infant comes with the head; for there is but this only means to save the child's life.'
Francois Mauriceau
The Diseases of Women with Child, and in Child-Bed. London: John Darby, 1663, p255

Prolapse of the umbilical cord is the classic obstetric emergency. It occurs when the membranes are ruptured and part of the cord lies below the presenting part of the fetus. Cord presentation is the same situation with intact membranes – a much rarer diagnosis. Over the past century the incidence of cord prolapse has decreased from about 1 in 150 to 1 in 500 deliveries; probably due to most malpresentations being delivered by caesarean section and more active management of the preterm fetus.[1-4] Similarly, in well-equipped hospitals, the perinatal mortality has fallen over the past 50 years from 50–60% to 2–15%.[2,4]

The risk to the fetus is the loss of umbilical blood flow to and from the placenta with consequent hypoxia due to physical compression of the blood vessels in the cord, or spasm of the blood vessels due to the colder temperature if the cord prolapses outside the vagina.

PREDISPOSING FACTORS

The following conditions may interfere with the close application of the fetal presenting part to the lower uterine segment and cervix and therefore predispose to cord prolapse.[4-8]

Fetal

- Malpresentations such as complete and footling breech, transverse and oblique lie.
- Prematurity: the premature fetus is more likely to lie in malpresentation and, in addition, the small size of the presenting part may facilitate prolapse of the cord.
- Fetal anomaly: the abnormal fetus is more likely to lie in an abnormal position and may have an irregular presenting part (e.g. anencephaly).
- Multiple pregnancy has a higher association with prematurity and malpresentations.

Maternal

- High parity, associated with lax uterine musculature and a high presenting part.
- Contracted pelvis.
- Pelvic tumours, such as a cervical fibroid.

Placental

- Minor degree of placenta praevia. The lower edge of the placenta elevates the fetal presenting part and the insertion of the umbilical cord is nearer the cervix and more prone to prolapse.

Amniotic Fluid

- Polyhydramnios is more often associated with malpresentation or a high presenting part. In addition, the cascade of a large volume of amniotic fluid when the membranes rupture increases the likelihood of washing down the cord.
- Prelabour rupture of the membranes.
- Amniotomy to induce or augment labour is often given as a risk factor, but provided it is appropriately carried out is no more likely to lead to cord prolapse than spontaneous rupture of the membranes.[9,10] Furthermore, should cord prolapse occur it is better that it is detected and managed as soon as possible.

Cord

- Long umbilical cord.

Obstetric Manipulation

- Manual or forceps rotation of the fetal head.
- Version.
- Amnioinfusion.

Many of the above factors are interrelated, with the main culprits being prematurity, malpresentations and multiple pregnancy.

DIAGNOSIS

On rare occasions, cord prolapse may be obvious with the dramatic appearance of a loop of umbilical cord at the introitus, usually shortly after spontaneous rupture of the membranes. The most common method of diagnosis is by vaginal examination and this should be carried out in all women with predisposing factors to cord prolapse. Thus, all women with breech presentations should have a vaginal examination immediately after spontaneous rupture of the membranes. Similarly, when fetal heart rate abnormalities are noted, particularly the cord compression pattern of variable or prolonged decelerations, a vaginal examination should be undertaken to exclude cord prolapse. Failure to perform vaginal examination in the presence of an abnormal fetal heart rate pattern is the commonest cause of delay in diagnosis and worsening of perinatal outcome.[8] A loop or loops of cord may be obvious on vaginal examination but, on occasions, the presentation can be quite subtle with a loop just beside and barely below the presenting part (Fig 18-1).

With the increased availability of ultrasound on labour wards, the diagnosis of cord presentation can be made in cases with predisposing factors before rupture of the membranes.[11] However, cord presentation on antenatal ultrasound examination reverted to the normal position during labour in about half the cases in one study.[12] Occasionally, loops of cord can be felt through the intact membranes below the presenting part.

MANAGEMENT

In general, the perinatal outcome is related to the detection–delivery interval, although with the application of the techniques outlined below, longer delays can be associated with good results.[8]

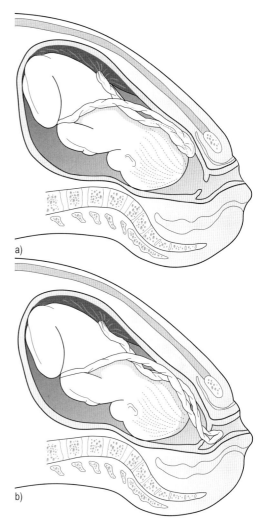

FIGURE 18-1 ■ (a) Occult cord prolapse. (b) Prolapsed cord.

Immediate Relief of Cord Compression

This is the first approach in all cases. If the cord has prolapsed outside the vagina it is gently cradled in the hand and replaced in the vagina. Even if the cord has only prolapsed into the vagina, similar gentle cradling should be performed to relieve pressure on the cord from the vaginal walls. The tips of the fingers are further advanced through the cervix to the presenting part to ensure that it is not compressing the cord against the cervix or bony pelvis. The cord must be handled as gently as possible as excessive manipulation may cause spasm of the vessels (Fig 18-2).

In addition to this manual replacement and protection of the cord the patient should be placed in the knee–chest position so that gravity

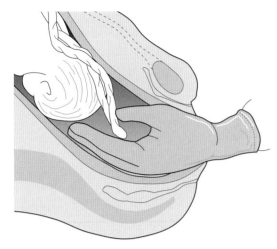

FIGURE 18-2 ■ Manual relief of cord compression.

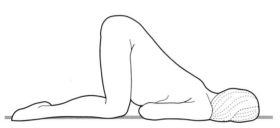

FIGURE 18-3 ■ Knee–chest position for immediate relief of cord compression.

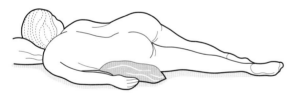

FIGURE 18-4 ■ Sims' lateral position.

also becomes an assistant (Fig 18-3). This position is undignified and exhausting to maintain for any length of time so that repositioning to the Sims' lateral position, with a pillow under one hip and the bed or trolley in Trendelenburg position is more practical (Fig 18-4). If the baby is viable, and delivery by immediate caesarean section is feasible, these manoeuvres are maintained while the patient is transferred to the operating theatre for delivery.

Fetal Assessment

Once cord compression has been relieved one must decide whether the fetus is viable. If the fetus is dead, too immature to survive, or has a lethal anomaly then intervention for fetal reasons is contraindicated and labour should be allowed to continue to vaginal delivery.

In most cases one can be reassured that the fetus is alive by palpating the pulsations in the prolapsed cord. This can be done by feeling the loop between two fingers or gently palpating it against the vaginal wall or presenting part. Take care to palpate in between contractions when any cord compression is released. If available a scalp electrode can be applied which, if it produces a normal tracing, allows a more orderly approach. An ultrasound transducer may also be used for this purpose. Even if cord pulsations cannot be felt the fetus may still be alive and this should be checked by ultrasound of the fetal thorax.[13]

The gestational age at which the infant is regarded as viable will depend on the level of neonatal care available.

A lethal anomaly may be known from the antenatal record or obvious on examination (e.g. anencephaly).

Delay in Transfer of Patient for Delivery

If umbilical cord prolapse occurs outside hospital or there is delay before the infant can be delivered the following approach can be used. After the initial attempts at cord decompression have been successful, the patient is guided to the Sims' lateral position, a Foley catheter placed and the bladder filled to approximately 500 ml.[14] This should elevate the presenting part and help relieve cord compression. One should check with the vaginal hand that this is the case, and if so the hand can be removed. A case can be made for filling the bladder in most cases at the time of diagnosis in case there is an unpredictable delay or, should the fetal heart be normal and stable, to allow time for spinal anaesthesia as opposed to rapid and more risky general anaesthesia.

Filling the bladder may also help inhibit uterine contractions. However, if uterine contractions start or continue, tocolysis with terbutaline may be indicated (see Chapter 28).

'In my experience, the best repositor is a thick roll of gauze. Quantities of this are pushed into the uterus well above the presenting part: the cord is entangled in the gauze. Now the gauze must be thick – thin gauze is of no use. I most strongly recommend this very simple device.'
    Munro Kerr
    Operative obstetrics. 4th edn. London: Balliere, Tindall and Cox, 1937, p207

'The late Dr. Mackenzie, than whom I have not known a man more intelligent in conversation, or more excellent in practice, informed me of another method which he has tried. Instead of attempting to replace the descended funis in the common way, he brought down as much more of it as would come with ease, and then enclosed the whole mass in a small bag made of soft leather, gently drawn together with a string, like the mouth of a purse. The whole of the descended funis, inclosed in this bag, was conveniently returned, and remained beyond the head of the child till this was expelled; and the bag containing the funis having escaped compression, the child was born living. But he very ingenuously told me, that he had afterwards made several other trials in the same manner without success.'

Thomas Denman
An Introduction to the Practice of Midwifery. New York: E. Bliss and E. White, 1825, p545–546

Replacement of Cord

Before the era of safe caesarean section many ingenious techniques were devised attempting, with varied success, to replace the cord behind the presenting part. In modern obstetrics there are only rare occasions when conditions favour this approach.[15] Should cord prolapse of a minor degree occur with a cephalic presentation it is occasionally feasible to manually replace the cord up above the head to the nuchal area of the fetus. Fetal heart rate monitoring should be carried out to ensure that any cord compression pattern does not recur. This technique is only rarely applicable and, unless successful with minimal handling of the cord, one should not persist.

Delivery

If cord prolapse occurs at full cervical dilatation with the presenting part in a position and station that allows safe vaginal delivery, breech extraction or vacuum/forceps assisted delivery may be undertaken. If not, caesarean section is the method of choice.

In many instances this requires general anaesthesia. However, if the above measures have been successful in relieving cord compression and the fetal heart is stable and monitored continuously, spinal anaesthesia may be feasible with less risk to the mother. If the vaginal hand is elevating the presenting part, a Foley catheter is placed to empty the bladder and, as the uterine incision is made, the hand is removed. If the full bladder technique has been used to elevate the presenting part, the catheter is opened and the bladder drained just before the caesarean section is started.

Simulation team training of labour ward personnel has been shown to reduce the diagnosis–delivery interval in cases of cord prolapse.[16]

While decisive speed is of the essence in this classic obstetric emergency, the calm and systematic approach outlined above will usually produce good perinatal results with least risk to the mother.

REFERENCES

1. Panter KR, Hannah ME. Umbilical cord prolapse: so far so good? Lancet 1996;347:74.
2. Murphy DJ, Mackenzie IZ. The mortality and morbidity associated with umbilical cord prolapse. Br J Obstet Gynaecol 1995;102:826–30.
3. Nizard J, Cromi A, Molendijk H, Arabin B. Neonatal outcome following prolonged umbilical cord prolapse in preterm premature rupture of membranes. Br J Obstet Gynaecol 2005;112:833–6.
4. Gannard–Pechin E, Rannah R, Cossa S, Mulin B, Maillet R, Riethmuller D. Umbilical cord prolapse: a case study over 23 years. J Gynecol Obstet Reprod (Paris) 2012;41:574–83.
5. Critchlow CW, Leet TL, Benedetti TJ, Daling JR. Risk factors and infant outcomes associated with umbilical cord prolapse: a population-based case-control study among births in Washington State. Am J Obstet Gynecol 1994;170:613–18.
6. Boyle JJ, Katz VL. Umbilical cord prolapse in current obstetric practice. J Reprod Med 2005;50:303–6.
7. Lin MG. Umbilical cord prolapse. Obstet Gynecol Surv 2006;61:269–77.
8. Royal College of Obstetricians and Gynaecologists. Umbilical Cord Prolapse. Green-top Guideline No. 50. London: RCOG; 2008.
9. Yla-Outinen A, Heinonen PK, Tuimala R. Predisposing and risk factors of umbilical cord prolapse. Acta Obstet Gynecol Scand 1985;64:567–70.
10. Roberts WE, Martin RW, Roach HH, Perry KG, Martin JN, Morrison JC. Are obstetric interventions such as cervical ripening, induction of labor, amnioinfusion or amniotomy associated with umbilical cord prolapse? Am J Obstet Gynecol 1997;176:1181–3.
11. Jones G, Grenier S, Gruslin A. Sonographic diagnosis of funic presentation: implications for delivery. Br J Obstet Gynaecol 2000;107:1055–7.
12. Ezra Y, Strasberg SR, Farine D. Does cord presentation on ultrasound predict cord prolapse? Gynaecol Obstet Invest 2003;56:6–9.
13. Driscoll JA, Sadan O, Van Gelderen CJ, Holloway GA. Cord prolapse – can we save more babies? Br J Obstet Gynaecol 1987;94:594–5.
14. Runnenbaum IB, Katz M. Intrauterine resuscitation by rapid urinary bladder installation in a case of occult prolapse of excessively long umbilical cord. Eur J Obstet Gynecol Reprod Biol 1999;84:101–2.
15. Barrett JM. Funic reduction for the management of umbilical cord prolapse. Am J Obstet Gynecol 1991;165:654–7.
16. Siassakos D, Hasafa Z, Sibanda T, Fox R, Donald F, Winter C, Draycott T. Retrospective cohort study of diagnosis-delivery interval with umbilical cord prolapse: the effect of team training. Br J Obstet Gynaecol 2009; 116:1089–93.

ANTEPARTUM HAEMORRHAGE

JCP Kingdom

Antepartum haemorrhage (APH) refers to bleeding from the genital tract after 20 weeks of gestation, which is 4–6 weeks below the lower limit of fetal viability. Establishing the cause of APH is important to distinguish scenarios at risk of substantial haemorrhage, such as major placenta praevia or abruption, from a range of possibilities that pose much lower risks (Table 19-1). Cases with serious underlying causes of vaginal bleeding, such as caesarean section scar pregnancy,[1] may present with vaginal bleeding before 20 weeks. Furthermore, the identification of a benign lower genital tract source of minor vaginal bleeding does not preclude an additional more serious uterine cause of APH. The two most serious causes are placental abruption and placenta praevia; the latter is becoming more common, due in part to a greater prevalence of: previous uterine surgery, assisted reproductive technologies, multifetal pregnancy and advanced maternal age.[2] Major abruption is much less common due to general advances in maternal health, including a large reduction in smoking, and improvements in antenatal care. Historically, the first description of placenta praevia in 1885 was by the Parisian physician, Paul Portal (1630–1703), who was the first to describe the attachment of the placenta to the lower uterine segment.

FIRST DESCRIPTION OF PLACENTA PRAEVIA

'I put my fingers into the orifice and felt the after birth which covered the orifice of the matrix from all sides and adhered in all its parts with the exception of the middle'.
   Paul Portal
   La Pratique des Accouchements Soutenue d'un Grand Nombre d'Observations. Paris: G. Martin, 1685.

The elegant, yet poignant, drawings of this disease from partially dissected dead women by the Scot, William Hunter (1718–1783), living in London, are a vivid reminder of the danger of placenta praevia, which still exists in many countries today.[3] The terms 'unavoidable ' referring to placenta praevia and 'accidental ' referring to placental abruption are attributed from 1775 to Edward Rigby (1747–1821) of Norwich, England. The historical background of placenta praevia has been documented.[4,5]

PLACENTA PRAEVIA

Placenta praevia occurs when the entire placenta, or in part, implants in the lower uterine segment after 20 weeks' gestation. The incidence varies by population but significant disease occurs in about 1/200 deliveries.[6] Perinatal mortality is increased almost twofold compared to non-praevia pregnancies adjusted for smoking, maternal age, parity and in vitro fertilization.[6] The risk factors for placenta praevia are summarized in Table 19-2. Some of these, in particular multiple previous caesarean deliveries and previous placenta praevia, confer recurrence risks of up to 5%. Finally, the increasing use of 18–20-week ultrasound examinations to assess fetal anatomy has increased the rate of diagnosis of asymptomatic minor degrees of placenta praevia.[7] An abnormally large placenta surface area predisposes to placenta praevia, the most common cause being multifetal pregnancy; amongst the rare causes, careful consideration of a succenturiate lobe in the lower segment is important, since it is associated with vasa praevia, which, when undiagnosed, may result in fetal mortality.[8] Twin pregnancies have a 50% greater risk of placenta praevia.[9]

Classification

The classical method describes four types, or degrees, of placenta praevia as illustrated in Figure 19-1. With additional descriptive terminology, these are as follows:
- Type 1 (low-lying): the lower edge of the placenta is inside the lower uterine segment but does not reach the internal cervical os.

- Type 2 (marginal): the lower edge of the placenta extends to but not across the internal os.
- Types 1 and 2 are commonly observed in asymptomatic women at the 18–20-week transabdominal fetal anatomy ultrasound examination. The distinction between the two, by transvaginal ultrasound, is unimportant at this stage, since in both instances, the likelihood of clinically significant placenta praevia in the third trimester is very small.
- Type 3 (partial): the lower edge of the placenta extends asymmetrically across the internal os; however, since the portion of the placenta covering the internal os is thin, it may pull away with minimal vaginal

bleeding during cervical effacement and dilation to permit safe vaginal delivery.
- Type 4 (complete or central): the placenta is almost centrally placed within the lower uterine segment.

With few exceptions the distinction between type 3 and 4 placenta praevia is not important in high-resource countries, because the risk/benefit

TABLE 19-1 Causes of Antepartum Haemorrhage

Site	Diagnosis
Uterine	Placenta praevia
	Abruption
	Placenta praevia increta
	Antepartum fetal death
Cervix	Cervical ectropion/congestion
	Cervical pregnancy
	Cancer of the cervix
Lower genital tract	Vulvo-vaginal varices
	Vulvo-vaginal infections
	Malignancies
	Trauma
Unclassified	Cervical effacement

TABLE 19-2 Risk Factors for Placenta Praevia

Category	Risk Factor
Maternal	Smoking
	Advanced maternal age
Obstetric history	High parity, twins
	Assisted reproductive technologies
	Previous placenta praevia
Uterine	Uterine surgery
	Caesarean sections
	Myomectomy
	Hysteroscopic surgery
	Septum
	Adhesions
Placental	Multifetal pregnancies
	Enlarged placenta
	High altitude
	Chronic fetal anaemia
	Abnormal placental development
	Succenturiate lobe (vasa praevia)
	Bi-lobar placenta
	Placenta membranacea

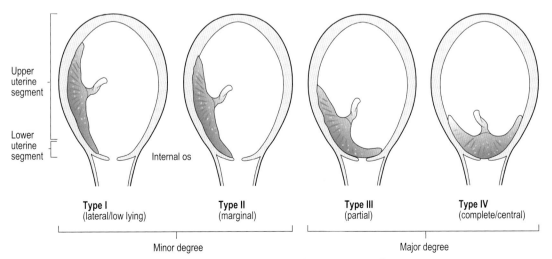

Upper uterine segment

Lower uterine segment

Internal os

Type I (lateral/low lying)   Type II (marginal)   Type III (partial)   Type IV (complete/central)

Minor degree   Major degree

FIGURE 19-1 ■ Classification of placenta praevia.

ratio of planned caesarean delivery outweighs that of attempting vaginal delivery. Exceptions would include: previous vaginal deliveries in a highly motivated and well-informed individual; and anticipation of a difficult caesarean, for example, due to morbid obesity. In other healthcare settings, especially those in which accurate transvaginal ultrasound imaging is not readily available to distinguish these types, the use of the term 'type 3' to describe transabdominal ultrasound findings implies that a proportion of women in labour with a small amount of placenta across the os can deliver safely by the vaginal route because during cervical effacement and dilation the small area of disrupted placenta may not bleed significantly.

The wide application of high resolution transabdominal and transvaginal ultrasound has largely obviated the need to describe four categories of placenta praevia, such that the disease is now commonly described as minor praevia (types 1 and 2) and major praevia (types 3 and 4) that respectively do not or do require elective caesarean delivery.

Physiology of the Lower Uterine Segment

In the non-pregnant state the uterus is comprised of just two parts, a corpus and cervix, the boundary between which is a fibro-muscular junction described originally by Danforth.[10] The lower uterine segment begins to form in the second trimester, once the gestation sac has fully occupied the uterine cavity; thereafter maternal tissue below the apex of the fetal membranes is considered the cervix and the junction is the internal os (Fig 19-2a). The lower uterine segment gradually forms, via myometrial growth and thinning, from the tissue above and below the internal os. As such, the cervix gradually shortens as pregnancy advances[11] while failure to do so increases the risk of caesarean section for dystocia.[12] Formation of the lower uterine segment provides one-third of uterine volume for fetal growth and is normally occupied by the fetal head from 34 weeks' gestation. Sonographically, the upper margin of the lower uterine segment is the reflection of the utero-vesical peritoneum at the upper edge of the semi-filled bladder (Fig 19-2a). In labour, the upper active uterine segment (the fundus) provides the driving force for labour, placental detachment and subsequent mechanical haemostasis. By contrast, the lower uterine segment is a passive structure in normal labour; at caesarean section for obstructed labour it may balloon out significantly and be a source of primary postpartum haemorrhage. In the labour and delivery setting, the lower uterine segment is defined pragmatically as that 6–8 cm portion of the uterine cavity palpable digitally in women with either regional or general anaesthesia following delivery of the placenta.

Placental 'Migration'

Gradual formation of the lower uterine segment is sometimes described as 'placental migration'. The forces underlying this phenomenon may cause the lower placental edge to bleed, even in women with type 1 or 2 praevia. Nevertheless, this migration means that at least 90% of low-lying placentas will resolve, leaving about 1 in 200 women with clinically significant placenta praevia after 34 weeks. The almost universal use of ultrasound at 19–20 weeks has the capacity to over-diagnose minor degrees of placenta praevia in asymptomatic women (Fig 19-2a). Advice on safe mode of delivery in this context can all too easily err on the side of caution and caesarean delivery; yet many options, described in Chapter 20, exist to manage postpartum haemorrhage effectively. The previous generally accepted standard was to recommend caesarean where the lower placental edge is <2 cm from the internal os in the third trimester.[13] However, the lower uterine segment continues to form, especially with cervical shortening and effacement from Braxton Hicks contractions. More recent evidence suggests that the majority of women with no other risk factors can achieve safe vaginal delivery if the lower placental edge is >1 cm from the internal os.[14] A flexible policy of serial transvaginal ultrasound in borderline situations can save some women from unnecessary caesarean delivery (Fig 19-2b,c).

Assessment of Vaginal Bleeding from Placenta Praevia

Around 80% of all women with major placenta praevia will have one or more bleeds before delivery. The first is a warning, or 'sentinel' bleed. Any subsequent bleeds are likely to be heavier. In general, major degrees of placenta praevia bleed earlier, more frequently and more heavily than do minor degrees. Nevertheless, even a complete placenta praevia may not bleed until either the onset of labour (if undiagnosed) or simply presentation with an oblique or transverse lie in the clinic after 34 weeks. Bleeding from placenta praevia is most commonly caused by disruption of small uteroplacental veins as the anchored placenta is gradually stretched. This maternal source of blood may escape through the decidua and enter the myometrium.

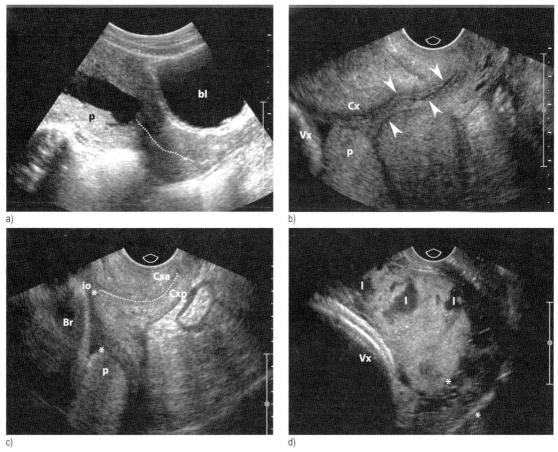

a)

b)

c)

d)

FIGURE 19-2 ■ Placenta praevia. (a) Ultrasound imaging of the lower uterine segment and saggital view at 18 weeks demonstrating a normal closed cervix (dashed line, length 46 mm) and a posterior placenta (p) that is 2.4 cm from the internal os. The maternal bladder (bl) is full. The lower uterine segment (LUS) is that part of the lower segment above the internal os and behind the bladder. Technically at this stage the lower edge of the placenta is within the LUS though it will migrate upwards as gestation advances. (b) Transvaginal ultrasound demonstrating posterior type 3 placenta praevia (p) at 22 weeks' gestation. Arrowheads indicate the cervical canal. Vx, vertex. (c) Corresponding transvaginal image at 28 weeks. Dashed line indicates the cervical canal. Note that the edge of the posterior placenta praevia (p) is now 2.4 cm (*–*) from the internal os (io). Cxa, anterior lip of cervix; Cxp, posterior lip of cervix; Br, breech. (d) Transvaginal ultrasound diagnosis of invasive placenta. Note multiple large lakes (l) in the placenta and expanded vascular myometrium beneath the placental tissue (*–*). Vx, vertex.

Thrombin, the local product of pathological haemorrhage, is a powerful myometrial irritant[15] and may explain why uterine contractions can accompany bleeding from placenta praevia. Maternal tocolysis may arrest ongoing APH and extend the duration of pregnancy.[16]

Transvaginal ultrasound may be useful to predict preterm birth in placenta praevia; at 32–33 weeks, a cervical length <30 mm conferred a threefold risk of subsequent delivery for haemorrhage and preterm birth.[17] A prominent marginal sinus at the lower edge also predicts the need for caesarean delivery due to vaginal bleeding.[18] Transvaginal ultrasound therefore provides useful predictors of recurrent bleeding and thus the need to remain in hospital if undelivered

following the sentinel bleed. Unexpectedly severe vaginal bleeding from a known minor placenta praevia may be due to a prominent marginal placental sinus where uterine venous blood drains out of the lower edge of the placenta. Transvaginal ultrasound is a valuable assessment tool in stable women following a sentinel bleed. Where vaginal bleeding with placenta praevia is seen, the rare accompaniment of gross haematuria should immediately raise the suspicion of associated invasive placentation (see below and Figures 19-2d and 19-9).

The importance of careful evaluation of women with a 'warning bleed' from placenta praevia was dramatically illustrated by Munro Kerr in an earlier edition:

Betke–Kliehauer (BK) test > 10 ml indicating a significant feto-maternal bleed is rare in placenta praevia[27] and would be an indication for delivery > 32 weeks. Likewise, cervical length < 30 mm on transvaginal ultrasound assessment confers a threefold increased risk of subsequent APH and preterm delivery < 37 weeks, which is presumably due to subclinical labour provoking bleeding.[17] The main elements of expectant management in hospital are as follows:

(a) Admission and bed rest with bathroom privileges
(b) Diagnose and treat anaemia
(c) Anaesthesia consultation
(d) Continuous cross-match of at least 2 units packed red cells
(e) Identify and arrange a date for elective caesarean and obtain consents – discuss and document type of surgery including desire for tubal ligation
(f) Rhesus-D-negative women with no antibodies should receive Anti-D.

When major placenta praevia is found in the context of an APH and a viable fetus, women are best advised to remain in hospital until delivery. If clinically stable, with no further bleeding, they can receive prophylactic daily heparin for thromboprophylaxis (especially if age > 40 and/or overweight, or have received a blood transfusion), otherwise they can be fitted with compression stockings. Women with minor placenta praevia, an isolated APH and no unusual considerations (such as poor ambulatory access to care) are often discharged home for ongoing antenatal care. Documenting a normal length cervix is relevant in this context.[17] The subset of women with recurrent APH should remain in hospital, following re-admission, until delivery. Despite the increased administrative pressure to limit antenatal admissions, in the context of placenta praevia decisions should err on the side of safety and always include the documented agreement of the woman.

6. *Follow-up of women with minor placenta praevia*: Where women remain undelivered for > 2 weeks in the context of minor (type 1 or 2) placenta praevia, repeat consideration should be given to the mode of delivery where vaginal delivery is feasible in the absence of placenta praevia. The modern cut-off for safe vaginal delivery of > 2 cm from the internal os[13] has been challenged by more recent prospective data, showing that two-thirds of women can deliver safely vaginally if the lower edge of the placenta is 1–2 cm from the internal os.[14] Since the cervix gradually shortens by effacement in the late second and third trimesters, a minor praevia in the context of a normal length (> 3 cm) cervix is very likely to pull back behind the fetal head, as a result of cervical effacement (Fig 19-2b,c), or during early normal labour. This apparent movement of the lower placental edge takes place even after 36 weeks; therefore even weekly assessments at this stage are worthwhile so as to avoid an unnecessary caesarean section.

7. *Fetal wellbeing assessment and placenta praevia*: Despite lower implantation, there is no convincing evidence that this results in any direct association with placental dysfunction.[28] Therefore the initial fetal health assessment in the context of placental praevia and an APH should be as follows: fetal biometry, amniotic fluid, umbilical artery Doppler, biophysical profile and a non-stress test. Additional Doppler studies should be reserved for specific indications: middle cerebral artery Doppler (if the fetus appears growth-restricted), uterine artery Doppler (if the fetus appears growth-restricted or the woman is hypertensive) and anterior lower segment colour Doppler (anterior praevia with previous caesarean section to rule out increta). Since placental function is normal in placenta praevia, fetal growth and tests of wellbeing should follow current advice.[29]

Vaginal Delivery in Placenta Praevia

The widespread availability of good-quality ultrasound means that most women with minor placenta praevia will have had discussions about mode of delivery with their obstetrician in the antenatal clinic setting. As such, the need to clarify the safety of attempting vaginal delivery in an acute setting is rare. Examples today would be either early normal labour with unusually heavy show and fresh bleeding vaginally, or presentation in labour between appointments where no final decision has been made on mode of delivery. In this context use of the 'double set-up' examination is valid, since this was the method used to make such decisions in the pre-ultrasound era in haemodynamically stable women. The components of the process are as follows: transfer to the operating room, co-care with anaesthesia, perform complete blood count

(CBC) and coagulation screen, cross-match two units of blood, staff present for immediate caesarean section. The major difference today in comparison with former times is that the majority of such procedures are done with a full top-up epidural. Women bleeding heavily would proceed faster through the above steps, with the exception of a general anaesthetic. It is useful to have a portable ultrasound machine at hand, which in acute circumstances may be helpful as follows: (1) the placenta may only be a minor praevia with an engaged fetal head – therefore proceed to vaginal examination as the bleeding may only be due to a rapidly dilating cervix; (2) there is major placenta praevia, but the fetus is a back-up transverse lie, mostly above the umbilicus – therefore use a midline skin entry and be mentally prepared to perform a classical caesarean section (see below).

Double set-up examination: Once the epidural is fully functional, the woman is examined abdominally, to determine lie, presentation and engagement. Any clinical doubts should be resolved using portable ultrasound prior to gowning, sterile preparation and adopting the lithotomy position. The procedure is abandoned in favour of caesarean in women with either transverse lie or (most) situations with breech presentation. Next, the bladder is catheterized with a Foley catheter and bag. A sterile finger is then inserted vaginally to palpate the fornices. This initial step is done to determine if thick placental tissue is present between the lower uterine segment and the fetal head. If the fetal head is easily palpated through a thin lower uterine segment it is then deemed safe to push the examining 1–2 fingers through the cervix, to explore the lower uterine segment for any intervening placental tissue. Blood clot and placental tissue may be difficult to distinguish, though placental tissue is firm and may have a gritty feel. If no placenta is found upon digital exploration of the inside of the lower uterine segment then labour can be safely induced with amniotomy and an oxytocin infusion. If placenta praevia is confirmed, or if there is active bleeding, a caesarean section is performed. If the cervix is long and closed, the examination is inconclusive – which is why portable ultrasound is important, so that the woman can leave the operating room with a clear plan for mode of delivery.

Monitoring in labour: Women attempting vaginal delivery with minor placenta praevia should have one-to-one nursing/midwifery care, in a labour room that is in immediate proximity to the operating room. Written informed consent should be obtained for care, including caesarean if needed as an emergency. Women should have large-bore IV access and two units of blood cross-matched, and be assessed by the anaesthetist and by the most senior on-call obstetrician. Pro-active care, using amniotomy and oxytocin infusion, is preferable since cervical effacement and dilation brings the placenta away from the leading edge of the cervix, while descent of the fetal head may compress the lower placental edge. Active bleeding in early labour is an indication for caesarean section, whereas new bleeding in more advanced labour may be a sign of advanced cervical dilatation and thus the possibility of vaginal delivery.

Postpartum considerations: Following successful vaginal delivery, the woman is at greater risk of primary postpartum haemorrhage because of increased bleeding from the lower uterine segment that is not capable of strong tetanic contractions. Prophylactic measures should be undertaken as described in Chapter 20.

Vaginal Delivery with Major (Type 3 or 4) Placenta Praevia

In modern obstetric practice, it is occasionally permissible to consider and attempt vaginal delivery when the placenta clearly covers the internal os. The most common situation is with the prenatal diagnosis of a major lethal abnormality (e.g. renal agenesis or skeletal dysplasia) or intrauterine fetal death, typically before 24 weeks of gestation. Assuming there are no other considerations (e.g. previous caesarean), the author's group have approached such cases using feticide and pre-induction Gelfoam embolization of the anterior divisions of the iliac arteries, followed immediately by a high-dose vaginal misoprostol regimen (600 μg every 4 hours) for induction of labour. Others have approached the challenge in a similar fashion.[30] We would generally not consider this approach after 28 weeks, due to the much greater risk of haemorrhage and the greater likelihood of achieving a lower segment caesarean section.

Abnormal Lie/Malpresentation in Early Labour with Minor Placenta Praevia

Given the potential danger of caesarean section in the pre-blood transfusion/antibiotic era, several techniques were developed to achieve maternal survival via vaginal delivery for the non-vertex fetus. These may remain applicable today when the fetus is dead, pre-viable or has a lethal anomaly and in remote areas with limited or unsafe facilities for caesarean section.

Bipolar podalic version: Rare circumstances exist where fetal manipulation and assisted vaginal delivery may be the safest maternal option in type 1–2 placenta praevia, though at the expense of fetal survival. The Braxton Hicks bipolar podalic version method was developed 150 years ago.[31] The technique demands that the cervix is >2 cm dilated and the placenta praevia does not cover the internal os – so that the gentle insertion of 1–2 fingers can be used to push up the fetal head between contractions while the external hand manipulates the breech in a downward direction into the pelvis (Fig 19-3). The fingers through the cervix then grasp a foot of the fetus (Fig 19-4) to bring that leg down through the cervix. In this way the breech is used to both dilate the cervix and tamponade the lower placental edge (Fig 19-5). Persistent traction is put on the breech to keep it firmly against the placenta: a bandage can be tied to the fetal ankle and a small weight, for example a bag of saline, is attached to provide sustained traction. For small immature fetuses, sponge forceps can be used to grasp a leg.

BRAXTON HICKS BIPOLAR VERSION

'Introduce the left hand, with the usual precautions, into the vagina, so far as to fairly touch the foetal head, even should it recede an inch. Having passed one or two fingers (if only one, let it be the middle finger) within the cervix, and resting them on the head, place the right hand on the left side of the breech at the fundus. Employ gentle pressure and slight impulsive movements on the fundus towards the left iliac fossa. In a very short time it will be found that the head is rising and at the same time the breech is descending. The foetus is now transverse; the knee will be opposite the os, and the membranes being ruptured it can be seized and brought into the vagina.'

BRAXTON HICKS BIPOLAR VERSION: USE IN PLACENTA PRAEVIA

'Anything which gave the practitioner some power of action was to be earnestly welcomed ... Turn, and if you employ the child as a plug the danger is over. Then wait for the pains, rally the powers in the interval, and let nature, gently assisted, complete the delivery.'
    John Braxton Hicks
    On a new method of version in abnormal labour. Lancet 1860; 2:28–30.

Cephalic traction: Vaginal delivery for cephalic presentation with bleeding from minor placenta praevia was described by John Willett using a specially designed T-forceps to grasp the scalp of the fetus and apply cephalic tamponade to the placenta[32] (Allis forceps or similar can be used). Having passed the forceps through the cervix and grasped the scalp, gentle traction is applied by means of a bandage tied to the handles of the forceps with a light weight hung over the end of the bed (Fig 19-6). The ensuing uterine contractions dilate the cervix to advance labour, while scalp traction provides tamponade on the lower separated edge of the placenta. Delivery is not to be forced by strong traction but should be accomplished by normal uterine contractions.

It is emphasized that the indications for these potentially dangerous techniques are very few. However, the degree of haemostasis produced by these techniques can be impressive and, on the rare occasions it is necessary, life-saving.

WILLETT'S SCALP FORCEPS

'The application of the forceps is easy and they can be applied to the scalp as soon as the os will admit a finger, thus ensuring early treatment ... a weight varying from 1lb to 2lb, hanging over the end of the bed, is applied to the handles by a tape. Nothing further is done until the head is in the vagina, when the forceps are removed and the patient is allowed to deliver herself without further interference'.
    John Willett
    The treatment of placenta praevia by continuous weight traction – a report of seven cases. Proc R Soc Med 1925; 18:90–94.

Technical Aspects of Caesarean Section for Placenta Praevia

The potential for rapid blood loss during caesarean section for major placenta praevia demands that senior staff should always attend. In addition to the surgical principles outlined in Chapter 13 the following should be considered specifically in the context of placenta praevia:

1. *Preoperative preparation*: A 'time out' procedure[33] should be conducted in the operating room, either following the establishment of regional anaesthesia (combined epidural-spinal is preferable for longer surgery) or prior to induction of general anaesthesia. At least two units of packed red blood cells should be in the operating room and checked. Prophylactic IV antibiotics should be given. Two large-bore IVs should be sited. The local 'code omega' protocol should ideally be on the wall near the anaesthetist.[22] If

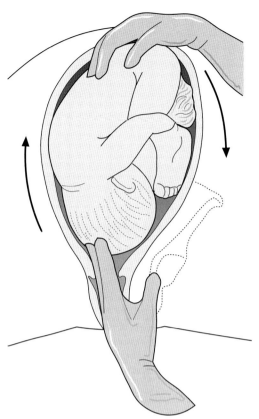

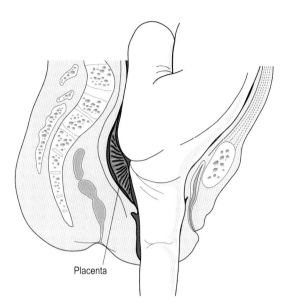

FIGURE 19-5 ■ Bipolar version: the leg of the fetus is pulled through the cervix so that the breech produces tamponade against the placenta and the lower uterine segment.

FIGURE 19-3 ■ Bipolar version: the fetal head is pushed up with the internal finger(s) and the external hand manipulates the breech down to the pelvis.

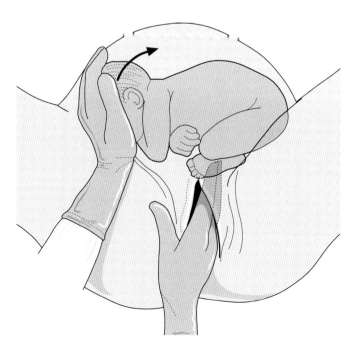

FIGURE 19-4 ■ Bipolar version: the fetus is turned by combined manipulation and the foot is grasped.

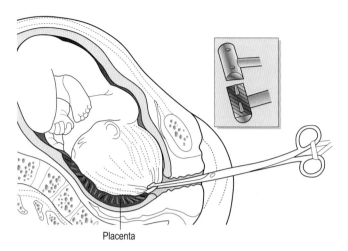

Placenta

FIGURE 19-6 ■ Application of Willett's scalp forceps.

the fetal lie is abnormal, or the woman is known to have fibroids, portable ultrasound at this stage is invaluable for the next step.

2. *Skin incision*: Subumbilical midline skin incision should be used for the following:
   (a) previous similar scar
   (b) major praevia with transverse lie and back-up (the fetus is then mostly above the umbilicus)
   (c) women with multiple previous caesareans and difficult access, multiple adhesions or previous bladder injury
   (d) rapid access under general anaesthetic for life-threatening APH.

   Pfannenstiel incision is adequate, however, for most controlled placenta praevia situations, especially when the fetus is in a longitudinal lie.

3. *Uterine incision*: In most cases with placenta praevia near term and a longitudinal lie, the lower uterine segment is sufficiently developed to allow the standard transverse lower segment incision to be performed. However, due to increased pelvic vascularity and a higher presenting part, a bladder flap need not be made, and access is made in the upper portion of the lower segment. There are, however, a number of situations in which a lower uterine segment incision is unwise and a classical uterine incision should be performed. These are as follows: (a) abnormal lie with a narrow poorly formed lower uterine segment – this will be easily recognized if the surgeon always uses his/her right hand to explore the uterus to determine the fetal attitude (lie, presentation and high vs. normal level of the presenting part); (b) extremely vascular lateral aspects

of the lower uterine segment; and (c) uterine abnormality or uterine distortion by fibroids. Taking a few moments to review the above is a useful mental strategy to anticipate how to best extract the fetus, assuming that excessive bleeding will instantly obscure visual guidance. If in doubt, a well-placed vertical incision is prudent as this will ensure easy and swift delivery of the fetus and placenta. Ultimately this approach will result in less blood loss than struggling with a transverse incision that either requires a central T extension to deliver the fetus, the risk of excessive bleeding from the uterine arteries or the formation of a broad ligament haematoma. Some authors advocate ligating large surface vessels on either side in the line of the proposed line of uterine incision before incising the uterus. A practical alternative is for the surgeon to compress the upper margin of the transverse uterine incision with the 2nd–4th fingers of his/her left hand on a rolled-up sponge, while the first assistant does the same on the lower margin – this approach also steadies the presenting part. The second assistant should hover a suction tip over the uterine incision to maintain vision during entry.

4. *Delivery of the fetus*: If the placenta praevia is either anterior or complete it is inevitable that placental tissue will be encountered immediately after incising the uterine muscle. No attempt should be made to cut through the placenta; rather, the right hand should separate the placenta either upwards or laterally to encounter the fetus palpable through the membranes. The surgeon's left hand is

used in conjunction to ideally attain a longitudinal lie. If the membranes are still intact they are ruptured by the first assistant, with persistent fundal pressure by the surgeon – remaining in control. The right hand of the surgeon either guides the fetal pole into the incision, or starts breech extraction. The surgical aspects of placenta praevia have been reviewed by Ward.[34]

5. *Intraoperative management of the third stage*: Following delivery of the fetus a bolus and infusion of oxytocin is given to promote a strong sustained contraction of the upper uterine segment. Often the uterus is exteriorized, but this is not essential and the uterine repair of an uncomplicated placenta praevia should take place in situ.[35] The following steps are suggested to minimize blood loss:

   (a) Put Green–Armytage clamps on actively bleeding vessels of the uterine incision

   (b) Ligate each uterine angle separately

   (c) Repair in the normal fashion if the lower uterine segment has minimal bleeding

   (d) If the lower uterine segment oozes significantly, the uterus should be exteriorized to perform compression. The author puts three large sponges behind, inside and in front of the lower uterine segment respectively, inserts the Doyen retractor anterior to these, his left hand behind the posterior sponge, then pushes the Doyen retractor with his right hand against his left hand – and holds this for 4 minutes timed 'by the wall clock'

   (e) Should bleeding of concern ('welling up') persist, the inside of the lower uterine segment is then explored, with suction to maximize visibility. Any sinusoids bleeding into the cavity are ligated with figure-of-eight 2/0 sutures under bimanual control. If the bleeding is generalized, a bladder flap should be developed and each uterine artery ligated with a strong No 1 figure-of-eight suture midway between the lateral margins of the uterine incision and the bladder angles.

Strategies for ligation of pelvic arteries in surgical postpartum haemorrhage are discussed in detail in Chapter 28, while additional medical therapies are discussed in Chapter 20. Massage and compression of the uterus, to await the effective action of second-line drugs is important, and gives the surgeon a sense of control. Meanwhile, discussions can continue with anaesthesia regarding estimated blood loss and need to commence blood transfusion. Additional surgical options to achieve adequate haemostasis include the placement of rectangular absorbable sutures through the lateral parts of the lower uterine segment cavity or the retrograde placement of a Bakri balloon, and are described in Chapter 28. In units with well-developed vascular interventional radiology (VIR), discussion of the feasibility to perform Gelfoam occlusion of both anterior divisions of the iliac arteries may avoid the necessity for caesarean hysterectomy.[36] Ultimately, a variety of factors (blood loss, patient stability, age, parity, practical ability to access VIR, consent for tubal ligation) contrive to determine if a caesarean hysterectomy should be performed. This is discussed in Chapter 28.

Jehovah's Witness Patients

Routine use of a blood transfusion consent form in tandem with operative consent will serve as a practical step to ensure that Jehovah's Witness patients are identified in advance. Discuss surgery and blood loss issues without extended family present, in order that specific informed consent is obtained; this is especially important when discussing surgery with women new to this faith via their partner. Current recommendations on management include safe transfer to a regional centre with a cell saver device that is capable of recycling intraoperative blood back into the woman.[37]

PLACENTAL ABRUPTION

Placental abruption refers to partial or complete separation of the normally situated placenta before delivery of the fetus. Since 1980 the population-based incidence in Finland of abruption has reduced by one-third, to approximately 1/300 deliveries.[38] In modern obstetric units maternal death is rare, although abruption increases the risk sevenfold above the general maternal mortality rate.[39] Maternal morbidity can be considerable though, and 10–20% of perinatal mortality is attributable to abruption.[39] The recent Finnish cohort study demonstrates the variety of social, medical and obstetrical risk factors for abruption:[38]

- advanced maternal age (incremental above age 30)

- hypertensive disorders, particularly severe pre-eclampsia and eclampsia
- increasing parity (≥3)
- smoking (doubles the risk)
- prolonged prelabour rupture of the membranes
- extreme preterm delivery (5–8% of deliveries 24–32 weeks)
- multifetal pregnancy (threefold increased risk)
- male pregnancy (55% cases)
- sudden decompression of an over-distended uterus, such as follows uncontrolled rupture of the membranes with polyhydramnios or after delivery of the first twin
- trauma: a fall, domestic violence, car accident or version; overall these are rare causes.

Classification

There are three types of abruption illustrated in Figure 19-7. The most common is revealed where the edge of the placenta separates and blood tracks down between the membranes and the uterine wall to escape through the cervix. In 5–10% of cases the bleeding is concealed, or retroplacental, where the haemorrhage remains trapped between the placenta and the uterus. In this scenario, the mother may complain of constant abdominal pain while hypovolaemic shock may occur and the fetus may either be dead, or exhibit signs of acute distress on fetal heart rate monitoring. Sometimes abruption has mixed features.

Pathophysiology

Placental separation is initiated by haemorrhagic disruption of vasculopathic decidual arterioles in the basal plate.[40] Progression of haematoma formation extends the separation, and may be compounded by uterine irritability causing labour since haemorrhage disperses through the myometrium and generates thrombin locally as a powerful contractile agent.[15] Abruption is usually an acute clinical diagnosis, but may be chronic and visible on ultrasound examination.[41] The haematoma adheres to the basal surface and thus facilitates a clinical diagnosis at the third stage of labour. In rare cases of concealed or mixed abruption, the retroplacental extravasation of blood through the myometrium may be so extensive as to reach the serosal surface, causing bruising and discoloration. This is apparent at the time of caesarean section and is known as the Couvelaire uterus, after Alexandre Couvelaire (1873–1948) of Paris who first described this as 'uteroplacental apoplexy'. In the past a Couvelaire uterus was often blamed as the cause of uterine atony and postpartum. In fact, in most cases this is due to the associated coagulopathy, which reflects the severity of the process. The combination of arteriolar spasm that accompanies the hypovolaemic shock of severe abruption, coupled with the renal burden of the products of disseminated intravascular coagulation, greatly increases the risk of renal tubular and cortical necrosis and subsequent renal failure.

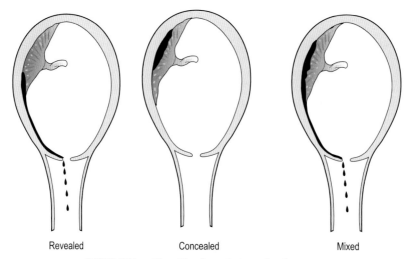

Revealed   Concealed   Mixed

FIGURE 19-7 ■ Classification of abruptio placentae.

Clinical Diagnosis and Management

The presentation of abruption can vary widely, from mild revealed bleeding in a stable patient to severe concealed abruption with acute, severe and unrelenting abdominal pain and profound hypovolaemic shock. In the latter situation the uterus is typically hard and tender and the fetus is either dead or exhibits a fetal hear rate pattern consistent with acute asphyxia. Labour has often become established by the time the patient reaches hospital. Initial assessment should focus on maternal resuscitation and collaborative teamwork. Most of the principles outlined above for placenta praevia equally apply to abruption, with a few specific differences that can be emphasized as follows:

1. *Acuity of disease*: Fetal distress and maternal shock can often be out of proportion with revealed blood loss and evolve with alarming speed. Patients with suspected abruption therefore require the full attention of senior staff. Major abruption with a viable fetus in early labour is best managed by a rapid combination of resuscitation, general anaesthesia and caesarean delivery.

2. *Potential for vaginal delivery*: Provided the fetus is vertex, there is always the potential for successful vaginal delivery in stable women labouring with a minor abruption, especially in multipara. A wise course of action is therefore to manage labour in or very close to an operating room, with amniotomy and attachment of a fetal scalp clip. Ob care with amniotomy is essential. Conversion to the lithotomy position at around 8cm, subsequent reflection of the cervix with a contraction, followed by pushing and use of vacuum or forceps to effect delivery when safe, are tips that may be useful to avoid a caesarean section as an abruption is evolving and causing progressive fetal distress.

3. *Potential for coagulopathy and PPH*: Extravasation of maternal blood into the myometrium, coupled with rapid progress in labour, are independent risk factors for postpartum haemorrhage. The management is generally as described for placenta praevia, except that more commonly the woman will have a vaginal delivery.

The emphasis is on ensuring that the uterus is empty and intact and repair of any vaginal trauma, leaving the anaesthetist to manage resuscitation and uterotonic drugs. In this setting use of a uterine tamponade balloon can buy time to correct any coagulopathy and to consider interventional radiology techniques as an alternative to laparotomy and caesarean hysterectomy. In most cases of moderate to severe abruption, under-transfusion is common. To avoid hypovolaemia patients require immediate IV crystalloid and blood transfusion to maintain tissue perfusion, especially renal perfusion, which may lessen the chance of disseminated intravascular coagulation (see Chapter 25).

COUVELAIRE UTERUS

'The uterine wall, in the zone of membranous insertion as well as the zone of placental insertion, was the site of a tremendous bloody infiltration separating the muscle bundles ... The ovaries were peppered with a punctiform bloody suffusion. The broad ligaments were infiltrated with blood. This was indeed a true case of utero-placental apoplexy'.
Alexandre Couvelaire
Traitement chirurgical des hémorrhagies utéro-placentaires avec décollement du placenta normalement inséré. Ann Gynécol 1911; 8:591–608

VASA PRAEVIA

Normal placental anatomy includes the insertion of the umbilical cord into the placental disc. In 1–2% of pregnancies the placental cord root is either marginal (on the edge – Fig 19-8a), or more rarely inserted into the fetal membranes and described as velamentous. In both instances, fetal-derived vessels may traverse portions of the membranes. These two situations place the pregnancy at risk of fetally derived vessels running in the membranes over the internal os, termed vasa praevia. The first occurs where the marginal or velamentous cord root is associated with the lower edge of a minor placenta praevia and the second, where fetally derived vessels run from the placental disc to a separate succenturiate lobe in the lower uterine segment.

Vasa praevia occurs in about 1/5000 unselected singleton pregnancies[42] though higher rates are observed in referral centres due to selection bias. Twins, especially monochorionic, are at increased risk due to the common association with velamentous cord; as such, universal screening is considered cost-effective in twins.[43] Undiagnosed, vasa praevia may present in labour with vaginal bleeding due to vessel rupture (especially the thin-walled larger veins, see Fig 19-8b–d) at either spontaneous or artificial rupture of the membranes. Fetal distress from vaginal bleeding is typically acute, severe, out of proportion to the amount of vaginal bleeding

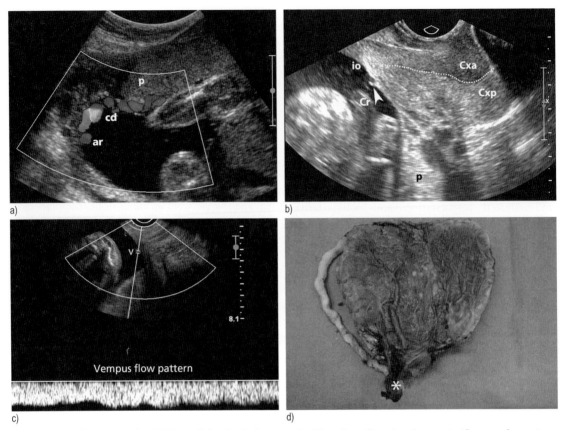

a)

b)

c)

d)

FIGURE 19-8 ■ Vasa praevia. (a) Transabdominal ultrasound with colour Doppler demonstrating a velamentous cord insertion (cd) at the placenta (p) with a chorionic plate artery (ar) running towards the inferior wall of the uterus. Transvaginal ultrasound is therefore indicated to find or exclude vasa praevia. (b) Transvaginal ultrasound showing minor posterior placenta praevia (p) that is 2.6 cm from the internal os (io). The dotted line indicates the cervical canal. Cxa, anterior lip of cervix; Cxp, posterior lip of cervix; Cr, free loop of cord. Arrowhead shows a vessel embedded in the amnion that is suspicious for vasa praevia. (c) Corresponding colour and pulsed Doppler view demonstrating continuous venous flow (v) from a fetal vasa praevia vein. (d) Consequences of failure to diagnose vasa praevia. Following amniotomy for induction of labour, vaginal bleeding led to acute fetal distress, emergency caesarean section and early neonatal death from consequences of hypovolaemic shock. The rupture point in the cord (asterisk) is shown in the velamentous cord.

and with no suggestive features of abruption. In this situation, immediate caesarean section under general anaesthesia followed by immediate transfusion of uncross-matched blood may save the infant from hypovolaemic shock, though many cases are fatal (Fig 19-8d). Prenatal diagnosis and planned elective caesarean delivery increase the chance of survival from 47% to 97%.[44]

Occasionally, fetally derived chorionic plate arteries may be felt pulsating in the bulging membranes in labour prior to amniotomy; in this case the woman should be transferred to the operating room to establish or refute the diagnosis by clinical methods (repeat vaginal examination between contractions when the membranes are soft, or amnioscopy) or transvaginal colour Doppler examination (Fig 19-8b,c).

Another presentation is variable decelerations with intact membranes, where cord presentation may be confused with vasa praevia on vaginal examination.

Rarely, vasa praevia may present more slowly following ruptured membranes in labour, with minor vaginal bleeding and progressive fetal tachycardia in otherwise normal labour.

The rapid bedside 'Apt test' quickly detects the presence of fetal haemoglobin in a small sample of collected vaginal blood, based on its resistance to denaturation by alkali compared with adult haemoglobin. A few drops of the vaginal blood are added to 10 ml of 0.1% sodium hydroxide. Adult haemoglobin will turn brown in the solution within 30 seconds but fetal haemoglobin, resisting denaturation by alkali, remains pink.[45]

Vasa praevia fulfils the criteria for an antenatal screening program that can be built into the 19–20 week fetal anatomical ultrasound examination, since planned elective caesarean is an effective treatment. In addition to screening for placenta praevia, the transabdominal ultrasound includes both a search for the placental cord root and a succenturiate lobe in the lower uterine segment. Transvaginal ultrasound is reserved for the small subset of women suspicious for vasa praevia (Fig 19-8a–c). Presently, one national guideline exists for vasa praevia.[8] A novel new treatment, to avoid an otherwise inevitable caesarean section, is fetoscopic laser ablation of the vasa praevia vessels.[46]

INVASIVE PLACENTA PRAEVIA

The term placenta accreta refers to excessive adherence of the placenta to the uterine wall. It can occur in the normally implanted site, though the most serious type is invasive placenta praevia, a rare and serious complication of pregnancy that occurs in about 1 in 5000 deliveries. The incidence of all types of placenta accreta is rising, mostly related to pregnancy with multiple prior caesarean deliveries. Advanced maternal age compounds the risk, since older women are at more risk of caesarean section, placenta praevia, dilatation and curettage for spontaneous miscarriage, myomectomy and pregnancy following endoscopic surgery for Asherman's syndrome.[47]

Risk factors in our recent series of 33 women with placenta praevia increta[48] are shown in Table 19-4. Common to all is injury to the endometrium that transforms to the decidua during implantation. When placental trophoblast makes contact with the decidua it stimulates the formation of a layer of fibrin deposits, Nitabuch's zone – this is the physiological plane of placental separation.[49] Deficient areas of decidua during implantation, especially in lower segment scars[50] predispose to praevia increta. Pathological placental adherence is patchy, because the underlying decidual damage is non-uniform.

The disease is classified histopathologically as:
accreta – loss of Nitabuch's zone and direct contact of placental villi with myometrium
increta – chorionic villi invade the (often deficient) myometrium
percreta – placental tissue erodes through the myometrium to the serosal surface of the uterus, or beyond (parametrium, bladder).
The variable pathology induces a wide spectrum of clinical presentation, ranging from a difficult manual removal of placenta and postpartum haemorrhage (focal accreta), through to a total

TABLE 19-4	Risk Factors for Placenta Praevia Increta	
Risk Factors		**Outcome (n=33)**
Previous caesarean sections		2 (0–4)
0		2 (6.1%)
1		11 (33.3%)
2		13 (39.4%)
3 or more		7 (21.2%)
Previous D&Cs		0 (0–4)
0		19 (57.6%)
1		10 (30.3%)
2 or more		4 (12.1%)
Asherman's syndrome		2 (6.1%)
Septal surgery		1 (3.0%)

Data presented as median (range) or *n* (%), as appropriate. Adapted from Walker MG, Allen L, Windrim RC, Kachura JR, Pollard L, Pantazi S, et al. Multidisciplinary management of invasive placenta previa. J Obstet Gynaecol Can 2013;35(5):417–25.

lack of placental separation at vaginal delivery, to an obvious 'increta reaction' on the lower surface of the uterus at laparotomy for planned caesarean hysterectomy.

> 'But when I endeavored to extract the placenta it had adhered so strongly to the cervix uteri that it was near an hour and half before I could remove it; nor then without separating the adhering part with my hands.'
>   Edward Rigby
>   An Essay on the Uterine Haemorrhage which Precedes the Delivery of the Full Grown Fetus: Illustrated with Cases. 6th ed. London: William Hunter, 1822

Screening for Placenta Praevia Increta

Women with a low-lying anterior placenta or obvious major placenta praevia at the 19–20 week fetal anatomy ultrasound should have a repeat ultrasound examination at 22 weeks to look for the signs of invasive placentation. The ultrasound features of placenta praevia increta are shown in Figure 19-9a,b. The placenta bulges into the back of the bladder due to progressive myometrial dehiscence. Transvaginal ultrasound may give clearer images and can also evaluate invasion of the cervix (Fig 19-2d). Magnetic resonance imaging (MRI) is not necessary for the diagnosis when ultrasound evaluation is performed and discussed amongst experienced staff.[51] The role of MRI is to define the extent

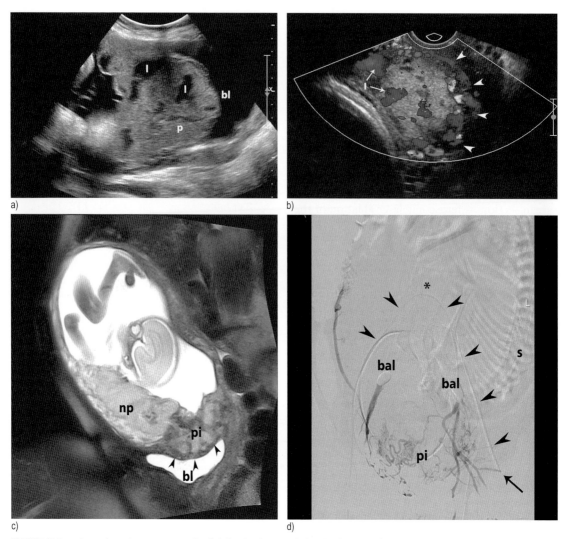

FIGURE 19-9 ■ Invasive placenta praevia. (a) Sagittal transabdominal view of the lower uterine segment demonstrating anterior placenta praevia (p) with the characteristic anterior 'bulge' into the bladder (bl) due to myometrial dehiscence. Note several large prominent lakes (l) suggesting placenta increta. (b) Corresponding transvaginal colour Doppler imaging demonstrating bladder wall vascularity (arrowheads) and venous flow within the lakes (l). (c) Sagittal magnetic resonance image. Contrast normal anterior placental tissue (np) with placenta increta (pi) above the bladder (bl) that contains dark placental bands corresponding to lakes seen on ultrasound. Arrowheads indicate increased bladder base vascularity. (d) Preoperative placement of internal iliac artery occlusion balloons (bal). Note fetal spine (s) on maternal left. Arrow indicates insertion point of catheter into the left femoral artery. Arrowheads indicate course to the right iliac artery, via the aortic bifurcation (asterisk). The test arteriogram shows proximal vessel occlusion and distal feeding of the placenta praevia increta (pi). Postoperatively the patient will return to interventional radiology for angiography and Gelfoam slurry embolization of any leaking branches of the anterior division of the internal iliac arteries.

of myometrial invasion, in particular to identify extrauterine placenta tissue that may involve vital structures, e.g. ureters (Fig 19-9c).

Surgical Strategies for Placenta Praevia Increta

Elective non-removal of the placenta: We[52] and others[53,54] have evaluated the potential value of elective non-removal of the placenta at delivery by classical caesarean section. Superficially, this is an attractive option since the surgery is technically easy, poses minimal risk of major haemorrhage and leaves the potential for future pregnancies. This procedure and ultrasound images of gradual spontaneous resolution have been described.[54] However, the risk of significant bleeding remains, with a protracted and uncertain period of resolution that can last more than 1 year.[52] Haemorrhage results from the formation of large arterio-venous fistulas in decaying placental tissue. Arterio-venous fistula formation resulted in emergency repeat laparotomy due to vaginal bleeding in 4/10 women in our series. Despite full resolution, two women requested tubal ligation. Based on this experience, we moved to the preferred option of planned caesarean hysterectomy in 2008.[48] Presently, the indications for conservative management are: (a) intraoperative diagnosis in a suboptimal setting for emergency caesarean hysterectomy and (b) patient choice, despite being fully informed of the risks versus benefits of definitive surgery (e.g. diagnosis after one previous caesarean).

Elective caesarean hysterectomy: Surgery should be scheduled at 34–35 weeks[55] balancing prematurity and risk of emergency surgery due to APH. Given the rarity of this diagnosis and the risk of haemorrhage, women requiring this surgery are best managed by regional teams comprising interested members of the contributing subspecialities.[53] These include surgical obstetrics (or maternal-fetal medicine), pelvic surgery, urology, obstetric anaesthesia, blood transfusion, pathology and critical care. In our recent prospective series of 33 cases, the progressive application of team-based elements of care significantly reduced serious morbidity.[48]

Important points to highlight are as follows:
1. *Consent*: Obtain consent for midline access, caesarean hysterectomy and (should the placenta separate spontaneously with acceptable bleeding) tubal ligation. Table 19-5 shows the major risks of surgery from our series that should be discussed preoperatively; 10% of women with placenta praevia increta did not need a caesarean hysterectomy.[48] We document cervical cytology results so as to retain the option of subtotal hysterectomy.
2. *Patient preparation*: We routinely place balloon catheters in the anterior divisions of the iliac arteries (Fig 19-9d) while others favour selective intraoperative ligation of the internal iliac arteries.[53] While intraoperative balloon inflation, following delivery of the fetus, results in variable degrees of arrest of bleeding, this strategy facilitates immediate postoperative angiography and Gelfoam embolization of aberrant branches of the anterior divisions of the internal iliac arteries. We place a 3-way urinary catheter for intraoperative methylene blue dye testing of bladder integrity. Ureteric catheters are a wise consideration, especially if lateral placental extension is suspected on MRI,

as they facilitate confident ureteric identification during dissection in the broad ligament. We inform intensive care in advance of the potential need for postoperative admission. We give preoperative antibiotics and do a 'time out' procedure.
3. *Anaesthesia*: Our preference is for regional epidural anaesthesia for several reasons: first, this gives analgesia for internal iliac catheter placement; second, the partner remains in the room during the operation for support so that both see the new-born; and third, the couple can be informed of progress. In our series, most women remained awake throughout surgery and did not move to intensive care postoperatively (Table 19-5).
4. *Surgery*: A general surgery environment is ideal for these cases, since other surgical specialities, in particular urology and vascular surgery, then have ready access to their equipment if called to assist. Once the uterus is exposed, we assess the external appearances of the lower uterus; in cases where the lower uterus bulges forwards with a major vascular reaction we make the decision, before performing a high midline uterine incision, to leave the placenta in situ, not to infuse oxytocin and to proceed immediately to caesarean hysterectomy. Typically the fundal incision retracts laterally and does not bleed excessively. Therefore, we clamp any bleeding sinusoids with Green–Armytage clamps and proceed with the dissection. We do not regard bladder dome injuries as serious and will repair small openings without consulting urology; indeed, opening the dome of the bladder to identify the trigone and/or catheterize a ureter can be a useful intraoperative strategy in the absence of ureteric catheterization. Once the bladder is dissected adequately and the cardinal ligaments are secured, we decide on the need for total versus subtotal hysterectomy, based on: difficulty with bladder dissection, haemostasis and perceived cervical length.
5. *Postoperative care*: Following postoperative angiography and Gelfoam embolization of both anterior divisions of the internal iliac arteries, one catheter is left overnight and, if stable, the woman is returned to the labour and delivery suite for one-to-one nursing. Epidural analgesia can be continued, which is a distinct advantage over patient-controlled narcotics after general anaestheisa. Where bladder repair or

TABLE 19-5 Intraoperative Course and Postoperative Complications

Complication	Outcome (n=33)
Mode of anaesthesia	
Regional	23 (69.7%)
General	4 (12.1%)
Conversion from regional to general	6 (18.2%)
Estimated blood loss (ml)	2000 (600–10000)
Bladder dome injury and repair	10 (30.3%)
Bowel or ureteric injury	0
Blood transfusion	
Intra-/postoperative pRBC required	24 (72.7%)
pRBC (units)	3.5 (0–20)
Other components required (FFP, cryoprecipitate, platelets)	11 (33.3%)
Primary surgery	
Classical caesarean section and removal of placenta	2 (6.1%)
Caesarean hysterectomy	31 (93.9%)
Subtotal	16 (48.5%)
Total	15 (45.5%)
Skin incision	
Pfannenstiel	3 (9.1%)
Midline	30 (90.9%)
Operative time (minutes)	107 (68–334)
Intensive care unit admission	5 (15.2%)
Length of postpartum stay (days)	5 (2–13)

Data presented as median (range) or n (%), as
  appropriate.
FFP, fresh frozen plasma; pRBC, packed red blood cells.
Adapted from Walker MG, Allen L, Windrim RC,
  Kachura JR, Pollard L, Pantazi S, et al.
  Multidisciplinary management of invasive placenta
  previa. J Obstet Gynaecol Can 2013;35(5):417–25.

ureteric stenting has been necessary, we arrange urology co-care for outpatient assessment.

6. *Blood transfusion*: Based on our experience of blood loss, we do not see the need to routinely deploy a cell saver (unless the woman is a Jehovah's Witness or has complex red cell antibodies). Normovolaemic haemodilution (crystalloid volume expansion immediately before skin incision) is a useful practical way to reduce red cell loss intraoperatively.

REFERENCES

1. Sinha P, Mishra M. Caesarean scar preganancy: A precursor of placenta percreta/accreta. J Obstet Gynaecol 2012;32:621–3.
2. Rosenberg T, Pariente G, Sergienko R, Wiznitzer A, Sheiner E. Critical analysis of risk factors and outcome of placenta previa. Arch Gynecol Obstet 2011;284:47–51.
3. Hunter W. Anatomy of the gravid uterus. London: Baskerville Press; 1774.
4. Baskett TF. Of violent floodings in pregnancy: evolution of the management of placenta praevia. In: Sturdee D, Olah K, Keane D, editors. The Yearbook of Obstetrics and Gynaecology. London: RCOG Press; 2001. p. 1–14.
5. Baskett TF. Edward Rigby (1747–1821) of Norwich and his essay on the uterine haemorrhage. J R Soc Med 2002;95:618–22.
6. Norgaard LN, Pinborg A, Lidegaard O, Bergholt T. A Danish national cohort study on neonatal outcome in singleton pregnancies with placenta previa. Acta Obstet Gynecol Scand 2012;91:546–51.
7. Blouin D, Rioux C. Routine third trimester ultrasound examination for low-lying or marginal placentas diagnosed at mid-pregnancy: Is this indicated? J Obstet Gynaecol Can 2012;34:425–8.
8. Gagnon R. Guidelines for the management of vasa previa. J Obstet Gynaecol Can 2009;31:748–53.
9. Weis MA, Harper LM, Roehl KA, Odibo AO, Cahill AG. Natural history of placenta previa in twins. Obstet Gynecol 2012;120:753–8.
10. Danforth DN, Ivy AC. The lower uterine segment: its derivation and physiological behaviour. Am J Obstet Gynecol 1949;57:831–8.
11. Bergelin I, Valentin L. Patterns of normal change in cervical length and width during pregnancy in nulliparous women: a prospective, longitudinal ultrasound study. Ultrasound Obstet Gynecol 2001;18:217–22.
12. Smith GCS, Celik E, To M, Khouri O, Nicolaides KH. Cervical length at mid-pregnancy and the risk of primary cesarean delivery. N Engl J Med 2008;358:1346–53.
13. Oppenheimer L. Society of Obstetrics and Gynaecologists of Canada Clinical. Practice Guideline: Diagnosis and Management of Placenta Previa. J Obstet Gynaecol Can 2007;29:261–6.
14. Vergani P, Ornaghi S, Pozzi I, Beretta P, Russo FM, Follesa I, et al. Placenta previa: distance to internal os and mode of delivery. Am J Obstet Gynecol 2009;201:e1–5.
15. O'Sullivan C, Allen NM, O'Loughlin AJ, Friel AM, Morrison J. Thrombin and PAR1-activating peptide: Effects on human uterine contractility in vitro. Am J Obstet Gynecol 2004;190:1098–105.
16. Towers CV, Pircon RA, Heppard M. Is tocolysis safe in the management of third-trimester bleeding? Am J Obstet Gynecol 1999;180:1572–8.
17. Stafford IA, Dashe JS, Shivers SA, Alexander JM, McIntire DD, Leveno KJ. Ultrasonographic cervical length and risk of hemorrhage in pregnancies with placenta previa. Obstet Gynecol 2010;116:595–600.
18. Ohira S, Kikuchi N, Kobara H, Osada R, Ashida T, Kanai M, et al. Predicting the route of delivery in women with low-lying placenta using transvaginal ultrasonography: Significance of placental migration and marginal sinus. Gynecol Obstet Invest 2012;72:217–22.
19. Baskett TF. Surgical management of severe obstetric hemorrhage: experience with an obstetric hemorrhage equipment tray. J Obstet Gynaecol Can 2004;26:805–8.

20. RCOG Guidelines. Royal College of Obstetricians and Gynaecologists 2012. Accessed 5 Nov 2012. Available at http://www.rcog.org.uk/womens-health/clinical-guidance.

21. Khalafallah A, Dennis A, Bates J, Bates G, Robertson IK, Smith L, et al. A prospective randomized, controlled trial of intravenous versus oral iron for moderate iron deficiency anaemia of pregnancy. J Internal Med 2010;268:286–95.

22. Burtelow M, Riley E, Druzin M, Fontaine M, Viele M, Goodnough LT. How we treat: management of life-threatening primary postpartum hemorrhage with a standardized massive transfusion protocol. Transfusion 2007;47:1564–72.

23. Fung KF, Eason E. Society of Obstetricians and Gynaecologists of Canada. Clinical Practice Guidelines: Prevention of Rh Alloimmunization. J Obstet Gynaecol Can 2003;25:765–73.

24. Roberts D, Dalziel SR. Antenatal corticosteroids for accelerating fetal lung maturation for women at risk of preterm birth. The Cochrane Collaboration 2010: 1–173.

25. Magee L, Sawchuck D, Synnes A, von Dadelszen P. Society of Obstetricians and Gynaecologists of Canada. Clinical Practice Guideline: magnesium sulphate for fetal neuroprotection. J Obstet Gynaecol Can 2011; 33:516–29.

26. Torrance HL, Voorbijb HAM, Wijnberger LD, vanBel F, Visser GHA. Lung maturation in small for gestational age fetuses from pregnancies complicated by placental insufficiency or maternal hypertension. Early Human Development 2008;84:465–9.

27. Wing DA, Paul RH, Millar RK. Usefulness of coagulation studies and blood banking in patients with symptomatic placenta previa. Am J Perinatol 1997;14:601–4.

28. Harper LM, Odibo AO, Macones GA, Crane JP, Cahill AG. Effect of placenta previa on fetal growth. Am J Obstet Gynecol 2010;203:330e1–e5.

29. Lausman A, McCarthy F, Walker M, Kingdom J. Screening, diagnosis, and management of intrauterine growth restriction. J Obstet Gynaecol Can 2012;34:17–28.

30. du Passage A, Le Ray C, Grange G, Cabrol D, Tsatsaris V. Termination of pregnancy and placenta previa, interest in performing feticide before the labour induction? J Gynecol Obstet Biol (Paris) 2011;40:149–55.

31. Hicks JB. On a new method of version in normal labour. Lancet 1860;2:28–30.

32. Willett JA. The treatment of placenta previa by continuous weight traction: a report of seven cases. Proc R Soc Med 1925;18:90–4.

33. Safe Surgery Saves Lives Frequently Asked Questions. World Health Organization, 2012. Accessed 5 Nov 2012. Available at http://www.who.int/patientsafety/safesurgery/faq_introduction/en/.

34. Ward CR. Avoiding an incision through the anterior previa at cesarean delivery. Obstet Gynecol 2003;102: 552–4.

35. Siddiqui M, Goldszmidt E, Fallah S, Kingdom J, Windrim R, Carvalho JCA. Complications of exteriorized compared with in situ uterine repair at cesarean delivery under spinal anesthesia: A randomized controlled trial. Obstet Gynecol 2007;110:570–5.

36. Kirby JM, Katchura JR, Rajan DK, Sniderman KW, Simons ME, Windrim RC, et al. Arterial embolization for primary postpartum hemorrhage. J Vasc Interv Radiol 2009;20:1036–45.

37. Placenta praevia, placenta praevia accreta and vasa praevia: diagnosis and management. Agency for Healthcare Research and Quality, 2011. Accessed 5 Nov 2012.

Available at http://www.guideline.gov/content.aspx?id=25668.

38. Tikkanen M, Riihimaki O, Gissler M, Luukkaala T, Metsaranta M, Andersson, et al. Decreasing incidence of placental abruption in Finland during 1980–2005. Acta Obstet Gynecol Scand 2012;91:1046–52.

39. Tikkanen M. Placental abruption: epidemiology, risk factors and consequences. Acta Obstetr Gynecol Scand 2010;90:14014–19.

40. Fitzgerald B, Shannon P, Kingdom J, Keating S. Rounded intraplacental haematomas due to decidual vasculopathy have a distinctive morphology. J Clin Pathol 2011;64:729–32.

41. Walker M, Whittle W, Keating S, Kingdom J. Sonographic diagnosis of chronic abruption. J Obstet Gynaecol Can 2010;32:1056–8.

42. Lee W, Lee VL, Kirk JS, Sloan CT, Smith RS, Comstock CH. Vasa previa: prenatal diagnosis, natural evolution and clinical outcome. Obstet Gynecol 2000;95: 572–6.

43. Cipriano LE, Barth WH Jr, Zaric GS. The cost-effectiveness of targeted or universal screening for vasa previa at 18–20 weeks of gestation in Ontario. BJOG 2010;117:1108–18.

44. Oyelese Y, Catanzarite V, Prefumo F, Lashley S, Schachter M, Tovbin Y, et al. Vasa previa: the impact of prenatal diagnosis on outcomes. Obstet Gynecol 2004;103:937–42.

45. Loendersloot EW. Vasa praevia. Am J Obstet Gynecol 1979;135:702–3.

46. Chmait RH, Chavira E, Kontopoulos EV, Quintero RA. Third trimester fetoscopic laser ablation of type II vasa previa. J Matern Fetal Neonatal Med 2010;23:459–62.

47. Fernandez H, Al-Najjar F, Chauveaud-Lambling A, Frydman R, Gervaise A. Fertility after treatment of Asherman's syndrome stage 3 and 4. Minimally Invasive Gynecol 2006;13:398–402.

48. Walker MG, Allen L, Windrim RC, et al. Multidisciplinary management of invasive placenta accreta. J Obstet Gynaecol Can 2013;35(5):417–25.

49. Craven CM, Chedwick LR, Ward K. Placental basal plate formation is associated with fibrin deposition in decidual veins at sites of trophoblast cell invasion. Am J Obstet Gynecol 2002;186:291–6.

50. Monteagudo A, Carreno C, Timor-Tritsch IE. Saline infusion sonohysterography in nonpregnant women with previous cesarean delivery: The 'Niche' in the scar. J Ultrasound Med 2001;20:1105–15.

51. Masselli G, Brunelli R, Casciani E, Polettini E, Piccioni MG, Anceschi M, et al. Magnetic resonance imaging in the evaluation of placental adhesive disorders: correlation with colour Doppler ultrasound. Eur Radiol 2008; 18:1292–9.

52. Amsalem H, Kingdom JCP, Farine D, Allen L, Yinon Y, D'Souza DL, et al. Planned caesarean hyterectomy versus 'conserving' caesarean section in patients with placenta accreta. J Obstet Gynaecol Can 2011;33: 1005–10.

53. Eller AG, Bennett MA, Sharshiner M, Masheter C, Soisson AP, Dodson M, et al. Maternal morbidity in cases of placenta accreta managed by a multidisciplinary care team compared with standard obstetric care. Obstet Gynecol 2011;117:331–7.

54. Wong VV, Burke G. Planned conservative management of placenta percreta. J Obstet Gynaecol 2012;32: 447–52.

55. Robinson BK, Grobman WA. Effectiveness of timing strategies for delivery of individuals with placenta previa and accreta. Obstet Gynecol 2010;116:835–42.

CHAPTER 20

POSTPARTUM HAEMORRHAGE

TF Baskett

> 'The dangerous efflux is occasioned by everything that hinders the emptied uterus from contracting ... in these cases such things must be used as will assist the contractile power of the uterus and hinder the blood from flowing so fast into it and the neighboring vessels.'
> William Smellie
> Treatise on the Theory and Practice of Midwifery. London: D. Wilson, 1752, p402–404

Every day about 1600 women die in childbirth and of these approximately 500 bleed to death.[1] Most of these are due to atonic postpartum haemorrhage (PPH) and more than 99% are in the developing world. The deaths are caused by the 'Three Delays': delay in seeking care, delay in reaching care, and delay in receiving care. While these 'delays' are most common in the developing world they are not unknown in countries with developed health services. The *United Kingdom Confidential Enquiry into Maternal Deaths* continues to emphasize that deaths due to PPH are often associated with treatment that is 'too little, too late' or 'major substandard care'.[1,2] While haemorrhage is only fifth or sixth among the leading causes of maternal death in developed countries, it accounts for the majority of cases that result in severe maternal or 'near-miss' obstetric morbidity.[3,4] Furthermore, reports from Australia and Canada show an increased incidence of PPH in those countries.[5,6]

This chapter will outline the causes and medical management of postpartum haemorrhage. Other aspects, including surgical management, are covered in separate chapters: retained placenta (Chapter 21); uterine inversion (Chapter 22); lower genital tract trauma (Chapter 23); uterine tamponade, uterine compression sutures, pelvic vessel ligation and embolization, and obstetric hysterectomy (Chapter 28).

PRIMARY POSTPARTUM HAEMORRHAGE

Primary PPH is defined as bleeding from the genital tract in excess of 500 ml in the first 24 hours after delivery. In most instances this haemorrhage occurs within the first few hours of delivery. Because the diagnosis is subjective the reported incidence varies widely from 2% to 10%.[7] Blood volume studies have shown that the normal woman loses about 500 ml at the time of spontaneous vaginal delivery, more with assisted vaginal delivery, and up to 1000 ml at caesarean section. In general, medical attendants tend to underestimate blood loss and patients overestimate it. Thus, when the attendant has estimated the blood loss to be more than 500 ml it is usually closer to 1 L, so the clinical definition is reasonable. However, it is important to remember that blood volume is related to body weight. Thus, the small, low-weight woman, particularly if she is anaemic, may tolerate poorly quite small blood losses (see Chapter 24).

Physiology of the Third Stage of Labour

Before discussing the causes and management of primary PPH it is necessary to understand the physiology of the third stage of labour, which lasts from delivery of the infant to delivery of the placenta. While this is the shortest of the three stages of labour it carries the greatest risk to the mother.

During pregnancy the myometrial fibres have been stretched considerably to accommodate the enlarged uterus and its contents. When the infant delivers the uterus continues to contract, leading to a dramatic shortening of these elongated fibres. The permanent shortening of the muscle fibres is achieved by retraction, a unique property of uterine muscle which, in contrast to contraction, requires no energy.

Placental separation is caused by the uterine contraction and retraction greatly reducing the site of placental implantation. The placenta is thus sheared from the uterine wall: analogous to a postage stamp stuck to the surface of an inflated balloon becoming detached when the balloon is deflated. When the placenta is completely separated from the implantation site the contractions continue its descent to the lower uterine segment, through the cervix and into the vagina.

Clinical Signs of Placenta Separation

The triad of clinical signs associated with placenta separation is as follows:

1. The uterus will be felt to contract and, as the placenta is sheared off the uterine wall and descends to the lower uterine segment, the uterine fundus changes from a broad and flat discoid shape to a more elevated, narrow and globular shape. This change from the discoid to globular configuration can be quite difficult to appreciate clinically except in the very thin. However, the uterus will be felt to harden as it contracts, rises in the abdomen and becomes ballotable.

2. A gush of blood often accompanies separation of the placenta from the uterine wall. This can be unreliable as bleeding may occur with only partial separation of the placenta and, even with complete separation of the placenta from the uterine wall, the blood may be contained behind the membranes and not be clinically apparent.

3. When the placenta has separated and descends to the lower uterine segment and through the cervix there is cord lengthening (8–15 cm) at the introitus. This is the most reliable sign.

The *mechanism of haemostasis* at the placental site is one of the physiological and anatomical marvels of nature. The muscle fibres of the myometrium are arranged in a criss-cross pattern and through this lattice-work of muscle fibres the blood vessels pass to supply the placental bed. When the uterine muscle contracts this lattice-work of fibres effectively compresses the blood vessels (Fig 20-1). This myometrial architecture is sometimes appropriately referred to as the 'living ligatures' or 'physiological sutures' of the uterus.

Management of the Third Stage of Labour

After the infant has been delivered, delayed cord clamping (after 2 minutes) is advocated to allow maximum transfusion to the fetus. Then the cord is divided and the necessary cord blood samples taken. Put very light tension on the cord to ensure there are no loops free in the vagina and then place the clamp on the cord at the level of the introitus, ensuring that real cord lengthening becomes clinically apparent. One hand cradles and 'guards the fundus' so that the changes associated with placental separation can be appreciated or to detect an atonic enlarging uterus filling with blood. When the clinical signs of placental separation are evident, assist delivery of the placenta by controlled cord traction. The abdominal hand moves to the lower part of the uterus just above the pubic symphysis and gently applies counter-pressure, pushing the uterus upwards and backwards while the other hand exerts steady downward traction on the cord. The distance between the suprapubic hand and the sacral promontory should be such as to

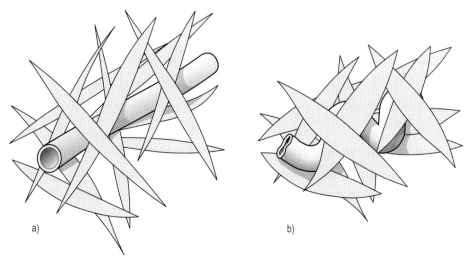

a)   b)

FIGURE 20-1 ■ Haemostatic mechanism after placental separation. The 'living ligatures' or 'physiological sutures' of the myometrium. a) Before myometrial contraction b) after contraction.

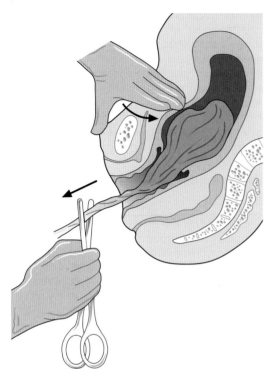

FIGURE 20-2 ■ Delivery of separated placenta by controlled cord traction.

prevent the possibility of uterine inversion (Fig 20-2).

There are two approaches, expectant and active, to the routine management of the third stage of labour:

- *Expectant management* involves observation while awaiting the physiological changes that bring about placental separation. This usually takes 10–20 minutes and is favoured by those who prefer limited intervention in the management of labour. Some will encourage suckling immediately after delivery to stimulate physiological oxytocin release.[8] Unfortunately, this physiologically attractive approach is not as effective at reducing PPH when compared with active pharmacological management.[9]

- *Active management* entails giving an oxytocic drug during or just after delivery of the infant in order to consistently cause the uterine contractions that lead to placental separation and haemostasis. Active management of the third stage of labour has evolved over the past half century and several randomized controlled trials have shown that it effectively reduces blood loss, need for therapeutic doses of oxytocic drugs, PPH and blood transfusion by 50–70% when compared with expectant

management.[10] The evidence and experience with active management is such that this has become the standard of care.[11] Expectant management is only followed at the express and informed request of the woman.

The choice of oxytocic for routine active management is usually between the cheaper injectable drugs, oxytocin and ergometrine, or a combination of both in the compound Syntometrine®. Of these, oxytocin is the cheapest, has the fewest side effects and does not cause retained placenta. It is, however, shorter-acting (15–30 minutes). Ergometrine is effective but has more side effects (see below), has a longer duration of action (60–120 minutes) and a slightly higher risk of causing retained placenta. Thus, oxytocin is the drug of first choice and is given as a dose of either 5 units intravenously or 10 units by intramuscular injection with delivery of the anterior shoulder or as soon thereafter as feasible.

> 'The uniform operation of the ergot to restrain uterine haemorrhage ... has frequently been prescribed, a little previous to the birth of the child, or immediately after, to the patients who have been accustomed to flow immoderately, at such times, and it has always proved an effectual preventive.'
> Oliver Prescott
> A Dissertation on the Natural History and Medical Effects of Secale Cornutum or Ergot. Andover: Flagg & Gould, 1813, p14

> 'In patients liable to haemorrhage, immediately after delivery ... ergot may be given as a preventive a few minutes before the termination of the labour.'
> John Stearns
> Observations on the secale cornutum or ergot, with directions for its use in parturition. Med Rec 1822; 5:90

The risk of atonic postpartum haemorrhage is greatest in the hour following delivery. However, the woman is susceptible to atonic haemorrhage over the next 2–3 hours. Thus, if oxytocin has been used for active management its short duration of action may necessitate the addition of oxytocin to the intravenous infusion for the next 2–3 hours. If ergometrine or Syntometrine® have been used the longer duration of action will usually suffice. In women with risk factors for more prolonged postpartum uterine atony (e.g. multiple pregnancy) longer-acting oxytocic drugs such as a prolonged oxytocin infusion and, in selected cases, prostaglandins or carbetocin may be necessary for adequate prophylaxis.

TABLE 20-1 **Characteristics of Oxytocic Drugs**

Drug	Dose and Route	Duration of Action	Adverse Effects	Contraindication
Oxytocin	5 units IV 10 units IM 20 units in 500 ml infusion	15–30 minutes	Insignificant hypotension and flushing. Water intoxication in high doses (>200 units)	None
Ergometrine	0.2–0.25 mg IV or IM	1–2 hours	Nausea, vomiting, hypertension, vasospasm	Pre-eclampsia/hypertension, cardiovascular disease
Syntometrine® (5 units oxytocin, 0.5 mg ergometrine)	1 ampoule IM	1–2 hours	Nausea, vomiting, hypertension, vasospasm	Pre-eclampsia/hypertension, cardiovascular disease
15-methyl PGF$_{2\alpha}$	0.25 mg IM or IMM 0.25 mg in 500 ml infusion	4–6 hours	Vomiting, diarrhoea, flushing, shivering, vasospasm, bronchospasm	Cardiovascular disease, asthma
Misoprostol	600 µg oral, sublingual 800–1000 µg, sublingual or rectal	1–2 hours	Nausea, diarrhoea, shivering, pyrexia	None
Carbetocin	100 µg IM or IV	1–2 hours	Flushing	None

IM, intramuscular; IMM, intramyometrial; IV, intravenous.
Adopted with permission from Baskett TF. Essential management of obstetric emergencies. 4th ed. Bristol: Clinical Press, 2004.

OXYTOCIC DRUGS

It is important to know the characteristics and side effects of the available oxytocic drugs, each of which has application in a variety of clinical circumstances (Table 20-1).

Oxytocin

Oxytocin is the cheapest and safest of the injectable oxytocic drugs. It induces the rapid onset of strong rhythmic uterine contractions which last for 15–30 minutes. The effect is mainly on the upper uterine segment. Oxytocin also produces a transient vascular smooth muscle relaxant effect which may lead to a mild, brief reduction in blood pressure because of the reduced total peripheral resistance. This hypotension is mild and clinically insignificant except in cases of cardiovascular instability.[12] The dose is 5 units intravenously by slow intravenous bolus, 10 units intramuscularly or 20 units in 500 ml crystalloid by intravenous infusion.

Ergometrine

Ergometrine was the first of the injectable oxytocics and has been in use for 75 years. It produces prolonged uterine contractions involving the upper and lower uterine segments with a duration of 60–120 minutes. Ergometrine produces contraction of smooth muscle throughout the body and this is particularly relevant in the vascular tree. Peripheral vasoconstriction, which in the normal woman is not clinically significant, can produce a severe rise in blood pressure in the hypertensive or pre-eclamptic woman. In such cases it is contraindicated. Ergometrine can also induce coronary artery spasm which is also of no significance in the healthy woman, but has been incriminated in very rare cases of myocardial infarction in susceptible women. Ergometrine-induced vasospasm is responsive to glyceryl trinitrate.

Because of its prolonged effect, ergometrine causes a slight increase in uterine entrapment of the separated placenta.[13] Compared with oxytocin this amounts to about an additional 1 in 200 cases requiring manual removal. Nausea and/or vomiting occur in 20–25% of women who receive ergometrine. The dose of ergometrine is 0.2–0.25 mg by intramuscular injection. Because of the vasopressor effect it is better not given intravenously, although if the indication is urgent it can be given as a slow intravenous bolus of 0.2 mg. The higher dose of 0.5 mg should not be given initially as the side-effect profile is increased, without a concomitant improvement in the uterotonic effect.

ERGOMETRINE

'Reckoned in the saving of human life, places it among the enduring achievements of medical science'
   Chassar Moir
   The obstetrician bids, and the uterus contracts. BMJ 1964; 110:1029

Syntometrine®

Syntometrine® comes in an ampoule combining oxytocin 5 units and ergometrine 0.5 mg. Given intramuscularly, oxytocin has its effect within 2–3 minutes while ergometrine takes 4–5 minutes. The side-effect profile of both drugs is combined and this may have the beneficial effect of the vasodilatation effect of oxytocin ameliorating, to some extent, the vasoconstricting effect of ergometrine. This combination provides the benefit of the short-acting oxytocin along with the more sustained uterotonic effect of ergometrine. It has the benefit, therefore, of providing more sustained oxytocic prophylaxis in the first 2 hours following delivery, thereby obviating the need for an intravenous infusion.[14]

15-Methyl Prostaglandin F2α

15-methyl $PGF_{2\alpha}$ or carboprost (Hemabate) is the 15-methyl analogue of the parent compound $PGF_{2\alpha}$. This is the most expensive of the injectable oxytocics. Its advantage is that, at a comparable dose, it has a strong uterotonic effect and fewer of the undesirable smooth muscle stimulation effects including nausea, vomiting, diarrhoea, vasospasm and bronchospasm. As a result it has supplanted the parent compound for this oxytocic indication. Other side effects which are usually not clinically significant are shivering, pyrexia and flushing. The duration of action is up to 6 hours and while, on the basis of cost and side effects, it is not recommended for routine prophylaxis it is a very useful agent when a prolonged oxytocic effect is required.

The dose is 0.25 mg and it can be given intramuscularly, intramyometrially or as a dilute intravenous infusion of 0.25 mg in 500 ml saline.[15] The quickest effect is usually attained by the intramyometrial route in which the 1 ml ampoule of 0.25 mg is diluted in 5 ml saline and injected transabdominally at two sites into the uterine fundus. 15-methyl $PGF_{2\alpha}$ can be given in cases of hypertension and asthma, although

these are relative contraindications. It is an excellent second line uterotonic agent if oxytocin and ergometrine have failed or if a long-term oxytocic effect is required.

Misoprostol

An analogue of prostaglandin E1, misoprostol is the cheapest oxytocic and the only one that can be given by the non-parenteral route. Misoprostol is used off-label as an oxytocic drug but has the endorsement of many national societies of obstetrics and gynaecology, has been added to the WHO list of Essential Medicines for the prevention of PPH and is increasingly chosen as the second-line uterotonic drug.[16] It has a long shelf life and is stable at extremes of temperature. This is in contrast with oxytocin and ergometrine which lose their potency unless stored in the dark at cool temperatures (0–8°C). Misoprostol can be given orally, sublingually, vaginally or rectally, depending on the clinical situation. It has a low side-effect profile with shivering, mild pyrexia and diarrhoea being the main associations. It has been shown to be more effective than placebo in the prevention of PPH but is slightly less effective than the injectable oxytocics.[17] However, the features mentioned above make it a drug of enormous potential for use in the developing world where obstetric facilities are limited, and where the majority of deaths occur.[18] It also has use as a second-line oxytocic drug when oxytocin and/or ergometrine have failed. The usual dose is 600 μg orally or sublingually, and in the case of haemorrhage, 800 μg sublingually or 1000 μg rectally.[16] Recent FIGO (International Federation of Gynaecology and Obstetrics) Guidelines on management of third stage of labour recommend 600 μg of misoprostol orally for prophylaxis of PPH and 800 μg sublingually for treatment of PPH.[19] The duration of effect of misoprostol is about 2 hours.

Carbetocin

Carbetocin is a long-acting synthetic analogue of oxytocin. The duration of action is 60–120 minutes. It is given as a single dose of 100 μg by intramuscular or intravenous injection. The side effects are similar to those of oxytocin, namely flushing and mild hypotension. Its purported advantage is that it provides a prolonged oxytocic effect compared with the parent compound oxytocin, obviating the need for an intravenous infusion of oxytocin for the 2 hours following initial active management of the third stage of labour.[20,21] It is more expensive than oxytocin but less so than 15-methyl $PGF_{2\alpha}$.

HISTORICAL BACKGROUND

The development of modern oxytocic drugs is of interest. Building on the observations by midwives and doctors in the previous four centuries that powdered ergot caused strong uterine contractions, Chassar Moir and the research chemist Harold Dudley set out to discover the active oxytocic component. In 1935, after 3 years of research, during which Moir tested many compounds for their oxytocic effect on the postpartum uterus, they isolated ergometrine – the active oxytocic alkaloid of ergot. Independently, and almost simultaneously, it was discovered in Chicago, Baltimore and Switzerland. Working under Sir Henry Dale's guidance in London, and recognizing the clinical importance of this first reliable and injectable oxytocic, Moir and Dudley published the full formula and method of production so that no patent or proprietary interest would be served.

In 1952 Vincent DuVigneaud at Cornell University, New York, identified and synthesized pure oxytocin. After the identification of the individual prostaglandins by Sune Bergstrom and his colleagues at the Karolinska Institute in Stockholm, the 15-methyl analogue of $PGF_{2\alpha}$ was applied to the treatment of PPH in the 1970s. By the 1990s misoprostol was being used for the prevention and management of PPH due to uterine atony. Thus, the modern era of oxytocic drug development started with the discovery of ergometrine in 1935, and has moved forward in approximately 20-year epochs over the last 75 years.[22,23]

CAUSES OF PRIMARY PPH

Uterine Atony

This is caused by anything that interferes with the ability of the uterus to contract and retract. It is the most common cause (80–85%). Although it can occur in low-risk cases, interference with uterine contraction and retraction is most likely in the following:

- Multiparity.
- Prolonged labour, particularly if it is associated with chorioamniotitis. The exhausted and infected uterus is vulnerable to uterine atony and may be unresponsive to oxytocic agents.
- Precipitate labour. In the other extreme of uterine action, the very rapid and efficient first and second stages of labour may be followed by uterine atony.
- Uterine over-distension: multiple pregnancy, macrosomia and polyhydramnios.
- Retained placenta or placental fragments.
- Retained blood clots. After delivery of the placenta the uterine fundus should be firmly massaged and an oxytocin drip kept running for 2–3 hours if there is any tendency for uterine relaxation. If not, a small amount of oozing from the placental site may occur, leading to clots in the uterus. As these accumulate they interfere with the ability of the uterus to contract and retract, leading to an insidious filling of the uterus with clots and blood, establishing a vicious cycle.
- Tocolytic drugs, such as glyceryl trinitrate or terbutaline and deep general anaesthesia, particularly with fluorinated hydrocarbons.
- Structural abnormalities of the uterus, including uterine anomalies and fibroids.
- Placenta praevia: the implantation site of the placenta is on the lower uterine segment which has limited ability to contract and retract.
- Inappropriate management of the third stage of labour with premature manipulation of the fundus and cord traction may lead to partial separation of the placenta and increased blood loss.

Genital Tract Trauma

See Chapter 23. This is the next most common cause accounting for the majority of the remaining 10–15% of cases and includes:

- lacerations of the perineum, vagina and cervix
- episiotomy
- uterine rupture
- vulvo-vaginal and broad ligament haematomas.

Other Causes

Other causes of primary PPH are uterine inversion (see Chapter 22) and coagulation disorders (see Chapter 25).

PREVENTION OF PRIMARY PPH

Women with risk factors for PPH should be delivered in hospitals with appropriate anaesthetic and obstetric personnel and available blood transfusion. In all women careful attention should be directed to details of safe management of the third stage of labour, including:

- Oxytocin is given with or shortly after delivery of the anterior shoulder.
- Avoid inappropriate manipulation of the uterine fundus ('fundus fiddling') and/or premature traction on the umbilical cord

before clear signs of placental separation are present.

- When the placenta is delivered, inspect it closely for completeness.
- Firmly massage the uterus to expel all clots that might interfere with contraction and retraction.
- Keep the uterus well contracted with an oxytocic for the next 2 hours, and longer in high-risk cases.
- Close surveillance, including attention to keeping the bladder empty and the uterine fundus well contracted for 2–3 hours following delivery.

MANAGEMENT OF PRIMARY PPH

The medical management of uterine atony will be covered here. The other causes and the surgical management of uterine atony are covered in other chapters. The immediate management of atonic postpartum haemorrhage is to enlist the normal physiological mechanism of uterine haemostasis – namely initiate uterine contraction and retraction. While getting the appropriate oxytocic drugs ready the hand should be used to apply firm but gentle fundal massage.

Oxytocic Drugs

It should be remembered that oxytocin administration down-regulates oxytocin receptors. Thus, if labour is augmented by oxytocin during the first and second stages of labour the receptors may be less responsive to oxytocin in the third stage of labour. In normal labour, oxytocin levels do not change in the third stage, but endogenous prostaglandin production increases. The myometrium has different receptors for each of the oxytocic drugs, so that if one drug is ineffective move quickly to the next choice. The following application and sequence of oxytocic drugs is recommended:

- Intravenous oxytocin 5 units and establish an infusion with 40 units of oxytocin in 500 ml crystalloid running rapidly enough to initiate and sustain uterine contractions.
- If this fails give ergometrine 0.2 mg slowly intravenously (provided there are no contraindications).
- The doses of oxytocin and ergometrine can be repeated. If oxytocin and ergometrine are ineffective do not delay in moving to the prostaglandins.
- In the presence of active haemorrhage the vaginal route for misoprostol is less appropriate –because the tablets are washed away by the haemorrhage. The preferred route is sublingual or oral 800 µg.[19] Because it is cheap and simple to administer many will move to misoprostol earlier in the sequence.
- 15-methyl prostaglandin $F_{2\alpha}$ 0.25 mg can be given by intramuscular or preferably by intramyometrial injection. This can be repeated up to four times if necessary. An alternative is an infusion of 0.25 mg in 500 ml crystalloid.
- Hypovolaemia should be actively treated with intravenous crystalloid, colloid, blood and blood products as required (see Chapter 24).

If uterine atony is unresponsive to fundal massage and the available oxytocic drugs, surgical techniques including uterine tamponade, uterine compression sutures, major vessel ligation and embolization, and even hysterectomy will have to be considered. These are all outlined in Chapter 28.

While preparations are being made for the surgical techniques *bimanual uterine compression* may be undertaken as a stop-gap measure. The vaginal hand forms a fist in the anterior fornix while the abdominal hand cups the posterofundal aspect of the uterus, pulling it down against the vaginal fist. The vaginal hand also elevates the uterus. In this way the uterine vessels may be attenuated and compressed to reduce the bleeding. The hands may also provide rotary massage to try and stimulate uterine contraction (Fig 20-3).

In desperate circumstances, while awaiting the muster of surgical instruments, *external aortic compression* can be tried. This involves the two

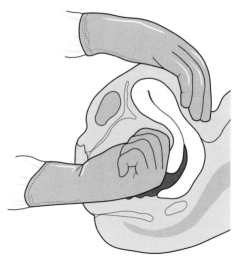

FIGURE 20-3 ■ Bimanual uterine compression.

hands lifting the fundus of the uterus up out of the pelvis; the lower hand then pushes upwards and backwards on the lower uterine segment while the other hand pushes the fundus firmly down onto the aorta. This may be of limited value if the uterus is very atonic, as it may not provide a firm enough compression pad. An alternative technique is to use the fist applied directly in the midline, just above the umbilicus and uterus, with the heel of the hand pressing down on the aorta.[24] This may be feasible due to the stretched abdominal muscles and separation of the rectus muscles, but is obviously a short-term measure.

Preparedness for PPH

Audit, education and simulation training by labour and delivery unit staff can reduce delay and improve outcomes in cases of obstetric haemorrhage.[25–27] For many of the surgical approaches to severe PPH (see Chapter 28) the necessary equipment may be rarely used and not readily to hand. It is therefore wise for each unit to have a PPH bundle or tray available beside the obstetric operating theatre which contains the necessary items for uterine and vaginal tamponade, uterine compression sutures and major vessel ligation.[28]

SECONDARY PPH

This is defined as abnormal bleeding from the genital tract between 24 hours and 6 weeks postpartum. It is much less common than primary PPH, occurring in about 1% of deliveries. The majority of cases occur within 3 weeks of delivery.

Causes

- Retained placental tissue is found in about one-third of cases.
- Intrauterine infection often co-exists with retained tissue.
- In many cases neither of the above can be clearly demonstrated but the patient will have a history of primary PPH and/or manual removal of the placenta at this delivery.
- Extremely rare causes also have to be considered, including: trophoblastic disease, chronic uterine inversion and the development of a pseudoaneurysm or arteriovenous sinus at the site of a healing caesarean section scar.

MANAGEMENT

If the bleeding is mild and settling, the uterus is not tender, is appropriately involuted, and there are no other signs of sepsis, initial observation is justified. Ultrasound may help this decision if it suggests that the uterus is empty and without retained placental tissue.[29]

Those patients with heavy bleeding, with signs of intrauterine sepsis and a subinvoluted uterus suggesting infected retained placental tissue should have uterine exploration under anaesthesia. Ultrasound may help confirm this decision but it is not always accurate so it should be overruled by clinical considerations. These cases require intravenous crystalloid, cross-match blood and broad-spectrum intravenous antibiotics to cover Gram-positive, Gram-negative and anaerobic organisms. Occasionally these patients can bleed severely and require transfusion.

Under anaesthesia the lower genital tract and cervix should be carefully inspected in case there is a laceration or discharging haematoma. Usually the cervix is open enough that the finger can enter and explore the uterine cavity. One may be able to detect and detach placental tissue from the uterine wall. This may be removed with sponge forceps followed by gentle suction curettage.

The tissue removed should be sent for histopathology to rule out trophoblastic disease. In septic cases a portion may be sent for culture and antibiotic sensitivity testing.[30]

The recently puerperal uterus is soft and very prone to perforation. One should be particularly cautious in cases delivered by caesarean section and avoid curetting the incised part of the uterus. Quite severe haemorrhage can be induced by curettage, as organized portions of placental tissue, some of which may be areas of partial accreta, are removed from the uterine wall opening up the partially thrombosed vessels. This bleeding is usually not responsive to oxytocic agents. On occasions, surgical management has to be considered including uterine tamponade, major vessel embolization and hysterectomy (see Chapter 28).

In cases following delivery by caesarean section the rare cases of pseudoaneurysm or arteriovenous sinus may be diagnosed and treated by uterine angiography and embolization.[31]

REFERENCES

1. Confidential Enquiry into Maternal and Child Health. Why Mothers Die 2000–2002. London: RCOG Press; 2004.
2. Confidential Enquiry into Maternal and Child Health. Saving Mothers' Lives 2003–2005. London: RCOG Press; 2006.

3. Baskett TF, Sternadel J. Maternal intensive care and near-miss mortality in obstetrics. Br J Obstet Gynaecol 1998;105:981–4.

4. Baskett TF, O'Connell CM. Severe obstetric maternal morbidity: a 15-year population-based study. J Obstet Gynaecol 2005;25:7–9.

5. Joseph KS, Rouleau J, Kramer MS, Young DC, Liston RM, Baskett TF. Investigation of an increase in postpartum haemorrhage in Canada. Br J Obstet Gynaecol 2007;114:751–9.

6. Ford JB, Roberts CL, Simpson JM, Vaughan J, Cameron CA. Increased postpartum haemorrhage rate in Australia. Int J Gynecol Obstet 2007;98:237–43.

7. Dildy GA, Paine AR, George NC, Velasco C. Estimating blood loss: can teaching significantly improve visual estimation? Obstet Gynecol 2004;104:601–6.

8. Chua S, Arulkumaran S, Lim I, Selamat N, Ratnam SS. Influence of breast-feeding and nipple stimulation on postpartum uterine activity. Br J Obstet Gynaecol 1994; 101:804–5.

9. Bullough CHW, Msuku RS, Karonde L. Early suckling and postpartum haemorrhage: controlled trial in deliveries by traditional birth attendants. Lancet 1989;2: 522–5.

10. Baskett TF. A flux of the reds: evolution of active management of the third stage of labour. J R Soc Med 2000;93:489–93.

11. World Health Organization. Recommendations for the prevention of postpartum haemorrhage. Geneva: WHO; 2007.

12. Davies GAL, Tessier JL, Woodman MC, Lipson A, Hahn PM. Maternal hemodynamics after oxytocin bolus compared with infusion in the third stage of labor: a randomized controlled trial. Obstet Gynecol 2005;105: 294–9.

13. Hammar M, Bostrom K, Borgvall B. Comparison between the influence of methylergometrine and oxytocin on the incidence of retained placenta in the third stage of labour. Gynecol Obstet Invest 1990;30:91–4.

14. Choy CMY, Lau WC, Tam WH, Yuen PM. A randomised controlled trial of intramuscular Syntometrine and intravenous oxytocin in the management of the third stage of labour. Br J Obstet Gynaecol 2002;109: 173–7.

15. Granstrom L, Ekinan G, Ulmsten U. Intravenous infusion of 15 methyl prostaglandin F2 alpha in women with heavy postpartum haemorrhage. Acta Obstet Gynecol Scand 1989;68:365–7.

16. Royal College of Obstetricians and Gynaecologists. Prevention and management of postpartum haemorrhage. Green-top Guideline No. 52. London: RCOG; 2009.

17. Gulmezoglu AM, Forna F, Villar J, Hofmeyer GJ. Prostaglandins for prevention of postpartum haemorrhage. Cochrane Database Syst Rev 2007;3:CD000494.

18. Alfirevic Z, Blum J, Walraven G, Weeks A, Winikoff B. Prevention of postpartum haemorrhage with misoprostol. Int J Gynecol Obstet 2007;99 (Suppl 2):s198–201.

19. Starrs A, Winikoff B. Misoprostol for postpartum haemorrhage: moving from evidence to practice. Int J Gynecol Obstet 2012;116:1–3.

20. Boucher M, Harbay GL, Griffin P. Double-blind randomised comparison of the effect of carbetocin and oxytocin on intraoperative blood loss and uterine tone of patients undergoing cesarean section. J Perinatol 1998; 18:202–7.

21. Leung SW, Ng PS, Wong WY, Cheung TH. A randomized trial of carbetocin versus syntometrine in the management of the third stage of labour. Br J Obstet Gynaecol 2006;113:1459–64.

22. Baskett TF. The development of prostaglandins. Best Pract Res Clin Obstet Gynaecol 2003;17:703–6.

23. Baskett TF. The development of oxytocic drugs in the management of postpartum haemorrhage. Ulster Med J 2004;73:2–6.

24. Riley DP, Burgess RW. External abdominal aortic compression: a study of a resuscitation manoeuvre for postpartum haemorrhage. Anaesth Intens Care 1994;22: 571–5.

25. Rizvi F, Mackey R, Barrett T, McKenna P, Geary M. Successful reduction of massive postpartum haemorrhage by use of guidelines and staff education. Br J Obstet Gynaecol 2004;111:495–1047.

26. Skupski DW, Lowenwirt IP, Weinbaum FI, Brodsky D, Danek M, Eglington GS. Improving hospital systems for the care of women with major obstetric haemorrhage. Obstet Gynecol 2006;107:977–83.

27. Brace V, Kernaghan D, Penney G. Learning from adverse clinical outcomes: major obstetric haemorrhage in Scotland, 2003–05. Br J Obstet Gynaecol 2007;114: 1388–96.

28. Baskett TF. Surgical management of severe obstetric haemorrhage: experience with an obstetric haemorrhage equipment tray. J Obstet Gynaecol Can 2004;26: 805–8.

29. Skinner J, Turner MJ. Postpartum exploration of the genital tract under general anaesthesia reviewed. J Obstet Gynaecol 1997;17:273.

30. Hoveyda F, Mackenzie IZ. Secondary postpartum haemorrhage: incidence, morbidity and current management. Br J Obstet Gynaecol 2001;108:927–30.

31. Lausman AY, Ellis CA, Beecroft JR, Simons M, Shapiro JL. A rare etiology of delayed postpartum haemorrhage. J Obstet Gynaecol Can 2008;30:239–43.

CHAPTER 21

RETAINED PLACENTA

AD Weeks

'I find it both amongst the ancients and moderns there have been different opinions and directions about delivering the placenta; some alleging that it should be delivered slowly, or left to come, of itself; others, that the hand should be immediately introduced into the uterus, to separate and bring it away ... So in my opinion we ought to go the middle way, never to assist but when we find it necessary: on the one hand, not to torture nature when it is self-sufficient, nor delay too long, because it is possible that the placenta should be sometimes, though seldom, retained several days'.
> William Smellie
> Treatise on the Theory and Practice of Midwifery. London: D Wilson, 1752, p239

The delivery of the placenta is the most dangerous point of pregnancy for the woman. Before delivery there is blood flow to the placental bed of around 500 ml per minute, and if the uterus does not contract as the placenta detaches, this flow will continue and the mother can exsanguinate within minutes. Great care is therefore taken to ensure that the placenta delivers cleanly and the uterus contracts immediately afterwards. The routine care is described below, followed by the management of delayed placental separation.

ROUTINE MANAGEMENT OF THE THIRD STAGE

It is now recognized that it is the oxytocic drug that prevents excessive blood loss – the other components of the 'active management package' appear to have little or no benefit.[1-4]

Oxytocic Drugs

Oxytocin 10 units intramuscularly is now accepted to be the first line oxytocic for routine management and is given immediately after delivery of the fetus.[1-3] The oxytocin/ergometrine combination (Syntometrine®) is slightly more effective but causes vomiting and hypertension. Oral misoprostol is a less effective alternative for use where oxytocin is unavailable.

Cord Clamping

The timing of cord clamping has been the topic of debate for over 200 years. There appears to be no maternal benefit of early cord clamping and it prevents around 90 ml of blood transferring to the baby from the placenta. Most authorities therefore suggest that the cord is not clamped until 2–3 minutes after birth.[1,3] For those babies who need immediate neonatal care this can either be received at the bedside (using a small resuscitation trolley if needed), or 'cord milking' can be employed. This involves squeezing the cord between finger and thumb and sliding the fingers along the cord for about 20 cm towards the fetus two or three times before clamping the cord. There are concerns that this technique could cause fetal cardiac overload and it is therefore not currently recommended.

'Another thing very injurious to the child, is the tying and cutting of the navel string too soon which should always be left not only until the child has repeatedly breathed, but till all pulsations in the cord cease. As otherwise the child is much weaker than it ought to be, a portion of the blood being left in the placenta, which ought to have been in the child.'
> Erasmus Darwin (British physician, philosopher and grandfather of Charles Darwin)
> *Zoonomia* 1794, Part I. London: J. Johnson

Controlled Cord Traction

Controlled cord traction is performed at the time of the first contraction following delivery of the baby. The birth attendant pushes the uterine body upwards with one hand while the other hand applies continuous traction on the umbilical cord to extract the placenta. A large recent trial has shown that this procedure has minimal effect on blood loss but shortens the length of the third stage slightly.[4]

Uterine Massage

Uterine massage is added to the active management package by some authorities, even though

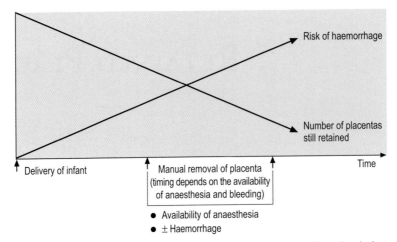

FIGURE 21-1 ■ Factors in decision and timing of manual removal of retained placenta.

there is little evidence for its benefit. After delivery of the placenta the fundus of the uterus is massaged every 15 minutes to ensure that the uterus is firmly contracted and not distending with clots.

RETAINED PLACENTA

With traditional or expectant management of the third stage of labour the placenta usually delivers within 10–20 minutes. With active management the placenta is commonly delivered within 5–10 minutes. In general, 90% of placentas deliver within 15 minutes, 96% within 30 minutes and 98% within 60 minutes. The incidence of retained placenta, therefore, depends on the time chosen. The rate is also higher in well resourced settings and has increased over time,[5] although the reason for this is unclear.

Once time passes without placental delivery, the risk of haemorrhage increases and the chance of spontaneous delivery of the placenta decreases. The time at which one declares the placenta retained and takes active steps for its removal depends on the facilities and personnel available for safe anaesthesia, as well as the presence or absence of haemorrhage. These considerations are illustrated in Figure 21-1.

Types of Retained Placenta

- *Trapped placenta*: The placenta has separated from the uterine wall but is retained in the uterus. Clinically the uterus is small and contracted, but the fundus high. Ultrasound examination shows a well-contracted uterus with the placenta retained in a bulging lower segment.[6]
- *Placenta adherens*: 'Adherence' of the placenta is due to failure of the myometrium

behind the placenta to contract. Until separation occurs, either partially or completely, these cases do not bleed excessively. Ultrasound shows the placenta within the uterine body attached to a thin, uncontracted myometrium.[6]
- *Placenta accreta*: This is usually detected at caesarean section, but can be found in small areas following vaginal delivery (see below). The management of placenta praevia accreta is discussed in Chapter 19.

Predisposing Factors[6]

- Retained placenta in previous pregnancy; the recurrence risk is 25%.[7]
- Poor myometrial contractility (causes placenta adherens): preterm labour (around 25% of all deliveries at 25 weeks have a retained placenta compared to only 3% at term),[8] uterine fibroids, labour induction or need for oxytocin augmentation.
- Disrupted myometrial–placental interface (causes partial accreta): pre-eclampsia, previous miscarriage and abortion, uterine anomaly (e.g. bicornuate uterus) or uterine scar (previous caesarean section, myomectomy, hysteroscopic surgery, curettage).
- Premature contraction of the lower segment (causes a trapped placenta): use of intravenous ergometrine for postpartum haemorrhage (PPH) prophylaxis.

'Since it is a verity indubitable, that the after birth remaining behind after the child is born, becomes a useless mass, capable of destroying the woman, we must take care that it be never left, if possible.'
Francois Mauriceau
The Diseases of Women with Child, and in Child-Bed. London: John Darby, 1683:p212

Management

In most cases of retained placenta, management consists of manual removal. However, the timing of this procedure depends on the availability of safe anaesthesia and also on the presence or absence of haemorrhage. If there is little or no bleeding most will delay for 30 minutes before preparing for manual removal, which is undertaken at around 1 hour postpartum. Just before induction of anaesthesia a pelvic examination should be carried out, as in a number of cases the placenta will deliver spontaneously while the resources for anaesthesia are being mustered.

If the woman has delivered with an existing regional anaesthetic in place, this delay is not necessary as the risks of anaesthesia have already been undertaken. On balance, waiting about 15 minutes in the absence of haemorrhage is reasonable.

In any case in which haemorrhage supervenes, manual removal should be carried out at once.

Technique of Manual Removal

General anaesthesia has the advantage of speed and will also assist by providing uterine relaxation. However, the additional risks of general anaesthesia to the mother make the choice of spinal anaesthesia better, provided there is no haemorrhage. With spinal anaesthesia, uterine relaxation may not occur and this can be provided by nitroglycerine if necessary (see Chapter 28).

With the patient in the dorsal lithotomy position and appropriate asepsis, one hand is placed on the abdomen to steady the fundus and push the uterus downwards. The well lubricated other hand follows the cord into the vagina and through the cervix. The lower uterine segment can be very thin and ballooned out, above which there is often a thick contraction ring at the junction of the upper and lower uterine segments (Fig 21-2). For the unwary operator this ballooned out lower uterine segment may be mistaken for the uterine cavity proper and the hand may be pushed through the thinned-out lower uterine segment. To avoid uterine rupture with the exploring hand, press down on the fundus of the uterus with the external hand. The fingers of the internal hand should be formed into a cone and slowly but firmly pushed upwards through the contraction ring. Uterine relaxation either by general anaesthesia or nitroglycerine may be necessary to allow the hand into the upper part of the uterine cavity. The fingers and thumb of the uterine

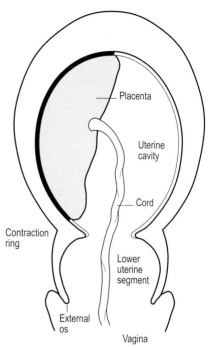

FIGURE 21-2 ■ A contraction ring has formed below the placenta at the junction of the upper and lower uterine segments. The thin, ballooned lower segment is vulnerable to perforation by the exploring hand during manual removal.

hand should be kept extended and used as one unit to advance along the umbilical cord to the lower margin of the placenta. This is recognized due to the different feel: while the membranes are smooth and slippery, the decidual layer is spongy and rough. With the correct layer identified, the placenta is detached by sweeping the hand from side to side within the plane of cleavage between the placenta and uterine wall. The external hand steadies the fundus to facilitate these internal manipulations (Fig 21-3). Once completely separated the placenta is grasped and removed slowly. The uterus is re-explored to ensure that there are no placental fragments remaining and that the uterine wall is intact.

Sometimes one will encounter accretic areas of placenta. Small pieces can be removed piecemeal and should not interfere with contraction and retraction of the uterus.

The cervix and vagina are examined and any lacerations sutured. An intravenous injection of 5 units of oxytocin followed by an infusion of 40 units in 1 L over 4 hours is established to maintain uterine contraction. A prophylactic dose of broad-spectrum antibiotic is given to prevent infection.

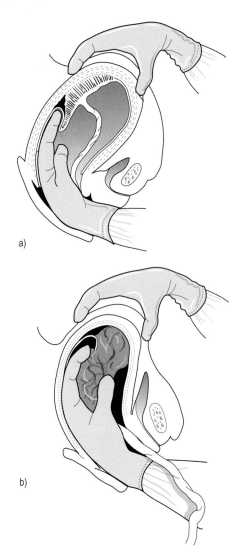

a)

b)

FIGURE 21-3 ■ (a) A sweeping movement separates the placenta. (b) The detached placenta is grasped and removed.

Intraumbilical Vein Injection of Oxytocics

In some studies intraumbilical vein injection of oxytocic drugs has been shown to aid spontaneous delivery of the placenta. Both oxytocin and prostaglandins have been used, but there is more experience with the former. Usually 20–50 units of oxytocin are mixed in 30 ml saline and injected through a catheter that has been threaded up the umbilical vein. The aim is to deliver high concentration oxytocin to the retroplacental myometrium which will then contract and shear off the placenta. Although the simplicity is attractive, two large WHO-sponsored randomized trials have failed to replicate the results of the smaller studies and the Cochrane meta-analysis does not support it.[9,10]

Tocolysis

In those cases in which the placenta is retained by a contraction ring or tight cervix, the use of acute tocolysis is logical. Recent randomized-controlled trials (RCTs) have suggested that sublingual glyceryl trinitrate tablets may be beneficial[11] and a definitive randomized trial is in preparation.

REFERENCES

1. National Collaborating Centre for Women's and Children's Health (NCCWCH). Intrapartum Care (NICE Guideline). London: RCOG Press; 2007.
2. Royal College of Obstetricians and Gynaecologists. Prevention and management of postpartum haemorrhage. Green-top Guideline No. 52. London: RCOG Press; 2009.
3. World Health Organization. WHO Recommendations for the prevention and treatment of postpartum haemorrhage. Geneva: World Health Organization; 2012.
4. Gülmezoglu AM, Lumbiganon P, Landoulsi S, Widmer M, Abdel-Aleem H, Festin M, et al. Active management of the third stage of labour with and without controlled cord traction: a randomised, controlled, non-inferiority trial. Lancet 2012;379:1721–7.
5. Cheung WM, Hawkes A, Ibish S, Weeks AD. The retained placenta: historical and geographical rate variations. J Obstet Gynaecol 2011;31(1):37–42.
6. Weeks AD. The retained placenta. Best Pract Res Clin Obstet Gynaecol 2008;22:1103–67.
7. Nikolajsen S, Løkkegaard EC, Bergholt T. Reoccurrence of retained placenta at vaginal delivery: an observational study. Acta Obstet Gynecol Scand 2013;92:421–5.
8. Dombrowski MP, Bottoms SF, Salah AAA, Hurd WW, Romero R. Third stage of labor: an analysis of duration and clinical practice. Am J Obstet Gynecol 1995; 172:1279–84.
9. Nardin JM, Weeks A, Carroli G. Umbilical vein injection for management of retained placenta. Cochrane Database Syst Rev 2011;(5):CD001337.
10. Weeks AD, Alia G, Vernon G, Namayanja A, Gosakan R, Majeed T, et al. Umbilical vein oxytocin for the treatment of retained placenta (Release Study): a double-blind, randomised controlled trial. Lancet 2010; 375:141–7.
11. Bullarbo M, Bokström H, Lilja H, Almström E, Lassenius N, Hansson A, et al. Nitroglycerin for management of retained placenta: a multicenter study. Obstet Gynecol Int 2012;3:321–7.

CHAPTER 22

ACUTE UTERINE INVERSION

TF Baskett

'The child was born about an hour before I came, and the midwife in attempting to bring away the placenta, had inverted the uterus; for upon examination, I found the whole body of the uterus with the placenta, adhering to the fundus, hanging out beyond the labia; there was a great profusion of blood, and the woman was dead before I came ... This case should be a caution to all practitioners how they attempt to bring away the placenta, and not to pull the string too rudely, lest they invert and draw out the uterus, by which the woman dies a martyr to their temerity and ignorance, as was too plainly the case in the precedent observation'.
   William Giffard
   Cases in Midwifry. London: Motte, 1734, p421–422

Acute uterine inversion is a rare but life-threatening complication of the third stage of labour. The incidence varies widely between 1 in 2000 and 1 in 50 000 deliveries, largely dependent upon the standard of management of the third stage of labour. Acute uterine inversion occurs within 24 hours of delivery; subacute between 24 hours and 4 weeks of delivery; and chronic uterine inversion presents after 4 weeks or in the non-pregnant state. Cases of subacute and chronic uterine inversion require surgical management and in this chapter we are concerned only with acute uterine inversion.

TYPES

- *Incomplete inversion* occurs when the fundus of the uterus has turned inside-out, rather like the toe of a sock, but the inverted fundus has not descended through the cervix.
- *Complete inversion* occurs when the inverted fundus has passed completely through the cervix to lie within the vagina or, less often, outside the introitus.

Uterine inversion is sometimes described in degrees:
- 1st degree = incomplete inversion
- 2nd degree = complete inversion in the vagina
- 3rd degree = complete inversion outside the introitus (Fig 22-1).

'A contracted uterus can be no more inverted than a stiff jackboot, but when it is soft and relaxed you may invert it'.
   William Hunter
   In: Andrews H R. William Hunter and his work in midwifery. BMJ 1915; 1:277–282

CAUSES

For the uterus to be inverted it must be relaxed and this, along with fundal insertion of the placenta, is an important predisposing condition. Additional factors are as follows:[1]
- Mismanagement of the third stage of labour involving fundal pressure and/or cord traction before placental separation and while the uterus is still relaxed. This can be implicated in the majority of cases, despite the manifest surprise of the accoucheur. When reviewing a series of cases of acute uterine inversion to establish the causes Munro Kerr (1908) wrote:

'In examining them it is very evident that in the majority of cases the occurrence has followed pressure from above or traction from below ... In looking over the series I was not a little surprised at the large proportion of cases in which traction on the cord was the cause'.

- Abnormally short umbilical cord, or functionally shortened by being wrapped around the fetal body, can, in theory, cause the fundus of the uterus to be pulled inside-out by traction on the cord as the fetus delivers. This is extremely rare but plausible cases have been described.
- Sudden rise in intra-abdominal pressure due to maternal coughing or vomiting. This may occur in a vulnerable situation with the uterus relaxed and fundal insertion of the placenta followed by sudden and strong propulsion on the uterine fundus caused by the acute rise in intra-abdominal pressure.

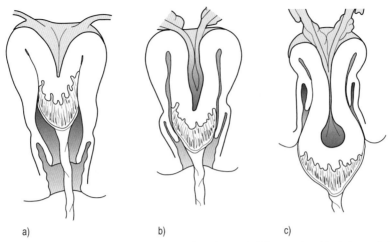

FIGURE 22-1 ■ Types of uterine inversion: (a) incomplete (1st degree), (b) complete (2nd degree), (c) complete (3rd degree).

- Morbid adherence of a fundally implanted placenta.
- Manual removal of the placenta. When separating a retained placenta from the uterine wall a portion may remain attached and as the placenta is withdrawn so too is the fundus of the uterus. This can occur with those who routinely and misguidedly undertake manual removal of the placenta at the time of caesarean section before the uterus has contracted.
- Connective tissue disorders, such as Marfan's syndrome, can predispose to acute uterine inversion.[2]

CLINICAL PRESENTATION

The diagnosis may be obvious and dramatic with a large boggy mass appearing at the introitus, with or without the placenta attached. While this is the most dramatic presentation it is also the least common. Other signs and symptoms are as follows:[3,4]

- Severe and sustained hypogastric pain in the third stage of labour.
- Shock that is initially out of proportion with apparent blood loss, due to the infundibulo-pelvic and round ligaments, ovaries and associated nerves being pulled into the crater of the inversion, which provides a strong vaso-vagal stimulus. Thus, the woman often becomes pallid and sweaty, with bradycardia, profound hypotension and even, on rare occasions, cardiac arrest. Within a short time, in the majority of cases, there is also marked haemorrhage and hypovolaemic shock.

- With complete inversion the uterus is not palpable per abdomen and the inverted fundus is either obvious at the introitus or on vaginal examination. In cases of incomplete uterine inversion, however, the fundus of the uterus may appear to be normal and only in thin women is it possible to feel the fundal dimple of the partial inversion.

MANAGEMENT

For acute uterine inversion to occur the myometrium and cervix must be relaxed. If the diagnosis is made immediately after it occurs, then that same degree of relaxation may allow immediate uterine replacement. Thus, if one is on the spot when the inversion happens, try immediate manual replacement. However, usually within 1–2 minutes the cervix and lower uterine segment clamp down and, along with increasing congestion, oedema and contraction of the inverted uterine fundus, this makes manual replacement without anaesthesia difficult, painful and usually impossible. If one attempt at immediate manual replacement of the uterus fails, move to the following sequence:

- Summon assistance (anaesthesia, nursing, obstetrician).
- Although the initial shock in these cases is usually of the neurogenic type, it is wise to

'Much of your success will depend upon your promptidude: the uterus should be returned quickly; but if there be much delay or violence, it may become impossible to do so'.
Edward W. Murphy
London Medical Gazette 1849; 8:751

be prepared for the haemorrhage and hypo-volaemia that will follow in most cases. Therefore, establish two wide-bore intravenous cannulae, rapidly run in 1–2 L of crystalloid, take blood for cross match of 4 units, and place a Foley catheter in the bladder.

- If pain is a dominant symptom, small doses of intravenous morphine may be given.
- *Anaesthesia* should be administered depending on the facilities and appraisal by the anaesthetist. If an epidural anaesthetic is already in place this may provide adequate analgesia. In those rare cases in which the patient is stable, not bleeding, and with normal vital signs some anaesthetists may give a spinal anaesthetic. In most patients, however, cardiovascular instability and shock make regional anaesthesia inappropriate. Thus, general anaesthesia is usually chosen, using one of the fluorinated hydrocarbons (sevoflurane or isoflurane) to aid uterine relaxation. In the past halothane was used effectively for this purpose, but it has been replaced because of its association with rare cases of myocardial irritability/arrhythmia and hepatotoxicity.
- If general anaesthesia does not produce adequate uterine relaxation, or if a regional anaesthetic has been used, tocolysis will be necessary.[5,6] The available drugs and technique are outlined in Chapter 28.
- *Manual replacement of the uterus* should be undertaken once anaesthesia and tocolysis have been established. If the placenta is still attached to the fundus do not remove it, as this will increase the blood loss. If the placenta is partially attached to the fundus it should be peeled off.

The uterine fundus, with or without the attached placenta, is cupped in the palm of the hand, the fingers and thumb of which are extended to feel the utero-cervical junction (Fig 22-2). The whole uterus is lifted up towards and beyond the umbilicus. Additional pressure is exerted with the fingertips to systematically and sequentially push and squeeze the uterine wall back through the cervix. This pressure may have to be sustained for 3–5 minutes to achieve complete replacement. Once the fundus has been replaced, keep the hand in the uterus while a rapid infusion of oxytocin is given to contract the uterus. When the uterus is felt to contract the hand is slowly withdrawn.

The sooner manual replacement is undertaken the more likely it is to succeed with relative ease. With suitable anaesthesia and tocolysis within 2 hours of the diagnosis, it is usually successful.

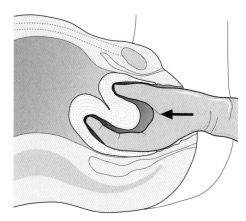

FIGURE 22-2 ■ Manual replacement of inverted uterus.

- If there is delay and/or manual replacement is unsuccessful try *O'Sullivan's hydrostatic replacement* technique.[7] Before using this procedure it is important to make sure that the uterus and vagina have no lacerations, and if these are found they should be sutured. The principle of this technique is to instil a large volume of fluid (3–5 L) into the upper vagina, thus distending the fornices, which serves to pull open the cervical ring, allowing replacement of the uterine fundus. Use 1 L bags of warmed saline with a pressure infuser. The intravenous tubing is guided into the posterior fornix by one hand which also cups the inverted fundus. The other hand seals the introitus around the wrist so that there is no egress of fluid (Fig 22-3). Alternatively, the tubing can be attached to a silastic vacuum extractor cup which is placed inside the introitus and may help provide a better seal.[8] For cases in which manual replacement has failed, O'Sullivan's technique can be remarkably and gratifyingly effective.[9]
- In rare delayed cases, manual replacement, with or without the hydrostatic technique, may be unsuccessful. In such cases *surgical replacement* will have to be undertaken. This involves laparotomy and *Huntington's operation* in which Allis or similar forceps are used to grasp the myometrium just inside the dimple of the inverted fundus.[10] Before using the Allis forceps the cervical ring may be stretched, either with the fingers or by opening the blades of a large forceps (Fig 22-4). Systematically and sequentially, using forceps on both sides, the inverted fundus is then withdrawn from the crater to fully correct the inversion (Fig 22-5). An alternative approach has been

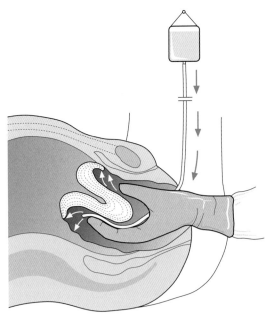

FIGURE 22-3 ■ Hydrostatic replacement of inverted uterus.

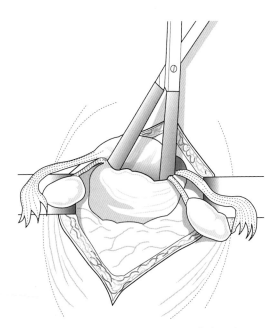

FIGURE 22-4 ■ Stretching the constriction ring.

undertaken using a soft silastic vacuum extraction cup instead of the potentially traumatic Allis forceps. The cup is placed through the dimple onto the uterine fundus, a vacuum created, and the inversion reduced by traction on the vacuum cup.[11]

On occasions the cervical ring is so tight that Huntington's technique is unsuccessful and merely causes tearing of the uterine muscle. In

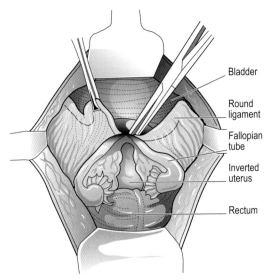

FIGURE 22-5 ■ Huntington's operation.

such cases *Haultain's operation* should be used.[12] This involves incision of the posterior cervical ring followed by withdrawal of the fundus using Allis forceps as described in the Huntington procedure. Once the fundus has been replaced the incision is sutured (Fig 22-6).

RECURRENT UTERINE INVERSION

Rarely, despite successful replacement and administration of oxytocic drugs, the acute inversion recurs. Two recent approaches to this problem have been proposed.[13,14] One is to manually replace the inversion again and keep the uterine fundus in place with insertion of an intrauterine tamponade balloon[13] (see Chapter 28). An alternative plan, for cases treated at laparotomy by the Huntington operation, is to maintain the uterine fundus in position with uterine compression sutures.[14]

- Whatever method of uterine replacement is used it should be followed by an oxytocic to keep the uterus well contracted for 8–12 hours. After the initial use of intravenous oxytocin to contract the uterus there is much to be said for using the longer-acting prostaglandins, such as 15-methyl $PGF_{2\alpha}$ or misoprostol for this purpose (see Chapter 20).
- A broad-spectrum antibiotic should be given for 24–48 hours because of the manipulation and the large uterine surface area which is traumatized and exposed to the vaginal bacterial flora.

The management of acute uterine inversion is summarized in Figure 22-7.

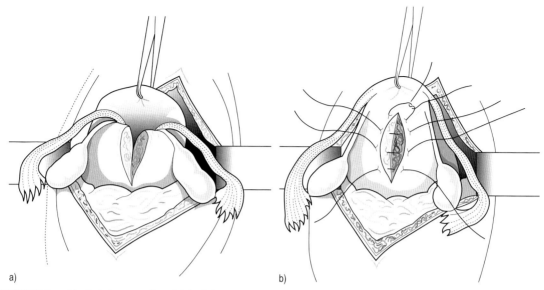

FIGURE 22-6 ■ Haultain's operation. (a) Incision of the posterior part of constricting ring. (b) Suturing uterine incision after reduction of the inversion.

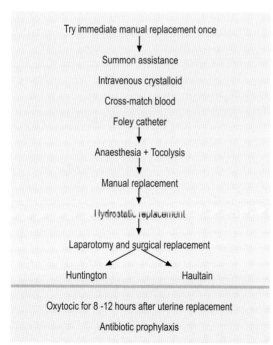

Try immediate manual replacement once

↓

Summon assistance

Intravenous crystalloid

Cross-match blood

Foley catheter

Anaesthesia + Tocolysis

Manual replacement

Hydrostatic replacement

↓

Laparotomy and surgical replacement

↙   ↘

Huntington   Haultain

Oxytocic for 8 -12 hours after uterine replacement

Antibiotic prophylaxis

FIGURE 22-7 ■ Management of acute uterine inversion.

Should acute uterine inversion occur in a setting without anaesthetic facilities, replacement will have to be undertaken with a combination of intravenous narcotic, inhalation analgesia, and combined pudendal and paracervical block, as available and feasible (see Chapter 27).

If manual replacement cannot be achieved O'Sullivan's hydrostatic technique should be used.

Acute uterine inversion presents a distinct risk of maternal death, particularly if facilities for anaesthesia and replacement are not available. It is almost completely preventable with careful and appropriate management of the third stage of labour.

REFERENCES

1. Baskett TF. Acute uterine inversion. A review of 40 cases. J Obstet Gynaecol Can 2002;24:953–6.
2. Quinn RJ, Mukerjee B. Spontaneous uterine inversion in association with Marfan's syndrome. Aust NZ J Obstet Gynaecol 1982;22:163–4.
3. Wendell PJ, Cox SM. Emergent obstetric management of uterine inversion. Obstet Gynecol Clin North Am 1995;22:261–74.
4. Achama S, Mohamed Z, Krishnan M. Puerperal uterine inversion: a report of four cases. J Obstet Gynaecol Res 2006;32:341–5.
5. Brar HS, Greenspoon JS, Platt LD, Paul RH. Acute puerperal uterine inversion: new approaches to management. J Reprod Med 1989;34:173–7.
6. Dommisse B. Uterine inversion revisited. S Afr Med J 1998;88:849–53.
7. O'Sullivan JV. Acute inversion of the uterus. BMJ 1945;2:282–4.
8. Ogueh O, Ayida G. Acute uterine inversion: a new technique of hydrostatic replacement. Br J Obstet Gynaecol 1997;104:951–2.
9. Mamani AW, Hassan A. Treatment of puerperal uterine inversion by the hydrostatic method. Report of five cases. Eur J Obstet Gynecol Reprod Biol 1989;32:281–5.
10. Huntington JL. Acute inversion of the uterus. Boston Med J 1921;184:376–80.

11. Antonelli E, Irion O, Tolck P, Morales M. Subacute uterine inversion: description of a novel replacement technique using the obstetric ventouse. Br J Obstet Gynaecol 2006;113:846–7.
12. Haultain FWN. Treatment of chronic uterine inversion by abdominal hysterotomy, with a successful case. BMJ 1901;2:74–6.
13. Majd HS, Pilsniak A, Reginald PW. Recurrent uterine inversion: a novel treatment approach using SOS Bakri balloon. Br J Obstet Gynaecol 2009;116:999–1001.
14. Matsubara S, Yano H, Taneichi A, Suzuki M. Uterine compression suture against impending recurrence of uterine inversion immediately after laparotomy repositioning. J Obstet Gynaecol Res 2009;35:819–23.

CHAPTER 23

LOWER GENITAL TRACT TRAUMA

AH Sultan · R Thakar

Perineal trauma after childbirth affects millions of women worldwide. Approximately 85% of women sustain some form of perineal trauma following vaginal delivery.[1] Short and long-term morbidity associated with perineal repair can lead to major physical, psychological and social problems affecting the woman's ability to care for her newborn baby and other members of the family. Perineal trauma may occur spontaneously during vaginal birth or when a surgical incision (episiotomy) is intentionally performed to enlarge the diameter of the vaginal outlet. Measures to reduce trauma to the lower genital tract, knowledge of anatomy of the pelvic floor and perineum, and techniques to repair trauma are integral components of obstetric care.

The overall risk of obstetric anal sphincter injury (OASIS) is 1% of all vaginal deliveries.[2] However 'occult' OASIS (i.e. defects in the anal sphincter detected by anal endosonography) has been defined in 33% of primiparous women following vaginal delivery.[3] The most plausible explanation for what was previously believed to be an occult OASIS is either an injury that has been missed, recognized but not reported or wrongly classified as a second degree tear.[4] With increased awareness and focused training, the clinical detection of OASIS has increased. In centres where mediolateral episiotomies are practised, OASIS occurs in 1.7% (2.9% in primiparae) compared to 12% (19% in primiparae) in centres practising midline episiotomy.[5]

ANATOMY

The perineum corresponds to the outlet of the pelvis and is somewhat lozenge shaped. Anteriorly, it is bound by the pubic arch, posteriorly by the coccyx, and laterally by the ischiopubic rami, ischial tuberosities and sacrotuberous ligaments. The perineum can be divided into two triangular parts by drawing an arbitrary line transversely between the ischial tuberosities. The anterior triangle, which contains the external urogenital organs, is known as the *urogenital triangle* and the posterior triangle, which contains the termination of the anal canal, is known as the *anal triangle*. The muscles of the pelvic floor and perineum are shown in Figure 23-1. The perineal body is composed of dense connective tissue to which is attached the bulbospongiosus muscle anteriorly, the superficial transverse perineal muscles laterally and the anal sphincter complex posteriorly. Also attached to the perineal body is the recto-vaginal septum and fascia. The anal sphincter complex consists of the external anal sphincter (EAS) and internal anal sphincter (IAS) separated by the conjoint longitudinal coat (Figure 23-2). The IAS is a thickened continuation of the circular smooth muscle of the bowel.[6]

PERINEAL TRAUMA

In order to standardize definitions of perineal tears, the following classification is recommended:[2]

- *First degree* – injury to perineal skin only
- *Second degree* – injury to perineum involving perineal muscles but not involving the anal sphincter
- *Third degree* – injury to perineum involving the anal sphincter complex:
  - 3a: Less than 50% of EAS thickness torn
  - 3b: More than 50% of EAS thickness torn
  - 3c: Both EAS and IAS torn
- *Fourth degree* – injury to perineum involving the anal sphincter complex (EAS and IAS) and anal epithelium.

If the tear involves only the anorectal epithelium with an intact anal sphincter complex this has to be documented as a separate entity of a button-hole tear and not a fourth degree tear.[2,3] If there is any doubt about whether the grade is a 3a or 3b, it should be classified as a 3b.

EPISIOTOMY

The traditional teaching that episiotomy was protective against more severe perineal lacerations has not been substantiated.[7] Thus, the

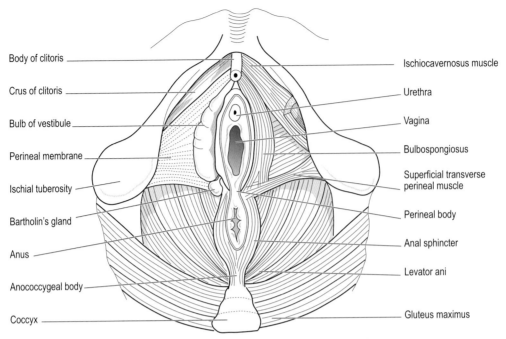

Body of clitoris

Crus of clitoris

Bulb of vestibule

Perineal membrane

Ischial tuberosity

Bartholin's gland

Anus

Anococcygeal body

Coccyx

Ischiocavernosus muscle

Urethra

Vagina

Bulbospongiosus

Superficial transverse perineal muscle

Perineal body

Anal sphincter

Levator ani

Gluteus maximus

FIGURE 23-1 ■ Muscles of the perineum and pelvic floor.

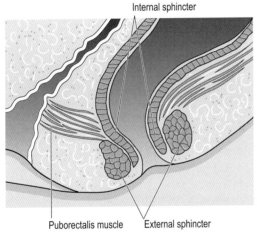

Internal sphincter

Puborectalis muscle   External sphincter

FIGURE 23-2 ■ Anal sphincter complex.

liberal use of 'prophylactic' episiotomy is no longer recommended. However, there are still valid reasons to perform an episiotomy:

- To reduce the occurrence of multiple lacerations in the presence of a thick or rigid perineum.
- To shorten the second stage in cases of fetal distress and where prolonged 'bearing down' may be harmful for the mother (e.g. severe hypertensive or cardiac disease).
- In selected cases of assisted vaginal delivery with forceps and, less frequently, for vacuum assisted delivery. Although there is increasing evidence from observational studies that routine mediolateral episiotomy during instrumental delivery reduces the risk of third and fourth degree tears, there are no randomized trials.
- To obtain more room for obstetrical manoeuvres such as those associated with shoulder dystocia, assisted breech delivery and delivery of the second twin.

FIRST DESCRIPTION OF EPISIOTOMY

'It sometimes happens ... that the head of the child ... cannot however come forward by reason of the extraordinary constriction of the external orifice of the vagina ... wherefore it must be dilated if possible by the fingers ... if this cannot be accomplished, there must be an incision made towards the anus with a pair of crooked probe-scissors, introducing one blade between the head and the vagina, as far as shall be thought necessary for the present purpose and the business is done at one pinch, by which the whole body will easily come forth'.
Fielding Ould
A Treatise of Midwifery in Three Parts. Dublin: Nelson and Connor, 1742, p145

There are two main types of episiotomy:

- *Midline episiotomy*. Two fingers are placed in the vagina between the fetal head and the perineum and, using straight scissors, the incision is made from the fourchette through the perineal body up to but not including the EAS. Advantages of the midline episiotomy are that it does not cut through the belly of the muscle, the two sides of the incised area are anatomically balanced making surgical repair easier, and blood loss is less than with mediolateral episiotomy. A major drawback is the propensity for extension through the EAS and into the rectum. For this reason many practitioners avoid the midline technique and it is not recommended in the UK.[8]

- *Mediolateral episiotomy*. The incision is made starting at the midline of the posterior fourchette and aimed towards the ischial tuberosity to avoid the anal sphincter. The incision is usually about 4 cm long. In addition to the skin and subcutaneous tissues the bulbocavernosus and the transverse perineal muscles are cut. Whether the incision is to the right or left depends on operator preference.

REPAIR OF PERINEAL TRAUMA

'But sometimes it happens by an unlucky and deplorable accident, that the perineum is rent, so that the privity and fundament is all in one ... Let it be strongly stitched together with three or four stitches or more, according to the length of the separation, and taking at each stitch good hold of the flesh, that so it may not break out ...'
　Francois Mauriceau
　The Diseases of Women with Childbed and in Childbed. Translated by Hugh Chamberlen. London: John Darby, 1683, p316

Episiotomy and Second Degree Tears

The principles involved in repairing both episiotomies and second degree tears are similar. First, it is essential to assess the full extent of trauma by doing a vaginal and rectal examination. Unless this careful appraisal is carried out, partial or complete tears of the anal sphincter can be missed. Although the repair of these tears was previously carried out using the interrupted technique, the continuous suturing technique for perineal skin closure has been shown to be associated with less short-term pain. Moreover, if the continuous technique is used for all layers (vagina, perineal muscles and skin), the reduction in pain is even greater.[9] The perineal muscles should be repaired using absorbable polyglactin material, which is available in standard and rapidly absorbable forms. A recent Cochrane review has shown that there are few differences in short-term and long-term pain, between standard and rapidly absorbing synthetic sutures but more women need standard sutures to be removed.[10]

Technique

- Using 2/0 absorbable polyglactin 910 material (Vicryl rapide®) the first stitch is inserted above the apex of the vaginal trauma to secure any bleeding points that might not be visible. The vaginal trauma is closed using a loose, continuous, non-locking technique making sure that each stitch is inserted not too wide, otherwise the vagina may be narrowed. Suturing is continued down to the hymenal remnants and the needle is inserted through the skin at the fourchette to emerge in the centre of the perineal wound (Fig 23-3a).
- The muscle layer is then approximated after assessing the depth of the trauma and the perineal muscles (deep and superficial) are approximated with continuous non-locking stitches. If the trauma is deep, two layers of continuous stitches can be inserted through the perineal muscles (Fig 23-3b).

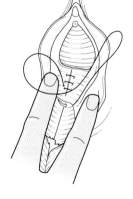
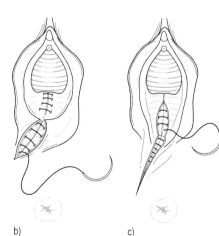

FIGURE 23-3 ■ Repair of episiotomy. (a) Loose, continuous non-locking suture to the vaginal wall. (b) Loose, continuous non-locking suture to the perineal muscles. (c) Closure of skin using a loose subcutaneous suture.

　　　　a)　　　　　　　　　　　b)　　　　　　　　　　c)

- To suture the perineal skin the needle is brought out at the inferior end of the wound, just under the skin surface. The skin sutures are placed below the skin surface in the subcutaneous tissue thus avoiding the profusion of nerve endings. Bites of tissue are taken from each side of the wound edges until the hymenal remnants are reached. A loop or Aberdeen knot is placed in the vagina behind the hymenal remnants (Fig 23-3c).
- A vaginal examination is carried out to ensure that the vagina is not narrowed and a rectal examination carried out to ensure that sutures have not been placed in the anal canal.[11]

Repair of Episiotomy Dehiscence

Breakdown of episiotomy repair occurs due to poor technique and/or infection. Small areas of breakdown, provided there is adequate drainage, can be treated by antibiotics and sitz baths. These minor breakdowns will then granulate and heal-in nicely in the ensuing days and weeks. More extensive breakdown of episiotomy repair can be treated initially with antibiotics and sitz baths and, when signs of active infection have subsided, a secondary repair can be undertaken.[12,13] This will require regional anaesthesia and careful surgical debridement of the wound. The principles of repair involve using the minimum number of sutures and knots. Interrupted skin sutures should be placed.

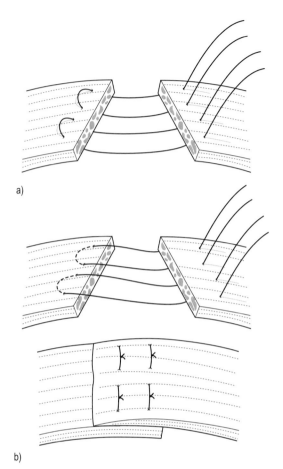

a)

b)

FIGURE 23-4 ■ Repair of third/fourth degree tear. (a) Repair of a fourth degree tear using the end-to-end repair technique of the external anal sphincter. (b) Repair of a fourth degree tear using the overlap repair technique of the external anal sphincter.

OBSTETRIC ANAL SPHINCTER TRAUMA (3RD AND 4TH DEGREE TEARS)

Technique

- Ideally the repair should be performed in the operating theatre with appropriate assistance, lighting, equipment and positioning.
- Regional anaesthesia, either spinal or epidural, is optimal as this allows relaxation of the sphincter and better identification and approximation of the separated ends of the muscle.
- The torn anorectal epithelium is closed with continuous 3/0 Vicryl suture (Fig 23-4a).
- The IAS tends to retract and can be identified lateral to the torn anal epithelium. It

should be repaired with mattress sutures using 3/0 PDS (Polydioxanone) or modern braided sutures such as 2/0 Vicryl (polyglactin – Vicryl®) (Figure 23-5b).
- The torn ends of the EAS are grasped using Allis forceps. It is not uncommon for the sphincter to be torn off to the side rather than in the midline. Therefore, one end of the sphincter may have retracted into a recess on one side. Having grasped each end of the torn muscle with Allis forceps, the muscle is mobilized.
- When the EAS is only partially torn (Grade 3a and some 3b) then an end-to-end repair should be performed using 2 or 3 mattress sutures instead of haemostatic 'figure-of-eight' sutures (Fig 23-4a). If there is a full thickness EAS tear (some 3b, 3c or fourth degree), either an overlapping or end-to-end method can be used with equivalent

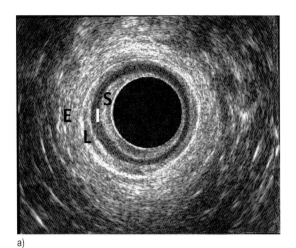

a)

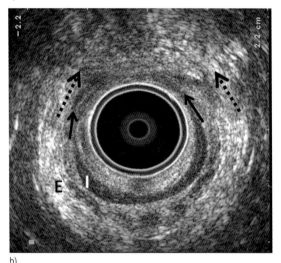

b)

FIGURE 23-5 ■ Endoanal ultrasound demonstrates postpartum disruption of external and internal anal sphincters. (a)The normal 4-layer pattern of the anal canal on axial endosonography in the normal orientation demonstrating the subepithelium (S), the internal sphincter (I), the conjoint longitudinal coat (L) and the external sphincter (E). (b) Endoanal ultrasound demonstrates postpartum disruption of external (broken black arrows) and internal anal sphincters (black arrows).

outcome (Fig 23-4b). The limited data available from the Cochrane review on the topic showed that compared to immediate primary end-to-end repair of OASIS, early primary overlap repair appears to be associated with lower risks of faecal urgency and anal incontinence symptoms and deterioration of anal incontinence over time. However, as the experience of the surgeon was addressed in only one of the three studies reviewed, it would be inappropriate to recommend one type of repair over the other.[14] After either technique of repairing

the external sphincter the remainder of the tear is closed using the same principles and suture material outlined in the repair of episiotomy.

- Broad-spectrum antibiotics are given intra-operatively (intravenously) and continued orally for 3 days.
- Stool softeners (Lactulose) should be prescribed for the first 10 to 14 days postpartum.
- All women who have had obstetric anal sphincter repair should be reviewed 6–12 weeks postpartum by a consultant obstetrician and gynaecologist. If a woman is experiencing incontinence or pain at follow up, referral to a specialist gynaecologist or colorectal surgeon for endoanal ultrasonography (Fig 23-5a, b) and anorectal manometry should be considered.[2]

LACERATIONS

In addition to perineal tears, lacerations of the vulva and vagina are common.

Periurethral and Periclitoral Lacerations

Small periurethral and periclitoral lacerations are common, particularly in the nulliparous woman when episiotomy is not performed and pressure from the delivering head is transferred to the anterior perineum by the intact posterior perineum. However, these lacerations are usually small and the edges come together when the woman's legs are positioned normally following delivery. If there is light bleeding, pressure with a pad for 1–2 minutes will usually arrest the bleeding. If there is significant bleeding these lacerations should be repaired with a fine continuous suture. It may be necessary to place a urethral catheter to guide the placement of sutures.

Vaginal Lacerations

Vaginal lacerations are common and usually involve the lower two-thirds of the posterolateral vaginal sulci. They may also occur as an extension of an episiotomy. Lacerations in the anterior sulcus of the vagina are less frequent, but can be associated with a narrow subpubic arch and elevation of the forceps before the occiput has descended completely below the symphysis pubis. Lacerations of the upper third of the vagina are rare and more often associated with forceps rotation delivery. This can produce

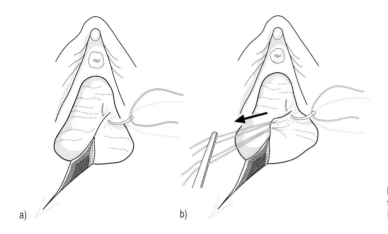

a)   b)

FIGURE 23-6 ■ Use of first suture as a tractor to expose apex of vaginal laceration.

crescentic lacerations high in the vaginal vault which can be difficult to expose.

One of the main problems with repair of vaginal lacerations can be exposure and access. Regional or general anaesthesia may be required. Assistance, retractors and good light are necessary. If you still cannot see the upper extent of the laceration place a suture as high as you can and use this as a tractor to bring the apex of the laceration into view (Fig 23-6). A continuous or, if very vascular, a continuous locking suture is used. In the case of extensive and high vaginal lacerations it may be necessary to pack the vagina tightly following suture for haemostasis and to avoid haematoma formation. If so, a Foley catheter is placed in the bladder and both this and the pack can be removed in 12–24 hours. In such cases broad-spectrum antibiotic coverage is advisable.

Cervical Lacerations

Cervical lacerations are relatively rare and in most cases do not bleed and require no treatment. The cervix can usually be inspected by applying ring (sponge) forceps to the anterior and posterior lips. If the posterior lip is not accessible apply one forcep to the anterior lip and a second one just lateral at the 2 o'clock position. The anterior forcep is then removed and 'leapfrogged' over the other forcep to the 4 o'clock position. In this manner the entire cervix can be closely inspected. Lacerations usually occur laterally and if they are less than 2 cm and not bleeding, they do not require a suture. If they are bleeding or large, place ring forceps on either side of the laceration and repair with a continuous locking suture (Fig 23-7). The cervix is extremely vascular and even with a continuous locking suture oozing may continue, while additional sutures only produce further bleeding points. In these cases apply

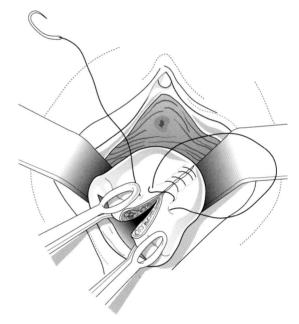

FIGURE 23-7 ■ Repair of cervical laceration.

ring forceps over the oozing areas and leave them in place for 4 hours, after which they can be removed. Surprisingly, this can be done with minimal disruption to the woman in the early postpartum period.

Annular Detachment of the Cervix

Annular detachment of the cervix is an extremely rare condition associated with cervical dystocia from a rigid or scarred cervix causing an annular detachment of the lower portion of the cervix in its entirety, such that a doughnut-shaped portion of the cervix is detached in front of the fetal head. In an earlier edition of this text Chassar Moir graphically described such a case:

'I recall the family doctor who came to the front door to greet the obstetrician. In his outstretched hand he held a detached cervix and in a scared voice he explained, "Just as I was about to put on the forceps this thing came away in my hand". Interestingly, this patient later came under my charge in a future confinement. Her cervix was minutely examined but showed no apparent abnormality'.

In modern obstetrics annular detachment of the cervix is virtually never seen but small 'bucket-handle' tears and small areas of detachment of the anterior lip of the cervix may occur with prolonged late first stage and second stages of labour. Unless it is bleeding this requires no treatment and, like Chassar Moir's case described above, the postpartum cervix looks normal.

HAEMATOMAS

Postpartum vulvo-vaginal haematomas can be classified as *vulval, paravaginal, broad ligament* and *retroperitoneal*. Predisposing causes include prolonged second stage of labour, instrumental delivery, pudendal nerve block and vulval varicosities. Haematomas may be associated with incomplete suturing of vaginal lacerations or episiotomy. In many cases there is no obvious trauma, the delivery is spontaneous and the vaginal epithelium overlying the damaged blood vessel is intact.

Clinical Presentation

- *Vulval* haematomas have an obvious clinical presentation with an acutely painful, tender, purple swelling in the area of the labium majus. These may extend into the lower vagina and into the ischiorectal fossa.
- *Paravaginal* haematomas are not visible externally and usually present with a combination of some or all of the following factors – pain, restlessness, inability to void and rectal tenesmus. A gentle one-finger vaginal examination will usually reveal the tender mass bulging into the vagina.
- *Broad ligament* and *retroperitoneal* haematomas occur when a vessel ruptures above the levator ani muscle. The bleeding extends into the supravaginal space between the leaves of the broad ligament and may track retroperitoneally, even as high as the kidneys. This type of haematoma may be associated with deep cervical lacerations extending into the lower uterine segment or with an occult rupture of the lateral

aspect of the lower uterine segment. Large broad ligament haematomas can be felt on bimanual examination and push the uterus to one side. Extensive broad ligament and retroperitoneal haematomas can cause profound hypovolaemic shock and may rupture into the peritoneal cavity. Diagnosis may be aided, if available, by ultrasound or MRI examination.

Management

Small vulval haematomas (≤ 5 cm) may be treated conservatively with analgesia, observation and ice packs. However, if the pain is not adequately controlled and if there is enlargement they have to be incised and evacuated. Paravaginal haematomas also need incision and evacuation. This requires regional or general anaesthesia. The incision is made over the area of maximum distension and the clot evacuated. Seek and ligate discreet bleeding points, although frequently none are found. Oozing areas may be oversewn with figure-of-eight sutures. Tamponade for 2–3 minutes should help identify any bleeding points or persistently oozing areas that require suture. The vagina is then tightly packed with gauze moistened with lubricating gel or antiseptic cream. A Foley catheter is placed in the bladder and both of these can be removed in 12–24 hours.

Broad ligament and retroperitoneal haematomas may be self-limiting and will absorb in the coming weeks. Provided the patient is stable they may be initially treated conservatively with intravenous crystalloid, cross-matched blood, analgesia and observation. If available, it is wise to muster the personnel and equipment for angiographic embolization of branches of the internal iliac arteries.[15,16] Should there be signs of progressive bleeding this can then be implemented and is often very effective. If angiographic embolization facilities are not available laparotomy is required and the haematoma is evacuated followed by ligation of bleeding points. A careful check should be made to confirm or deny uterine rupture as the source of the haematoma. This may require repair of the uterine rupture, or even hysterectomy.

REFERENCES

1. McCandlish R, Bowler U, van Asten H, Berridge G, Winter C, Sames L, et al. A randomised controlled trial of care of the perineum during second stage of normal labour. Br J Obstet Gynaecol 1998;105:1262–72.
2. Royal College of Obstetricians and Gynaecologists. Management of third and fourth degree perineal tears following vaginal delivery. Guideline No. 29. London: RCOG Press; 2007.

3. Sultan AH, Kamm MA, Hudson CN, Thomas JM, Bartram CI. Anal sphincter disruption during vaginal delivery. N Engl J Med 1993;329:1905–11.

4. Andrews V, Thakar R, Sultan AH. Occult anal sphincter injuries: myth or reality. Br J Obstet Gynaecol 2006;113:195–200.

5. Sultan AH, Thakar R. Third and fourth degree tears. In: Sultan AH, Thakar R, Fenner D, editors. Perineal and anal sphincter trauma. London: Springer-Verlag; 2007. p. 33–51.

6. Thakar R, Fenner DE. Anatomy of the perineum and the anal sphincter. In: Sultan AH, Thakar R, Fenner DE, editors. Perineal and anal sphincter trauma. London: Springer-Verlag; 2007. p. 1–12.

7. Carroli G, Mignini L. Episiotomy for vaginal birth. Cochrane Database Syst Rev 2009;1:CD000081.

8. Intrapartum Care. NICE Clinical Guideline. Guideline 55; Sept 2007. Available at http://www.nice.org.uk/CG055

9. Kettle C, Hills RK, Ismail KMK. Continuous versus interrupted sutures for repair of episiotomy or second degree tears. Cochrane Database Syst Rev 2007;4:CD000947.

10. Kettle C, Dowswell T, Ismail KM. Absorbable suture materials for primary repair of episiotomy and second degree tears. Cochrane Database Syst Rev. 2010;6:CD000006.

11. Kettle C, Fenner D. Repair of episiotomy, first and second degree tears. In: Sultan AH, Thakar R, Fenner D, editors. Perineal and anal sphincter trauma. London: Springer; 2007. p. 20–32.

12. Ramin SM, Ramus RM, Little BB, Gilstrap LC. Early repair of episiotomy dehiscence associated with infection. Am J Obstet Gynecol 1992;167:1104–7.

13. Arona AJ, Al-Marayati L, Grimes DA. Early secondary repair of third and fourth degree perineal lacerations after outpatient wound preparation. Obstet Gynecol 1995;86:294–6.

14. Fernando R, Sultan AH, Kettle C, Thakar R, Radley S. Methods of repair for obstetric anal sphincter injury. Cochrane Database Syst Rev 2006;3:CD002866.

15. Chiu HG, Scott DR, Resnik R. Angiographic embolization of intractable puerperal hematomas. Am J Obstet Gynecol 1989;160:434–8.

16. Fargeaudou Y, Soyer P, Morel O, Sirol M, Le Dref O, Budiaf M, et al Severe primary postpartum hemorrhage due to genital tract laceration after operative vaginal delivery: successful treatment with transcatheter arterial embolization. Eur Radiol 2009;19:197–203.

CHAPTER 24

HAEMORRHAGIC SHOCK

TF Baskett · VS Talaulikar

> 'It is clear that when patients are in this condition, trembling upon the very brink of destruction, there is but little time for you to think what ought to be done; these are moments in which it becomes your duty not to reflect, but to act. Think now, therefore, before the moment of difficulty arrives. Be ready with all the rules of practice, which those very dangerous cases require'.
> James Blundell
> The Principles and Practice of Obstetricy. London: E. Cox, 1834, p336

Obstetric haemorrhage is the leading direct cause of maternal death in the developing world and remains a major cause of death and severe maternal morbidity in the developed world. 'Substandard care' and 'too little too late' have been repeatedly highlighted as significant factors contributing to many maternal deaths. A number of the complications discussed in this book are associated with obstetric haemorrhage and thus the pathophysiology, clinical features and management of hypovolaemic shock will be discussed here.

PHYSIOLOGICAL CHANGES IN PREGNANCY

Part of the physiological adaptation to pregnancy includes an increase of about 40% in the circulating blood volume. This accommodates the increased utero-placental circulation and also prepares the woman, to some extent, to withstand haemorrhage at delivery. This is necessary because the 'normal' blood loss at vaginal delivery and caesarean section is about 500 ml and 1000 ml respectively, and such loss is accommodated well by the normal pregnant woman. However, obstetric haemorrhage is often rapid and may be poorly tolerated by the woman who is anaemic, dehydrated after prolonged labour, or with the reduced blood volume and contracted intravascular space associated with pre-eclampsia/eclampsia.

An additional important consideration is the size of the woman and therefore her circulating blood volume. In the non-pregnant woman the formula to calculate blood volume is about 70 ml/kg or her weight in kilograms divided by 14. Thus, the circulating blood volume of a 50 kg woman and an 80 kg woman would be about 3500 ml and 5600 ml, respectively. In pregnancy, with the 40% increase in blood volume, the formula is approximately 100 ml/kg; so in the same 50 kg and 80 kg weight categories the blood volume would be 5000 ml and 8000 ml respectively – a difference of 3 L. The woman of small stature who is anaemic may withstand poorly even a blood loss of 1000–1500 ml, which the larger, non-anaemic woman would tolerate with relative impunity.

PATHOPHYSIOLOGICAL RESPONSE TO HAEMORRHAGE

Severe haemorrhage associated with hypotension causes an increased release of catecholamines and stimulation of the baroreceptors leading to increased sympathetic tone, with the following results:

- Increased cardiac output due to an increase in the rate and force of myocardial contraction
- Maintenance of blood flow to the critical organs (heart and brain) by selective peripheral arteriolar constriction reducing blood flow to all the other organs.
- Venous constriction causing, in effect, an autotransfusion from these capacitance vessels.
- As a result of the peripheral vasoconstriction the reduced hydrostatic pressure in the capillaries causes them to imbibe extracellular fluid in an attempt to augment the intravascular volume. Increased levels of aldosterone and antidiuretic hormone cause sodium and water retention by the kidneys.

These mechanisms are aimed at improving cardiac output, sustaining the blood pressure, restoring the intravascular volume and maintaining tissue perfusion. At this stage, provided the haemorrhage is arrested and the circulation restored, the shock is completely reversible without sequelae. However, if the blood loss continues, the above mechanisms fail to sustain adequate circulation, leading to reduced tissue perfusion, tissue hypoxia, metabolic acidosis, cell damage and ultimately cell death. The hypoxic metabolites damage the capillary cells leading to more loss of intravascular volume as fluid leaks through the damaged capillary walls. Persistent hypoperfusion of peripheral organs may cause damage to the lung ('shock lung', adult respiratory distress syndrome), the kidney (acute tubular and cortical necrosis), the liver and to the pituitary (Sheehan's syndrome).

As the diastolic blood pressure falls, coronary artery perfusion is compromised, leading to myocardial hypoxia and failure. Such extensive hypoxic tissue damage and release of metabolites may initiate disseminated intravascular coagulation (see Chapter 25).

CLINICAL FEATURES

In the early phase of blood loss, peripheral arteriolar constriction will sustain normal maternal blood pressure but may lead to a reduction in utero-placental perfusion. Thus, abnormalities of the fetal heart rate may serve as an early warning sign of maternal vascular decompensation.

The classic early signs of haemorrhagic shock are changes in the vital signs with tachycardia, hypotension, tachypnoea and air hunger. In addition to these vital signs one can monitor the skin, brain and kidney for clinical manifestations of hypovolaemia as these are end-organs sensitive to reduced perfusion and hypoxia. The clinical manifestations of hypoperfusion and hypoxia in these end-organs are as follows:

- Skin: sweating, cold, pallor, cyanosis. A clinically useful sign of skin perfusion is the capillary refill time. This is easily assessed by compressing a finger nail for 5 seconds; if normal, the colour in the nail bed returns within 2 seconds.
- Brain: alteration in mental state including restlessness, anxiety, aggression, confusion and coma.
- Kidney: oliguria and anuria.

Hypovolaemic shock can be classified into three categories:

- *Mild*: 10–25% loss of blood volume. In cases of mild hypovolaemic shock there is tachycardia and possibly mild hypotension along with decreased perfusion of non-vital organs and tissue such as skin, fat and skeletal muscle. Provided bleeding stops at this stage the circulation is well compensated, will respond to intravenous crystalloid alone and does not require blood replacement.
- *Moderate*: 25–40% loss of blood volume. With moderate shock there is decreased perfusion to the vital organs due to peripheral vasoconstriction and this is usually manifest by tachycardia, hypotension, tachypnoea, cool skin and oliguria. This requires intravenous crystalloid and blood replacement.
- *Severe*: >40% loss of blood volume. This is life threatening, with all of the clinical manifestations of shock present in their most extreme form. A working guide to the presence of severe haemorrhagic shock is when the radial pulse is impalpable, which means the systolic blood pressure is less than 70 mmHg – at which level perfusion to the vital organs (heart, brain and kidney) is critically reduced. Loss of more than 50% of blood volume results in loss of consciousness. These patients require immediate blood replacement and urgent measures to stop the bleeding.

MANAGEMENT

When excessive blood loss is encountered the first task is to identify the source and stop the bleeding. While it is also important to mobilize blood transfusion, this should not detract from efforts to immediately stem the haemorrhage. The principles of management of haemorrhagic shock are simple – maintain and restore the circulating blood volume to sustain tissue perfusion and oxygenation. The simple 'Rule of 30s' and the 'Shock index' are useful background guides to treatment:

Rule of 30s:

- Up to 30% of blood volume can be lost without major haemodynamic changes
- Keep the haematocrit above 30%
- Keep the urinary output above 30 ml/hour
- If systolic blood pressure falls by 30 mmHg, pulse rate rises by 30 beats/minute, respiratory rate increases to more than 30 breaths/minute, this indicates moderate shock leading to severe shock.

Shock index:

- Heart rate divided by the systolic blood pressure
- The normal value is 0.5–0.7
- With significant haemorrhage it increases to 0.9–1.1. A shock index of over 0.9 indicates need for intensive therapy.

Visual estimation of blood loss by the clinician is often inaccurate. Thus, clinicians should also assess the rate of bleeding and associated changes in the woman's haemodynamic status to guide appropriate management.

The individual principles of management are as follows:

Protect the airway and administer oxygen by face mask (10–15 L/minute). In severe shock with an unconscious patient, intubation and ventilation will be necessary.

During resuscitation undelivered pregnant women should be placed in the left lateral tilt (15–30°).

Keep the patient warm and warm all intravenous fluids. Platelet and other coagulation factor functions are inhibited by the cold.

Two portals of venous access in the arms are required. If normal venous access is unsuccessful, cut-down of the antecubital or saphenous vein of the ankle will have to be established. Intravenous cannulae should be of 14 gauge – the flow through a cannula is proportional to the diameter, such that crystalloid can be infused twice as fast through a 14-gauge compared with an 18-gauge cannula.

Intravenous crystalloid is the first choice for fluid resuscitation in hypovolaemia. The crystalloid chosen is one of the isotonic solutions – Ringer's lactate, Hartmann's solution or 0.9% saline. Crystalloids provide short-term expansion of the intravascular space but are soon excreted by the kidneys and rapidly distributed to the extracellular fluid, such that 80% of the volume is lost to the circulation. The key is rapid transfusion of warmed crystalloid solution at a volume approximately 2–3 times the estimated blood loss. Crystalloid has no powers of coagulation or of oxygenation but is very valuable as a short-term volume expander. As such, it may be all that is required in women with mild hypovolaemic shock in whom the blood loss is promptly arrested. If not, it has value in maintaining the circulating blood volume until blood products are available for transfusion. Better to have an anaemic circulating blood volume perfusing the tissues than no perfusion. It is possible that future trials will show that hypertonic saline may be advantageous in the initial management of acute hypovolaemic shock.

The colloids are an alternative solution to crystalloids. These include the human derivatives, albumin 5% and plasma protein fraction (plasmanate) or the artificial colloids, hydroxyethyl starches (pentaspan) and the gelatins (gelofusine, haemaccel). The previously used dextrans (macrodex, rheomacrodex) are no longer recommended because they adversely affect platelet function, interfere with subsequent blood cross-match tests and can, rarely, initiate severe anaphylactoid reactions. The colloids have the advantage of remaining longer in the intravascular space but are also rapidly distributed to the extracellular fluid in large amounts. In the case of crystalloid this fluid is usually reabsorbed quite rapidly, whereas colloid will persist and may, for example, exacerbate pulmonary oedema by drawing further fluid into the extracellular tissues. The combination of pre-eclampsia and hypovolaemic shock renders these women very susceptible to overload with either crystalloid or colloid due to the combination of vasospasm and reduced intravascular capacity, hypoproteinaemia and increased capillary permeability. Thus, women with severe pre-eclampsia/eclampsia and hypovolaemic shock require cautious administration of crystalloid or colloid and may need central venous pressure and pulmonary artery wedge pressure monitoring to guide safe restoration of blood volume.

In general, crystalloid is the initial infusion of choice and 2–3 L should be given rapidly. If blood is still unavailable and more than 3 L of crystalloid is necessary to sustain the circulation then colloid may be given. If albumin is chosen it is very viscous and should be drawn up with a wide-bore needle and added to saline so it can be infused rapidly.

In moderate and severe haemorrhage the oxygen-carrying capacity of blood is essential in addition to restoration of the intravascular volume. Packed red blood cells have a haematocrit of 70–80% and these are transfused for their oxygen-carrying capacity, while simultaneously transfused crystalloid or colloid provides the volume. Each unit of packed red cells is expected to increase the haemoglobin by 1 g/dl and the haematocrit by 3%. Packed red cells have a high viscosity and it is best to add 50–100 ml isotonic saline to each unit to facilitate rapid transfusion. In an extreme emergency 2 units of O Rh-negative blood (the universal donor blood) can be transfused. However, O Rh-negative donors may have anti-A, anti-B antibodies in their plasma which can react with A or B cells of a non-type O recipient. There is almost always time (15 minutes) to ascertain the patient's ABO and Rh type so that type-specific blood can be given without cross-match. In most cases it is possible to both type and screen for irregular antibodies with a short (20 minute) saline cross-match. It is essential that the transfused blood is warmed. There are a number of electric blood warmers with thermostats suitable for this purpose. If these are not available, additional intravenous tubing can be coiled in a basin of water warmed to 37–40°C. It is important that the water should not exceed this temperature otherwise haemolysis of the blood can occur. Thus, the temperature in the basin should be monitored by a thermometer and one usually needs to add warm water frequently as the heat loss to the cold blood is considerable. If equipment is limited the temperature in the water basin can be assessed by the elbow, in the same way that one tests the bath water for a baby. Generally speaking, however, if laboratory facilities exist for blood transfusion the equipment for blood warming is also available.

The avoidance of hypothermia is extremely important. Transfusion of cold intravenous fluids will cause shivering, which increases oxygen consumption. In addition, the activity of coagulation factors, citrate, lactate and potassium metabolism are all negatively affected by hypothermia. At its most extreme, blood transfused at a temperature <30°C can cause ventricular fibrillation and cardiac arrest.

Although autologous transfusions appear safe in pregnancy they are recommended only for patients with rare blood types and/or alloimmunization to rare antibodies who are at high risk of bleeding and for whom immediate availability of allogeneic blood products may be limited. Intraoperative cell salvage has been successfully used in obstetrics and may be considered in high-risk cases where facilities permit. There is emerging evidence for the use of tranexamic acid (1 g intravenously) in the management of postpartum haemorrhage to minimize blood loss and reduce the requirement for blood transfusion.

Dilutional coagulopathy generally begins to operate after 4–5 units of packed cells have been transfused. Thus, as a working rule, 1–2 units of fresh frozen plasma should be transfused for every 5 units of packed cells. Furthermore, for every 15 units of packed red cells 5 units of platelets should be given.

MONITORING PROGRESS

It is important to involve senior staff early on in cases of haemorrhagic shock. In addition, when available, guidance from a haematologist is advisable. Depending on the amount of blood loss and the facilities available the following monitoring may be necessary:

- Vital signs of blood pressure, pulse, respiration and temperature.
- Indwelling urinary catheter to assess oliguria and the desired goal of keeping urinary output >30 ml/hour.

- Haemoglobin, haematocrit, platelets, urea, electrolytes and coagulation profile should be performed at regular intervals, remembering that these do not reflect the acute changes but may be useful to show trends over the longer term.
- Auscultation of the lung bases for signs of pulmonary oedema.
- Pulse oximetry, which provides a useful continuous assessment of pulse rate and oxygen saturation.
- If undelivered, continuous fetal heart rate monitoring is advisable. As mentioned before, in general terms if the fetus is well oxygenated then so is the mother.
- More sophisticated invasive monitoring may be required in selected cases and include arterial blood pressure, central venous pressure and pulmonary artery wedge pressure (Swan–Ganz). This is particularly so in cases of severe pre-eclampsia/eclampsia associated with hypovolaemia.

FIRST SUCCESSFUL HUMAN BLOOD TRANSFUSION BY DR JAMES BLUNDELL, DESCRIBED BY HIS COLLEAGUE, DR WALLER

'The vein in the bend of the arm was laid bare, and an incision of sufficient extent to admit the pipe of the syringe was made into it...The syringe used by Dr. B. was similar to the common injecting syringe, and contained two ounces... The blood was drawn from the patient's husband into a tumbler, and Dr. B. stood ready with his syringe to absorb it instantly, in fact, while it was flowing: it was then immediately introduced into the orifice in the vein, and cautiously injected. No effect appeared to be produced by the first injection of two ounces, but towards the end of the second there was an approach to syncope; the pulse fell a little; there was sighing...'
C Waller
Case of uterine haemorrhage, in which the operation of transfusion was successfully performed. Med Phys J 1825; 54:273–277

'After floodings, women sometimes die in a moment, but more frequently in a gradual manner; and over the victim, death shakes his dart, and to you she stretches out her helpless hands for the assistance which you cannot give, unless by transfusion. I have seen a woman dying for two or three hours together, convinced in my own mind that no known remedy could save her: the sight of these moving cases first lead me to transfusion'.
J Blundell
The Principles and Practice of Obstetricy. London: E. Cox, 1834, p337

STOP THE BLEEDING

As already emphasized, in parallel with the above treatment, measures should be taken to arrest the haemorrhage. These are described in the appropriate chapters on haemorrhagic complications elsewhere in this book.

BIBLIOGRAPHY

American College of Obstetricians and Gynecologists. Educational Bulletin No. 235. Hemorrhagic shock. Washington DC: ACOG; 1997.

Baskett TF. Preparedness for postpartum haemorrhage: an obstetric haemorrhage equipment tray. In: Arulkumaran S, Karoshi M, Keith LG, Lalonde AB, B-Lynch C, editors. A comprehensive textbook of postpartum haemorrhage. 2nd ed. Duncow: Sapiens Publishing; 2012.

Bose P, Regan F, Paterson-Brown S. Improving the accuracy of estimated blood loss at obstetric haemorrhage using clinical reconstructions. Br J Obstet Gynaecol 2006;113:919–24.

Dildy GA, Scott JR, Saffer CS, Belfort MA. An effective pressure pack for severe pelvic hemorrhage. Obstet Gynecol 2006;108:1222–61.

Hofmeyr CJ, Mohala BKF. Hypovolaemic shock. Best Prac Res Clin Obstet Gynaecol 2001;15:645–62.

Miller S, Hamza S, Bray EH, Lester F, Nada K, Gibson R. First aid for obstetric haemorrhage: the pilot study of the non-pneumatic anti-shock garment in Egypt. Br J Obstet Gynaecol 2006;113:424–9.

Patel A, Goudar SS, Geller SE. Drape estimation vs. visual assessment for estimating postpartum hemorrhage. Int J Gynecol Obstet 2006;93:220–4.

Prata N, Mbaruku G, Campbell M. Using the kanga to measure postpartum blood loss. Int J Gynecol Obstet 2005;89:47–50.

Rady MY, Smithline HA, Blake H, Nowak R, Rivers F. A comparison of shock index and conventional vital signs to identify acute critical illness in the emergency department. Ann Emerg Med 1994;24:685–90.

Rees GAD, Willis BA. Resuscitation in late pregnancy. Anaesthesia 1998;43:347–9.

Santoso JT, Saunders BA, Grosshart K. Massive blood loss and transfusion in obstetrics and gynaecology. Obstet Gynaecol Surv 2005;60:827–37.

Shevell T, Malone FD. Management of obstetric hemorrhage. Semin Perinatol 2003;27:86–104.

Skupski DW, Lowenwirt P, Weinbaum FI, Brodsky D, Danek M, Eglinton GS. Improving hospital systems for the care of women with major obstetric hemorrhage. Obstet Gynecol 2006;107:977–83.

Society of Obstetricians and Gynaecologists of Canada. Clinical Practice Guidelines No 115. Haemorrhagic shock. J Obstet Gynaecol Can 2002;24:504–11.

Su LL, Chong YS. Massive obstetric haemorrhage with disseminated intravascular coagulation. Best Pract Res Clin Obstet Gynaecol 2012;26:77–90.

Yazer MH. The blood bank 'black box' debunked: pretransfusion testing explained. Can Med Assoc J 2006;174:29–32.

Younes RN, Aun F, Ching CT, Goldenberg DC, Franco MH, Miura FK et al. Prognostic factors to predict outcome following the administration of hypertonic/hyperoncotic solution in hypovolemic patients. Shock 1997;7:79–83.

Young P, Johanson R. Haemodynamic, invasive and echocardiographic monitoring in the hypertensive parturient. Best Prac Res Clin Obstet Gynaecol 2001;15:605–22.

CHAPTER 25

DISSEMINATED INTRAVASCULAR COAGULATION

TF Baskett • VS Talaulikar

> 'Is there such a disease as acquired haemophilia? ... I believe there is such an affection as a temporary haemophilia, but the demonstration of the same, I admit, presents no little difficulty'.
> Joesph B DeLee
> Am J Obstet Dis Women Child 1901; 44: 785–792

Haemostasis is a dynamic balance between coagulation and fibrinolysis. Normal pregnancy is accompanied by profound changes in both of these systems. In addition to the increased blood volume there is a rise in most of the procoagulant factors and a relative suppression of fibrinolysis.[1] These changes help prepare the woman to restrict blood loss at delivery and to produce haemostasis in the large and vascular uterine 'wound' following placental separation. As a result of these physiological changes the pregnant woman is rendered more vulnerable to the whole spectrum of coagulation disorders, ranging from venous thromboembolism to disseminated intravascular coagulation.

CAUSES

The definition of disseminated intravascular coagulation (DIC) is a systemic thrombohaemorrhagic disorder found in association with well-defined clinical situations and laboratory evidence of procoagulant activation, fibrinolytic activation, inhibitor consumption and biochemical evidence of end-organ damage or failure.[2] DIC is always secondary to another condition that provokes clotting within the vascular compartment. There are three main mechanisms by which obstetric conditions may activate the coagulation system:[3]

1. Release of thromboplastins from placental and decidual tissue into the maternal circulation. This may happen with dramatic suddenness in cases of amniotic fluid embolism and abruptio placentae. It can occur at the time of surgical intervention for placenta praevia accreta, ruptured uterus and trophoblastic disease. In patients with intrauterine fetal death or missed abortion, release of thromboplastins into the maternal circulation is delayed and less consistent. In such cases about 25% will develop DIC some 5–6 weeks after fetal demise. Fetal death and missed abortion are now rare causes of DIC because, with ultrasound, the diagnosis is usually made early and the pregnancy terminated before DIC can develop.

2. Endothelial damage exposes the underlying collagen to plasma and procoagulants. Such endothelial damage may be caused insidiously by pre-eclampsia/eclampsia, HELLP (Haemolysis, elevated liver enzymes and low platelets) syndrome, acute fatty liver or by sepsis. Another cause of endothelial hypoxia and damage is haemorrhagic shock with delayed restoration of the circulating intravascular volume. This is now one of the commonest causes of DIC in obstetrics.

3. Red blood cell/platelet injury may occur with incompatible blood transfusion reactions leading to the release of phospholipids and initiation of the coagulation cascade.

PATHOPHYSIOLOGY

Normal haemostasis is a complex and dynamic balance between coagulation, which leads to fibrin formation, and the fibrinolytic system, which disposes of fibrin once its haemostatic function has been fulfilled. In DIC there is excessive and widespread coagulation which leads to consumption and depletion of the coagulation factors, resulting in haemorrhage.[4] In response to this widespread coagulation and

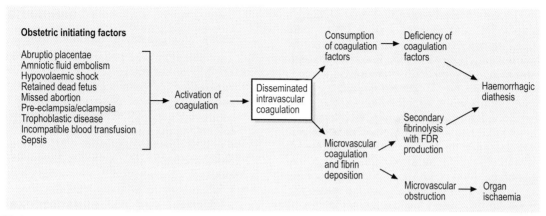

FIGURE 25-1 ■ Causes and pathophysiology of disseminated intravascular coagulation. (Adapted from Baskett TF. Essential management of obstetric emergencies. 4th ed. Bristol: Clinical Press Ltd, 2004, with permission of Clinical Press Ltd.)

deposition of fibrin in the microvasculature the fibrinolytic system is activated. As plasminogen is converted to plasmin it breaks down the fibrin to form fibrin degradation products (FDP). FDP have anticoagulant properties as they inhibit both platelet function and the action of thrombin, serving to aggravate the coagulopathy. While the haemorrhagic diathesis is the dominant pathology in most cases, extensive microvascular thrombosis can also occur, leading to organ ischaemia and infarction. This can be a secondary factor, along with hypovolaemic shock, in the causation of renal cortical necrosis, lung damage and Sheehan's syndrome. The causes and pathophysiological features of DIC are outlined in Figure 25-1.

CLINICAL PRESENTATION

It is common for the main clinical features to be those of the obstetric complication that has triggered the DIC. Clinical manifestations of the DIC *per se* will depend upon its severity. These will range across the spectrum from no clinical manifestations with only haematological changes of DIC (↓ platelets, ↑ FDP); relatively subtle clinical signs such as bruising, epistaxis, purpuric rash, and oozing from venepuncture sites; to the dramatic torrential postpartum haemorrhage (PPH) and bleeding from all operative sites.

DIAGNOSIS

Diagnosis is aided by recognition of the obstetric initiating causes of DIC. Certain haematological tests are useful in the diagnosis and, if available, it is appropriate to enlist the aid of a haematologist. Depending upon the level of sophistication of the hospital laboratory some tests may be unavailable. In addition, the process of DIC is so dynamic that results, as they become available, may not reflect the current status. Bedside whole-blood clotting tests are not helpful as their accuracy is limited unless controlled laboratory conditions are applied.[5]

The most rapid and useful screening tests are the platelet count (low and falling), activated partial thromboplastin time (which is usually prolonged when clotting factors are severely depleted), prothrombin time (usually prolonged) and the thrombin time, which is usually prolonged and is one of the more valuable tests. Fibrinogen levels are increased in normal pregnancy to 400–650 mg/dl; with DIC this level falls but may still be in the normal non-pregnant range. In severe DIC the fibrinogen levels usually fall below 150 mg/dl. Fibrin degradation products such as D-dimer can be unreliable for diagnosis in pregnant women as their levels are often increased in normal pregnancy.

The diagnosis of DIC in pregnancy is therefore primarily clinical, supported by the coagulation profile.[6] Letsky has suggested a three-stage severity system based on the degree of haemostatic compensation allied to the blood levels of coagulation factors.[5]

MANAGEMENT

With awareness of the initiating obstetric causes it may be possible to treat these before there is progression to severe DIC. An obvious example of this is the evacuation of the uterus in cases of fetal death and missed abortion. Cases of severe pre-eclampsia and/or HELLP syndrome may have haematological changes of mild DIC with low platelets and elevated FDPs. These cases should be stabilized and delivered before the clinical manifestations of DIC become apparent.

In most obstetric situations DIC develops rapidly and prompt treatment is required. The initial treatment of haemorrhage is the same whether DIC is a contributing factor or not. Thus, the principles of managing hypovolaemic shock outlined in the preceding chapter are relevant. While it is important to send the appropriate bloods for haematological testing and to involve the consultant haematologist, the minute-by-minute management will not be influenced by these tests. The principles of management are as follows:

Treat the Obstetric Cause

As DIC is always secondary to an initiating cause it is obvious that the obstetric trigger must be promptly treated in order to cure the DIC. In most cases this entails emptying the uterus and controlling the surgical or obstetric haemorrhage.

Maintain Circulation

While treating the obstetric cause, and therefore removing the trigger and ultimately curing the DIC, it is necessary to sustain the patient's circulation and maintain organ perfusion. These management principles have been outlined in Chapter 24 and include oxygen, rapid infusion of crystalloid, colloid and blood transfusion. An effective circulation is also essential to help clear the FDP, which is largely achieved by the liver. FDP compound the DIC as they interfere with platelet function, have an antithrombin effect and inhibit the formation of firm fibrin. They also interfere with myometrial function and possibly with myocardial function as well. Thus, the clearance of FDP is a very important part of the recovery from DIC.

Replacement of Procoagulants

Because of the risk of infection, fresh whole blood, which would be ideal, is not available. Packed red blood cells are deficient in platelets and other procoagulants, particularly factors V and VIII. Thus, it is essential in cases of severe haemorrhage complicated by DIC to add procoagulants using the following guidelines:

- Fresh frozen plasma (FFP) has all of the clotting factors present in the plasma of whole blood, without the platelets. These clotting factors are not in concentrated form however, so it is difficult to raise the circulating levels. The traditional rule is to give 1 unit of FFP after 5 units of blood and thereafter give 1 unit for every 2 units of blood transfused. However, recent experience in trauma cases suggests that early correction of coagulopathy leads to improved outcomes. Clinicians should consider administering 1 unit of platelets and 1 unit of FFP for every unit of blood transfused in cases of massive haemorrhage with evidence of coagulopathy.[7]

- Cryoprecipitate is rich in fibrinogen, in addition to von Willebrand factor and factors VIII and XIII. It is usually reserved for cases with severe hypofibrinogenaemia (<100 mg/dl).

- Platelets deteriorate quite rapidly in stored blood and are not present in FFP. In a woman with persistent bleeding and severe thrombocytopaenia (<30 000) platelet transfusion is indicated. One unit of platelets will raise the count by approximately 5000–10 000.

- Antithrombin is rapidly consumed in DIC and, under the guidance of a haematologist, antithrombin concentrate may be given if the levels are low.[8]

- Recombinant activated factor VIIa was originally used in haemophilia but has recently been applied to obstetric haemorrhage with DIC.[9–13] It combines with the local tissue factor at the site of haemorrhage to enhance thrombin generation and stabilize fibrin formation. It is expensive and has a short half-life. The Royal College of Obstetricians and Gynaecologists guideline recommends that in the face of life-threatening PPH, and in consultation with a haematologist, rFVIIa may be used as an adjuvant to standard pharmacological and surgical treatment.[14] The suggested dose is 90 µg/kg, which may be repeated in the absence of clinical response within 15–30 minutes. Fibrinogen should be above 1 g/L and platelets greater than 20×10^9/L before rFVIIa is given.

It is emphasized that most cases of obstetric haemorrhage and DIC occur in previously healthy young women. Such women have a great ability to recover rapidly and completely once the initial obstetric cause of haemorrhage and DIC is removed, provided their circulating blood volume can be sustained to ensure adequate tissue perfusion. If this can be achieved the liver will usually remove the harmful FDP and replace most of the other desirable coagulation factors within 24 hours. Platelets may continue to fall in the next 24 hours, but as long as there is no haemorrhage they do not need to be replaced at this stage.

REFERENCES

1. O'Riordan MN, Higgins JR. Haemostasis in normal and abnormal pregnancy. Best Prac Res Clin Obstet Gynaecol 2003;17:385–96.
2. Bick RL. Disseminated intravascular coagulation: a review of etiology, pathophysiology, diagnosis, and management: guidelines for care. Clin Appl Thromb Hemost 2002;8:1–31.
3. Baskett TF. Disseminated intravascular coagulation. In: Essential management of obstetric emergencies. 4th ed. Bristol: Clinical Press Ltd; 2004. p. 242–5.
4. Lurie S, Feinstein M, Mamet Y. Disseminated intravascular coagulation in pregnancy: thorough comprehension of etiology and management reduces obstetricians' stress. Arch Gynecol Obstet 2001;263:126–30.
5. Letsky EA. Disseminated intravascular coagulation. Best Prac Res Clin Obstet Gynaecol 2001;15:623–44.
6. Rattray DD, O'Connell CM, Baskett TF. Acute disseminated intravascular coagulation in obstetrics: a tertiary centre population review (1980 to 2009). J Obstet Gynaecol Can 2012;34:341–7.
7. Pacheo LD, Soade GR, Gei AF, Hankins GD. Cutting-edge advances in the medical management of obstetrical hemorrhage. Am J Obstet Gynecol 2011;205:526–32.
8. Bucur SZ, Levy JH, Despotis GJ. Use of antithrombin III concentrate in congenital and acquired deficiency states. Transfusion 1998;38:481–98.
9. Zupanic SS, Sololic V, Vishovic T, Sanjug J, Simic M, Kastelan M. Successful use of recombinant factor VIIa for massive bleeding after caesarean section due to HELLP syndrome. Acta Haematol 2002;108:162–3.
10. Branch DW, Rodgers GM. Recombinant activated factor VII: a new weapon in the fight against hemorrhage. Obstet Gynecol 2003;101:115–16.
11. Bouwmeester FW, Jonkhoff AR, Verheijen RHM, van Geijn HP. Successful treatment of life-threatening postpartum hemorrhage with recombinant activated Factor VII. Obstet Gynecol 2003;101:1174–6.
12. Pepas LP, Arif-Adib M, Kadir RA. Factor VIIa in puerperal hemorrhage with disseminated intravascular coagulation. Obstet Gynecol 2006;108:757–61.
13. Sobieszczy KS, Breborowicz GH. Management of recommendations for postpartum haemorrhage. Arch Perinat Med 2004;10:1–4.
14. Royal College of Obstetricians and Gynaecologists. Prevention and management of postpartum haemorrhage. Clinical Guideline No. 52. London: RCOG; 2009.

CHAPTER 26

AMNIOTIC FLUID EMBOLISM

DJ Tuffnell

'Pulmonary embolism by the particulate matter contained in amniotic fluid which gained entrance to the maternal circulation has been demonstrated by us at autopsy in 8 cases in which it seemed to be the cause of death ... Having gained entrance to the maternal venous system, the emboli would be carried to the first filter bed, in these instances the lungs, and would lodge in vessels corresponding to their size. Sudden showers of foreign particulate material lodging in the lungs may produce severe systemic reactions resembling shock or anaphylactoid reactions'.

C. C. Steiner and P. E. Lushbaugh
Maternal pulmonary embolism by amniotic fluid as a cause of obstetric shock and unexpected death in obstetrics. JAMA 1941; 117:1245–1254, 1340–1345

Amniotic fluid embolism (AFE) is rare (2–3.3/100 000 deliveries) but is a potentially catastrophic complication of pregnancy. Despite its rarity, it has such a high fatality rate that it accounts for 7–10% of direct maternal deaths in the developed world. However, more recent series show a reducing maternal mortality. This may be due to improving care or to milder cases being identified. Maternal mortality is 20–35% and perinatal mortality 13.5–32%.[1-3]

Whilst individual cases have been reported in association with most interventions the larger series consistently show certain risk factors. Induction of labour is associated with a three- to fourfold increase in risk,[1,4] multiple pregnancy with a 10-fold increase[1] and older women also have an increased risk.[1] Caesarean section is associated with an eightfold increased chance of an amniotic fluid embolism occurring after the birth of the baby, so the caesarean section is associated with the AFE rather than being performed as a result of the AFE.[1] Ethnic minority groups may also be more vulnerable. Many cases present immediately postpartum but very rarely the manifestations may be delayed for 1–2 hours after delivery.[5]

PATHOPHYSIOLOGY

It is not uncommon for amniotic fluid and fetal squames to enter the maternal circulation without ill effect. In certain susceptible women, however, it seems that the presence of fetal cells and/or other components of amniotic fluid may trigger a complex pathophysiological cascade similar to that seen with anaphylaxis and septic shock.[6,7] The initial pathophysiological mechanism is of acute pulmonary vascular obstruction and hypertension leading to cor pulmonale. This is quite transient and soon followed by left ventricular failure leading to profound hypotension and shock. An acute inflammatory response disrupts the pulmonary capillary endothelium and alveoli leading to a ventilation–perfusion imbalance – resulting in severe hypoxia, convulsions and coma.[8] If the patient survives for more than 1 hour it is virtually inevitable that she will develop disseminated intravascular coagulation due to the activation of coagulation factors by the amniotic fluid (which contains tissue factor) and fetal cells, in addition to the profound shock.

DIAGNOSIS

The clinical diagnosis is based on the sudden development of acute respiratory distress and cardiovascular collapse in a patient in labour or recently delivered. In some cases the signs and symptoms occur within minutes of the triggering event, such as amniotomy or caesarean section.

The current criteria for defining a case in the UK are:[1]

Either

In the absence of any other clear cause, acute maternal collapse with one or more of the following features:
- Acute fetal compromise
- Cardiac arrhythmias or arrest
- Coagulopathy
- Convulsion
- Hypotension
- Maternal haemorrhage

- Premonitory symptoms, e.g. restlessness, numbness, agitation, tingling
- Shortness of breath

Excluding women with maternal haemorrhage as the first presenting feature in whom there was no evidence of early coagulopathy or cardiorespiratory compromise

Or

Women in whom the diagnosis was made at postmortem examination by finding fetal squames or hair in the lungs.

The differential diagnosis includes other acute catastrophes that may present with similar features. These would include cardiac causes (myocardial infarction, cardiomyopathy, heart failure secondary to volume overload, valvular disease), respiratory (pulmonary oedema secondary to volume overload, acute asthma, pulmonary embolus), infectious (severe sepsis, chest, chorioamnionitis, endocarditis), pregnancy complications (pre-eclampsia and eclampsia, HELLP (Haemolysis, Elevated Liver enzymes and Low Platelets) syndrome, ante- and postpartum haemorrhage) and others (anaphylaxis, air embolus, local anaesthetic toxicity).

The clinical features and context should help differentiate between these causes but, in any event, the initial management – cardiopulmonary resuscitation – may be required for all of these conditions. The initial clinical diagnosis of AFE, then, is really a combination of the above clinical features without any of the other obvious clinical causes.

MANAGEMENT

With AFE many women die shortly after presentation. Those that survive the initial event have a good prospect for survival. This means specialist assistance from anaesthesia, intensive care and haematology is often vital. The following management principles may improve survival:

- Early institution of effective cardiopulmonary resuscitation (CPR).
- If CPR is not effective within 5 minutes deliver the fetus. Perimortem caesarean section improves the effectiveness of CPR

for the mother by reducing oxygen requirement, improving venous return and by making the mechanics of CPR easier.

- Supportive care will include intubation and ventilation, possibly inotropic support with dopamine and correction of coagulopathy. Although hydrocortisone and heparin have both been suggested there are few reports of their use and none showing any benefit.
- Recently, plasma exchange and haemofiltration have been used in isolated cases with some benefit to help clear or 'wash out' the effects of the amniotic fluid in the circulation.[9]

Unfortunately, the initial hypoxic insult may be so profound that a number of the survivors suffer permanent neurological damage. Haemorrhage can only be controlled by hysterectomy in around 25% of cases.[1] Similarly, the outlook for the fetus undelivered at the time of diagnosis is very poor unless it can be delivered within 5–10 minutes.

REFERENCES

1. Knight M, Tuffnell D, Brocklehurst P, Spark P, Kurinczuk JJ, on behalf of the UK Obstetric Surveillance System. Incidence and risk factors for amniotic fluid embolism. Obstet Gynecol 2010;115:910–17.
2. Roberts C, Algert C, Knight M, Morris J. Amniotic fluid embolism in an Australian population-based cohort. Br J Obstet Gynaecol 2010;117:1417–21.
3. Kramer MS, Rouleau J, Liu S Bartholomew S, Joseph KS; Maternal Health Study Group of the Canadian Perinatal Surveillance System. Amniotic-fluid embolism incidence risk factors and impact on perinatal outcome. Br J Obstet Gynaecol 2012;119:874–9.
4. Kramer MS, Rouleau J, Baskett TF, Joseph KS. Amniotic-fluid embolism and medical induction of labour: a retrospective, population-based cohort study. Lancet 2006; 368:1444–8.
5. Clark SL, Hankins GDV, Dudley DA, Dildy GA, Porter TF. Amniotic fluid embolism: analysis of the national registry. Am J Obstet Gynecol 1995;172:1158–69.
6. Benson MD. Anaphylactoid syndrome of pregnancy. Am J Obstet Gynecol 1996;175:749.
7. Benson MD, Kobayashi H, Silver RK, Oi H, Greenberger PA, Terao T. Immunologic studies in presumed amniotic fluid embolism. Obstet Gynecol 2001;95:510–14.
8. Clark SL. New concepts of amniotic fluid embolism: a review. Obstet Gynecol Surv 1990;45:360–8.
9. Kancko Y, Ogihara T, Tajima H, Mochimaru F. Continuous hemofiltration for disseminated intravascular coagulation and shock due to amniotic fluid embolism: report of a dramatic response. Intern Med 2001;40: 945–7.

CHAPTER 27

ANALGESIA AND ANAESTHESIA

A Addei · TF Baskett

> 'No greater boon has ever come to mankind than the power thus granted to induce a temporary but complete insensibility to pain'.
>   Howard Wilcox Haggard
>   Devils, drugs, and doctors. the story of the science of healing from medicine-man to doctor. London: William Heinemann (Medical Books) Ltd, 1929.

INTRODUCTION

Labour is an intense and painful experience for most women, many of whom find it worse than they expected. For the woman having her first baby there is often additional fear and anxiety about the unknown.

Maternal pain and stress increase maternal sympathoadrenal activity which may lead to inco-ordinate uterine action, reduced uteroplacental perfusion, increased fetal oxygen requirements and adverse fetal effects.[1]

There are two schools of thought around how women might cope with the pain of labour. The first suggests that in the 21st century there is no need to suffer unnecessarily during labour and that effective analgesia is available and should be offered. The second sees pain as part of the experience of birth and advocates that women should be supported and encouraged to 'work with the pain' of labour. Whatever the woman's viewpoint, it is fundamental that she should be treated with respect and as an individual. Effective forms of pain relief are not necessarily associated with greater satisfaction with the birth experience and, conversely, failure of a chosen method can lead to dissatisfaction. The challenge for healthcare professionals is to recognize and respond appropriately to changes in the woman's stance during labour.[2]

Pain management strategies include non-pharmacological interventions (that aim to help women cope with pain in labour) and pharmacological interventions (that aim to relieve the pain of labour). Most methods of non-pharmacological pain management are non-invasive and appear to be safe for mother and baby; however, their efficacy is unclear, due to limited high-quality evidence. There is more evidence to support the efficacy of pharmacological methods, but these have more adverse effects.[3]

PAIN PATHWAYS

In the first stage of labour the origin of pain is from effacement and dilatation of the cervix and formation of the lower uterine segment. These painful impulses pass through the hypogastric plexus to the lumbar sympathetic chain and, via the dorsal horn, to T10, T11, T12 and L1 at the spinal cord level. The nociceptive information passes from the dorsal horn via the spinothalamic tract through the brain stem and medulla to the posterior thalamic nuclei. From here fibres pass to the somatic sensory cortex and thence to the frontal cortex. These pathways help regulate the associated responses to pain, such as anxiety, adverse reaction and learned behaviour.

In the second stage of labour, in addition to the uterine contractions, pain results from stretching of the pelvic floor and perineum. These painful stimuli enter the spinal cord via the somatic pudendal nerves: S2, S3 and S4.

METHODS OF PAIN RELIEF

Analgesia provides a varying amount of relief for a painful condition. Anaesthesia provides total relief of pain which is necessary for a surgical operation.

Non-Pharmacological Methods

Most of these techniques rely on counter-stimulation as the basis for their success.

Prepared Childbirth

The so-called 'natural childbirth' movement started in the early part of the 20th century in response to the 'twilight sleep' era at the beginning of the century with its excessive use of narcotics and sedatives. The basis of childbirth preparation is that women who are properly prepared can control the pain of labour themselves and either do without or reduce their need for pharmacological pain relief. There have been a number of prominent, often consumer-led, movements following the lead of Grantly Dick Reid in Britain, Velvoski in Russia and Lamaze and Le Boyer in France. In addition to these specific techniques many regions and hospitals will provide antenatal classes with information about the various methods of pain relief in labour (both non-pharmacological and pharmacological) as well as infant care classes, with the overall aim of engendering confidence in the couple.

NATURAL CHILDBIRTH

'It is not generally recognized that in childbirth there is an "emotional labour" which is as definite and important as its physical counterpart. This must be understood if parturition is to be conducted as a physiological performance...Is a woman pained and frightened because her labour is difficult, or is her labour difficult and painful because she is frightened?...Pain is the mental interpretation of harmful stimulus, and fear the intensifier of stimulus-interpretation. The biological purpose of each is protective. The physiological reaction to each is tension'.

Grantly Dick Read
Natural childbirth. London: Heinemann, 1933

Continuous Support

No woman in labour should be left alone. In addition to the trained nurse or midwife many women will have social support in the form of their male partner or other family member and some will choose to have a specially trained lay person (sometimes known as a doula). These personnel can provide reassurance, encouragement and explanation during labour. In addition, they may help guide counter-stimulation techniques such as touch, massage, change of position, baths, ambulation, music, etc. Cultural factors may dictate the personnel and techniques used for support to the woman in labour.

Hypnosis

This often requires extensive antenatal training sessions and individual receptivity to hypnosis varies. In some cases the hypnotherapist also needs to be present during labour. When

successful, the results of hypnosis are very impressive; however, the time and personnel commitment required are such that this is not practical for the majority of women.

Transcutaneous Electrical Nerve Stimulation (TENS)

This consists of a small, battery-driven pulse generator which is connected to two pairs of electrodes on either side of the spine overlying the dermatomes, T10 to L1, and attached to the skin with adhesive tape. When activated it causes a tingling sensation in the skin under the electrodes. The strength of the stimulus can be adjusted by the control generator. It is said to be most helpful in early labour with back pain and may stimulate the release of endorphins. The woman can remain ambulant but TENS equipment may interfere with electronic fetal heart rate monitoring using a fetal scalp electrode.

Intradermal Injection of Water

Using a 1 ml syringe and a 25-gauge needle, injections of 0.05–0.1 ml of sterile water are injected into the skin in four sites: one on each side over the posterior iliac spines and one each just medial and below the upper sites. This causes intense stinging for about 30 seconds and may provide amelioration of back pain for 45–90 minutes. It is thought to act by counter-irritation, possible release of endorphins or, according to the gate-control theory of pain, the intense superficial sensory stimulation may inhibit pain signals in the deeper, slower nerve fibres. In general this technique may give short-term relief from backache but rarely influences the total analgesia requirements.

Acupuncture

This and related procedures may have application in societies which have practitioners skilled in this technique and in women who are knowledgeable and receptive to this method.

Pharmacological Methods

Inhalation Analgesia

The safest and most practical agent for inhalation analgesia is nitrous oxide. The aim is to administer subanaesthetic concentrations of nitrous oxide providing analgesia without loss of consciousness and with retention of protective laryngeal reflexes. Nitrous oxide is absorbed from and excreted by the lungs. It crosses the placenta but is also eliminated efficiently and there are no untoward neonatal effects. It has no effect on uterine contractility. The exact mode of action is unknown but it works at the level of the brain, producing analgesia in low doses and anaesthesia with higher and sustained doses.

FIRST USE OF NITROUS OXIDE/ OXYGEN INHALATION ANALGESIA IN LABOUR

'The woman should be coached to exhale deeply and then inhale as much gas as possible...It is important to begin the first anaesthesia early in order to obtain good pain relief; a late start will prevent the deep inhalation and, thus render the effect incomplete...Thereafter the inhalation is begun at one-half to one minute prior to the anticipated next contraction. Two to five breaths of the gas mixture usually suffice to produce the desired effect'.
Stanislav Klikovich
Über das Stickstoffoxydul als Anaestheticum bei Geburten. Arch Gynäk 1881; 18:81–108

The advantage of nitrous oxide inhalation analgesia is that it is cheap, safe and simple to administer. In one-third to one-half of women it provides helpful, albeit incomplete, analgesia. It is most effective for short-term (1–2 hours) pain relief. As such, it is of most benefit in the multiparous woman in the late first stage of labour, in whom analgesia is usually required for the last hour or so before and during the second stage of labour. It is also of benefit as an adjunct to local anaesthetic techniques, such as infiltration of the perineum and pudendal block for instrumental vaginal delivery, assisted breech and twin delivery, and suture of genital tract lacerations.

Technique of Administration. There is a variety of equipment for self-administration of nitrous oxide. The simplest and most commonly used is a pre-mixed gas cylinder of 50% nitrous oxide and 50% oxygen (Entonox). An alternative is a blender apparatus that produces the appropriate 50/50 concentration from separate cylinders via hospital gas lines (Nitronox, Midogas).

The breathing circuit is connected to a face mask or mouthpiece. Within the breathing circuit is a demand valve which only opens when the user applies negative pressure with strong inhalation. For this to occur the user has to retain enough consciousness to keep the seal of the mouthpiece or face mask intact. If the woman becomes drowsy, and long before protective laryngeal reflexes are lost, her grip on the apparatus will break the seal and not permit further inhalation of gas. This protective mechanism is one of the most important safety features of the self-administered apparatus.

There is a latent period from when the woman starts inhalation until there is sufficient gas tension in the central nervous system to produce analgesia. This time lag is approximately 30–40 seconds. In the first stage of labour, uterine contractions are palpable about 20 seconds before the woman feels pain. The most important point, therefore, for those assisting the woman in labour is to palpate the uterine contraction and get her to start the inhalation so that some concentration of the gas is effective before the pain becomes intense. This is an essential practical point that is often overlooked. An alternative, if the contraction pattern is regular and predictable, is to guide the inhalation of nitrous oxide by the clock so that it starts about 30–40 seconds before the contraction. If nitrous oxide is to be used as an adjunct to local anaesthesia for painful procedures, it can be administered continuously until satisfactory analgesia is provided. Once again, the safeguard of self-administration by the woman should prevent anaesthesia and loss of protective reflexes.

Narcotic Analgesia

Over the past century parenteral administration of narcotics has been one of the most frequently used methods of pain relief in labour. For the past 50 years the most commonly used narcotic has been meperidine (demerol, pethidine). In many countries, midwives have autonomous use of meperidine in labour and it is this practical point that has accounted for its widespread use. Unfortunately, narcotics by intramuscular injection are not very effective at providing adequate pain relief in labour. The half-life of meperidine is about 2–3 hours and it rapidly crosses the placenta. The maximum fetal tissue uptake occurs about 2–3 hours after maternal administration and the half-life in the neonate is about 12 hours. Thus, the neonate is at greatest risk for respiratory depression 2–3 hours after meperidine administration to the mother. Maternal side effects include nausea, vomiting, hypotension, pruritis, respiratory depression and sedation. All narcotics may reduce the baseline variability of the fetal heart rate. In addition to neonatal depression there is altered neonatal behaviour for the first 12–24 hours and impairment of breast feeding.

FIRST USE OF ETHER AND CHLOROFORM INHALATION ANALGESIA IN LABOUR

'Whilst this agent has been used extensively, and by numerous hands, in the practice of surgery, I am not aware that anyone has hitherto ventured to test its applicability to the practice of midwifery. I am induced, therefore, to hope that the few following hurried and imperfect notes, relative to its employment in obstetric cases may not at the present time prove uninteresting to the profession'.
   James Young Simpson
   Ether inhalation in parturition. Edinb Mon J Med Sci 1847; 74:639–640

   'This new anaesthetic agent is chloroform... as an inhaled anaesthetic agent, it possesses, I believe, all the advantages of sulphuric ether, without its principle disadvantages... greatly less quantity of chloroform than of ether is required to produce the anaesthetic affect... Its action is much more rapid and complete, and generally more persistent... The inhalation and influence of chloroform... far more agreeable and pleasant than those of ether'.
   James Young Simpson
   On a new anaesthetic agent, more efficient than sulphuric ether. Lancet 1847; 2:549–551

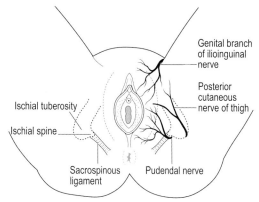

FIGURE 27-1 ■ Cutaneous nerve supply of the perineum.

There are individual circumstances in which the use of narcotic analgesia can be adjusted to the woman's requirements:

- Meperidine can be given by intramuscular or subcutaneous injection (the latter route gives more reliable absorption) in a dose of 50–150 mg depending on the patient's size. This can be useful in the anxious woman early in established labour. The effect is maximal in 45–60 minutes and lasts about 3 hours. An antiemetic administered at the same time reduces nausea and vomiting.
- Intravenous narcotic provides quick pain relief for the woman who has uncontrolled and distressing pain. Remifentanil has superseded meperidine and fentanyl as the opioid of choice for intravenous analgesia if epidural analgesia is unavailable or contraindicated. Remifentanil is a synthetic opioid with direct agonist action specifically on mu-opioid receptors. Its rapid hydrolysis by non-specific blood and tissue esterases to an inactive metabolite results in a very short duration of action. The pharmacodynamic profile of remifentanil is characterized by a rapid onset of action and short latency to its peak effect. The context sensitive half-life is 3–4 minutes and the elimination half-time ranges from 10 to 20 minutes. Most of an intravenous dose is excreted in the urine as the carboxylic acid

metabolite. The metabolism of remifentanil is independent of renal and hepatic function and there is no accumulation during repeat bolus injection. Placental transfer of remifentanil does occur but in the neonate it appears to be rapidly metabolized, redistributed or both.[4] Remifentanil is set up via a pump as patient controlled analgesia (PCA) by an anaesthetist.

Local Anaesthesia

The use of local anaesthetic for infiltration and regional blocks is of great value for obstetric operative procedures. It is important to know the dose and potential toxicity of local anaesthetics. The most commonly used is lidocaine (lignocaine) and the dose is 3–4 mg/kg plain solution, and 7–8 mg/kg with added epinephrine (adrenaline). A 1% solution of lidocaine contains 10 mg/ml, and the dose for a 70 kg woman should, therefore, not exceed 250 mg or 25 ml.

The local anaesthetic should be allowed to take effect and tested before proceeding. Incomplete anaesthesia may be supplemented with inhalational analgesia.

Local Infiltration

The cutaneous nerve supply of the perineum is shown in Figure 27-1. For perineal and lower vaginal lacerations, direct infiltration of the involved areas is performed by advancing the needle and injecting and aspirating, to avoid intravascular injection, as the needle is advanced and withdrawn. Before the performance of episiotomy the site of the proposed incision and the adjacent areas of the fourchette and labia are infiltrated to reduce both the pain of incision and distension of the perineum.

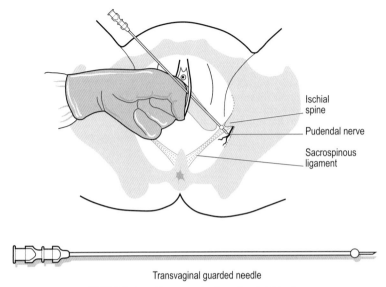

Ischial spine

Pudendal nerve

Sacrospinous ligament

Transvaginal guarded needle

FIGURE 27-2 ■ Transvaginal pudendal block.

As an adjunct to pudendal block the site of the proposed episiotomy can be infiltrated as well as the areas of the lower labia supplied by the posterior cutaneous nerve of the thigh and the genital branch of the ilio-inguinal nerve.

Pudendal Block

If epidural or spinal anaesthesia is not available or is contraindicated, pudendal block is a safe and useful technique for low assisted vaginal delivery with forceps or vacuum and for the manipulations necessary for assisted breech delivery and delivery of the second twin. Pudendal block can be performed by two techniques:

- *Transvaginal* – this is the technique of choice as it is less painful and more accurate than the transperineal route. Using a 20 ml syringe with 1% lidocaine the needle guard is guided medial and just below the ischial spine. Use the left index and middle fingers to guide to the left side and the right hand to guide to the right ischial spine (Fig 27-2). If the special needle guard is not available it is possible to guide a bare spinal needle to the spine if the point is firmly shielded between the fingers – this requires great care to avoid personal injury when making the final manipulation of the needle point through the sacrospinous ligament. After aspiration 5–8 ml of local anaesthetic is injected around the pudendal nerve.
- *Transperineal* – this method is much more painful and less accurate than the transvaginal route and is only used if the presenting part is so low as to preclude the

transvaginal technique. The skin is infiltrated with local anaesthetic half way between the anus and the ischial tuberosity. With one index finger in the vagina the ischial spine is palpated and a 10 cm spinal needle is advanced through the infiltrated skin and guided towards the ischial spine and sacrospinous ligament. Aspiration and infiltration around the pudendal nerve follows.

To supplement an incomplete block, use the remaining local anaesthetic, starting at the fourchette and fan out with local infiltration to the perineum, site of the episiotomy and lower aspect of the labia.

Paracervical Block

This is a very simple and effective method of pain relief in the first stage of labour when other conservative methods fail and epidural analgesia is not available. Fetal bradycardia can occur following paracervical block and there have been several cases of intrauterine death. The rapid absorption of local anaesthetic from the very vascular paracervical tissues may lead to high fetal levels and cause myocardial and central nervous system depression. If modified techniques with less toxic local anaesthetics are developed it may become safer in the future, but at present its use in labour with a viable fetus cannot be recommended. It may, however, be useful in cases of labour with a dead or non-viable fetus and it can also be useful in cases requiring intrauterine manipulation following delivery, such as manual removal of retained placenta and acute uterine

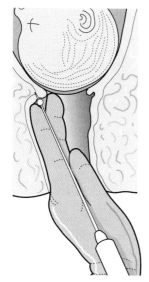

FIGURE 27-3 ■ Paracervical block.

inversion if epidural, spinal or general anaesthesia is not available.

The technique is simple, using a specially designed needle and guard, such that the needle protrudes only 3–5 mm from the guard. Between 3 and 4 o'clock and 8 and 9 o'clock 5–10 ml of local anaesthetic is injected into each lateral fornix where the cervix reflects off from the vagina (Fig 27-3). Frequent aspiration is essential as the paracervical space is extremely vascular.

Local Anaesthesia for Caesarean Section

Depending upon available facilities and personnel, or lack thereof, there may be occasions when caesarean section needs to be performed under local anaesthesia. Inhalation analgesia with nitrous oxide may be used to augment the local anaesthetic.

Make up 100 ml 0.5% lidocaine to which 0.5 ml of 1 in 200 000 epinephrine (adrenaline) has been added. Using a 20 ml syringe, the principle is to 'inject as you go':

- 15–20 ml along the line of the proposed skin incision
- 10–15 ml under the rectus sheath and adjacent rectus muscle
- 10–15 ml in the extraperitoneal tissue and transversalis fascia

- The peritoneum is then opened
- 10 ml in the utero-vesical peritoneal fold – this fold is then incised and the uterine muscle exposed
- The uterine muscle is relatively insensitive to incision but the muscle may be infiltrated with 10–15 ml before incision
- Once the infant has been delivered the mother should be given intravenous morphine.

The above methods of pain relief with the exception of remifentanil PCA can be administered or guided by an obstetrician. Administration of epidural, spinal or general anaesthesia is beyond the scope of this book.

REFERENCES

1. Reynolds F. Labour analgesia and the baby: good news is no news. Int J Obstet Anesth 2011;20:38–50.
2. Intrapartum care. Care of healthy women and their babies during childbirth. National Collaborating Centre for Women's and Children's Health. Commissioned by the National Institute for Health and Clinical Excellence. London: RCOG Press; 2007.
3. Jones L, Othman M, Dowswell T, Alfirevic Z, Gates S, Newburn M, et al. Pain management for women in labour: an overview of systematic reviews (Review). The Cochrane Library 2012, Issue 3. doi: CD009234.pub2.
4. Douma MR, Verwey RA, Kam-Endtz CE, van der Linden PD, Stienstra R. Obstetric analgesia: a comparison of patient-controlled meperidine, remifentanil, and fentanyl in labour. Br J Anaesth 2010;104:209–15.

BIBLIOGRAPHY

Baskett TF. Edinburgh connections in a painful world. J R Coll Surg Edin Irel 2005;3:99–107.

Hodnett ED, Lowe NK, Hannah ME, Willan AR, Stevens B, Weston JA, et al. Effectiveness of nurses as providers of birth labor support in North American hospitals. A randomized controlled trial. JAMA 2002;288:1373–81.

Hodnett ED. Pain in women's satisfaction with the experience of childbirth: a systematic review. Am J Obstet Gynecol 2002;186S:160–72.

Kuczkowski KM. Neurologic complications of labor analgesia: facts and fiction. Obstet Gynecol Surv 2003;59: 47–51.

Pang D, O'Sullivan G. Analgesia and anaesthesia in labour. Obstet Gynaecol Reprod Med 2008;18:87–92.

Rosen MA. Paracervical block for labor analgesia: a brief historic review. Am J Obstet Gynecol 2002;186S:127–30.

Rosen MA. Nitrous oxide for relief of labour pain: a systematic review. Am J Obstet Gynecol 2002;186S:110–26.

Simkin PP, O'Hara MA. Non-pharmacologic relief of pain during labor: a systematic review of five methods. Am J Obstet Gynecol 2002;186S:131–59.

Waldenström U, Hildingsson I, Ryding EL. Antenatal fear of childbirth and its association with subsequent caesarean section and experience of childbirth. Br J Obstet Gynaecol 2006;1132:638–46.

CHAPTER 28

PROCEDURES AND TECHNIQUES

CERVICAL CERCLAGE

AA Calder

Among the catalogue of procedures designed to improve pregnancy outcome cervical cerclage is one of the most controversial. Its purpose is clear, namely to prevent or reduce the incidence of miscarriage from a presumed diagnosis of 'cervical incompetence'. On the face of it this seems entirely logical if the obstetrician believes that the cervix is likely to fail in its duty of remaining long and closed to retain the fetus in utero until the time is right for delivery. However, our ability to make a secure diagnosis of the condition is fraught with difficulty and our 'belief' may be built on false premises. The condition remains poorly understood and for upwards of 50 years investigators have striven to devise a reliable means of diagnosis. The clinician has often had to fall back on the clinical history of the pattern of previous pregnancy losses but even when there is seemingly compelling evidence of cervical incompetence uncertainty remains as to the best remedy amid a disappointing lack of persuasive evidence of benefit.

None of this appears to have discouraged clinicians from employing this intervention. Indeed it has often been grossly over used. In its simplest form it may seem a relatively harmless procedure but it is by no means without risk and needs to be employed with careful circumspection. One may sympathize with the clinician who, faced with a woman who has endured a succession of harrowing pregnancy losses, feels compelled to do something rather than nothing; but this is fuelled by an unfortunate paradox. The more sutures inserted in women who do not in fact have the condition, the better may the results appear to be because many of those women will have a good outcome despite the intervention. Furthermore they are likely to believe that the intervention saved the pregnancy. It is therefore imperative that the clinician should make an honest appraisal of each case before embarking on a procedure which, although seemingly innocuous, may in some cases expose the woman to serious risks.

SURGICAL PROCEDURE

The surgical options range from the comparatively straightforward insertion of a suture around the portio vaginalis of the cervix to insertion of one at the level of the fibro-muscular junction between the uterine corpus and cervix (Fig 28-1). The latter is clearly a much more elaborate intervention, requiring a laparotomy. Not only does this cause pain and discomfort to the woman, but it requires a higher degree of experience and skill of the operator, and carries more serious implications for the subsequent management of the pregnancy. This will almost certainly mandate delivery by caesarean section.

A transvaginal approach is most commonly employed. Because of the manner in which effacement of the cervix occurs (see Chapter 1) it will be obvious that a suture placed too low on the portio vaginalis will be worse than useless. It is therefore important to place it as high as possible and this requires that effective traction be applied to the cervix. It used to be fashionable to employ sponge holding forceps for this in the belief that they would be atraumatic but experience has shown that they tend to slip off and to avulse the cervical epithelium in the process. A single tooth vulsellum is greatly to be preferred and while this may result in some bleeding this should not be significant. The advantage of an effective grip on the ectocervix greatly outweighs any concern about bleeding. The suture should be placed as high as feasible and some clinicians feel justified in opening the anterior vaginal fornix and pushing up the bladder in order to achieve as high a placement as is possible by a transvaginal approach.

TIMING

Although some clinicians have considered inserting a suture between pregnancies this has little or nothing to commend it. In the first place, it may interfere with conception and secondly there is no merit in the presence of a suture in a

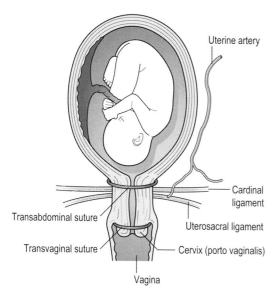

Uterine artery

Cardinal ligament

Transabdominal suture

Uterosacral ligament

Transvaginal suture

Cervix (porto vaginalis)

Vagina

FIGURE 28-1 ■ Diagram illustrating the sites of placement of transabdominal and transvaginal cervical supporting sutures respectively.

woman destined to miscarry in the first trimester. Such miscarriages cannot be prevented by cervical cerclage. The appropriate timing for insertion of an elective suture is between 10 and 14 weeks' gestation after an ultrasound scan has confirmed that the pregnancy is progressing normally.

Assuming the pregnancy has progressed satisfactorily it is usual to remove transvaginal sutures at around 37 weeks. In the event of spontaneous miscarriage or antepartum haemorrhage the suture may have to be removed earlier. In the case of transabdominal sutures it is usually possible to divide them with scissors introduced through the posterior fornix in the midline. This begs the question why this should not also be done at 37 weeks but it is considered better to deliver such pregnancies abdominally. The suture may then be left in place where it may serve again in a subsequent pregnancy.

MATERIALS AND MANAGEMENT

In past decades an exotic catalogue of different suture materials has been used including strips of the woman's own fascia lata, tantalum wire and all manner of synthetic, non-absorbable materials. We feel there is no need to employ any other material than mersilene tape, which serves well regardless of the route of insertion. It has become conventional to cover the insertion period and subsequent few hours with an inhibitor of prostaglandin synthesis such as indomethacin and that particularly applies in the

case of a decision to attempt a 'rescue' suture when the cervix has already dilated and allowed the amniotic sac to bulge into the vagina. When this occurs in the absence of uterine contractions an attempt of this sort may be worthwhile. It may seem that the cervix is already irrevocably dilated and delivery imminent, but this is by no means always so. With the sac filling the vagina it is easy to assume that the cervix is fully dilated but often there has been an 'hour glass' prolapsing of the sac through an only partially dilated cervix. In such circumstances strategies such as employing a steep head-down tilt, a balloon to persuade the sac back into the uterus and perhaps transabdominal amniocentesis to reduce the amniotic fluid volume may improve the prospects of success. Such cases are fraught with difficulty because an attempt at rescue may result in rupture of the membranes, leaving the clinician to feel that conservative management might have been preferable, but one has to consider all the risks and try to arrive at a balanced decision.

RISKS

It is important to stress the danger if labour should become established with a suture still in place and the woman must be advised that, if that should happen, its prompt removal is essential. The risks include further damage to the cervix if the suture tears out or rupture of the uterus. The latter is a particular hazard if there is a previous caesarean scar. There have also been cases reported of annular detachment of the cervix and of delivery through the posterior vaginal fornix bypassing the cervix. A special warning should be highlighted of a circumstance where a second higher suture has been inserted because the original one has been deemed inadequate but left in place. We know of an instance in which a suture was later removed without recognizing that the other remained in place; a disastrous outcome was only narrowly avoided. This also highlights the need for accurate and prominent recording in the case records of the presence of sutures and their location, together with clear instructions about their subsequent management.

BIBLIOGRAPHY

Anthony GS, Robbins JB, Cameron AD, Calder AA. Cervical cerclage in Scotland – fifty years on. Scot Med J 2009;54:42–5.

Benson RC, Durfee RB. Transabdominal cervico-uterine cerclage during pregnancy for the treatment of cervical incompetency. Obstet Gynecol 1965;25:145–55.

Drakeley AJ, Roberts D, Alferevic Z. Cervical cerclage for previous pregnancy loss in women. Cochrane Database Syst Rev 2003;1:CD003253.

McDonald IA. Suture of the cervix for inevitable miscarriage. J Obstet Gynaecol Br Emp 1957;64:346–50.

Royal College of Obstetricians and Gynaecologists. Cervical cerclage. Green-top Guideline No. 60. London: RCOG; 2011.

Shirodkar VN. A new method of operative treatment for habitual abortion in the second trimester of pregnancy. Antiseptic 1955;52:299–300.

ACUTE TOCOLYSIS

TF Baskett • S Arulkumaran

In certain obstetric complications, rapid uterine relaxation is required for their successful resolution. Until relatively recently acute uterine tocolysis required the institution of general anaesthesia with halogenated agents and involved rapid sequence induction and tracheal intubation with its associated maternal risks. The recent application of β-adrenergic drugs, oxytocin antagonists and nitroglycerine to achieve rapid uterine relaxation has obviated the need for general anaesthesia in these circumstances.

FIRST USE OF UTERINE TOCOLYSIS

'I found it impossible to get my hand into the uterus to deliver the placenta. Bearing in mind the remarkable power which nitrite of amyl possesses in relaxing tension in the blood-vessels, I determined to test its action on the uterine spasms. The patient had three drops of the nitrite of amyl given her on a handkerchief to inhale. During the inhalation, the ring of muscular fibres around the os interna, which had been so rigid as to be absolutely undilatable, steadily yielded, until I could pass the whole hand into the uterus…'

  Fancourt Barnes
  Hour-glass contraction of the uterus treated with nitrate of amyl. BMJ 1882; 1:377

NITROGLYCERINE

Nitroglycerine is an ester of nitric acid and exerts its relaxant effect on smooth muscle by the formation of nitric oxide. The drug is rapidly metabolized by the liver so that the half-life is only 2 minutes. It has a low molecular weight of 227 and therefore crosses the placenta, but no adverse fetal or neonatal effects have been described in either animal studies or humans. In addition to uterine tocolysis the smooth muscle relaxation effect causes peripheral vasodilatation and reduced venous tone. Provided there is no hypovolaemia this causes only a mild and clinically insignificant hypotension. However, if there is associated hypovolaemia, rapid infusion of intravenous crystalloid is necessary to avoid acute and severe maternal hypotension. The peripheral vasodilation responds to epinephrine (adrenaline) and the uterine relaxation responds to oxytocin.[1]

BETA-ADRENERGIC DRUGS

The biggest experience with this group of drugs has been with ritodrine, terbutaline and hexoprenaline. These selective β-2 receptor agonists have the main effect of relaxing arteriolar and uterine smooth muscle. These drugs are given subcutaneously or by slow intravenous injection diluted in saline; they do not inhibit uterine activity when given as nebulizers. They may cause mild hypotension and tachycardia and there have been isolated reports of atrial fibrillation. These agents cross the placenta and may cause a mild transient fetal tachycardia. They abolish uterine activity for 15–30 minutes, and their effect can be reversed by β-blockers.[2]

ATOSIBAN

Atosiban is a synthetic analogue of oxytocin that acts as an oxytocin antagonist by binding to myometrial cell oxytocin receptors. The half-life is about 12 minutes and it crosses the placenta, but umbilical vein levels are only 10% of those in the maternal uterine vein.[3] The advantage of atosiban is that it has fewer cardiovascular side effects compared with the β-adrenergic agents. Atosiban has been used mainly in attempts to suppress preterm labour but it may also have an application for acute tocolysis in intrapartum fetal distress.[4]

INDICATIONS

Rapid uterine relaxation may be necessary in the following clinical situations.

Excessive Uterine Action

Excessive uterine action in labour is defined as more than five uterine contractions in a 10-minute period averaged over 30 minutes (tachysystole) or contractions exceeding 2 minutes in duration (hypertonus).[5] This uterine hyperstimulation is most likely to occur in response to oxytocic drugs, either oxytocin or, more likely, the longer acting prostaglandins used for cervical ripening and induction of labour. Although less common, tachysystole and uterine hypertonus can occur in spontaneous labour and more so with pathological conditions such as placental abruption.[2,6,7]

Breech Delivery

Unless the uterus is relaxed there may be difficulty with delivery of extended arms and/or the after-coming head of the preterm breech. This can occur with both vaginal and caesarean delivery but is more likely with the latter. The fetal breech, trunk and legs may be easily delivered through the uterine incision because of their smaller diameter, but the unrelaxed uterine muscle may clamp down around the fetal head, leading to delay, asphyxia and potential trauma. This is particularly likely in the preterm breech, but can also occur with the term fetus.[8]

External Cephalic Version

Short-term uterine relaxation may help facilitate external cephalic version of breech presentation at term.[9] In this context the beta-adrenergic drugs are more effective than nitroglycerine, because of their longer duration of action.[10]

Intrapartum Version of Fetal Malpresentations

Uterine relaxation is usually necessary to safely and effectively carry out both external cephalic and internal podalic version at both vaginal and caesarean delivery of the second twin (see Chapter 17). With regional anaesthesia uterine relaxation is often inadequate and additional tocolysis is necessary.

Cord Prolapse

If uterine contractions interfere with cord decompression after cord prolapse, acute tocolysis may be needed. This is more likely if there is an anticipated delay in the diagnosis-to-delivery interval (see Chapter 18).

Shoulder Dystocia

In rare cases of shoulder dystocia that cannot be resolved with the traditional manoeuvres, cephalic replacement may be considered (see Chapter 12). In this situation, replacement of the head is facilitated by uterine relaxation, which may also help restore the utero-placental circulation and fetal oxygenation.

Retained Placenta

Acute tocolysis may aid relaxation of a contraction ring and allow spontaneous delivery of the separated but retained placenta.[11] On other occasions, tocolysis may be necessary to facilitate the manual removal of a non-separated placenta, in which a contraction ring prevents manual access.

Acute Uterine Inversion

Manual replacement of acute uterine inversion may be possible using acute tocolysis, obviating the need for general anaesthesia.[12]

In many of the above situations, regional anaesthesia in the form of epidural or spinal analgesia may be in effect. However, these regional techniques, while providing excellent analgesia, do not provide uterine relaxation, so that additional tocolysis may be necessary.

ADMINISTRATION OF TOCOLYTICS

Nitroglycerine

This can be given by the sublingual or intravenous routes. Sublingual administration is via an aerosol spray in doses of 400 µg. However, the mucosal absorption is not as predictable or precise as the intravenous route and the latter is usually chosen for acute tocolysis.

Nitroglycerine comes in an ampoule containing 5 mg in 1 ml solution. If this is added to a 100 ml bag of normal saline it produces a solution of 50 µg per ml. Draw up 20 ml into a syringe – this allows the precise titration of 50 µg per ml administered. Nitroglycerine is rapidly degraded and its effect is usually obvious within 90 seconds and lasts for a further 1–2 minutes. At the time of its administration intravenous crystalloid should be running rapidly, particularly if there is any question of hypovolaemia. The dose is titrated depending on the initial response and the clinical situation.[13,14] For cases of fetal entrapment a rapid response is necessary and one usually starts with a dose of 200 µg, repeating this at about 2-minute intervals until appropriate uterine relaxation is achieved. In cases with retained placenta or acute uterine inversion, hypovolaemia should be corrected and smaller initial doses (100 µg) may be given.

In all cases in which oxytocin or prostaglandins have been previously administered, higher doses of nitroglycerine may be required.

Terbutaline

It is most commonly given as 250 µg subcutaneously, but can be given intravenously in 5 ml saline, slowly over 5 minutes.[15,16] The antagonist to terbutaline is propranolol 1–2 mg IV.

Ritodrine

This is given as 6 mg mixed in 10 ml normal saline and administered intravenously over 3 minutes.

Hexoprenaline

Give 5 µg in 10 ml normal saline intravenously over 5 minutes.

Atosiban

Mix 6.75 mg of atosiban in 5 ml normal saline and give intravenously over 1 minute.[4]

For rapid short-lived tocolysis necessary to deal with malpresentations and third stage complications, nitroglycerine is the drug of choice. For more sustained uterine relaxation needed with uterine hypertonus or external cephalic version atosiban or terbutaline are more appropriate.

REFERENCES

1. Lau IC, Adaikau PC, Arulkumaran S, Ng SC. Oxytocics reverse the tocolytic effect of glyceryl trinitrate on the human uterus. Br J Obstet Gynaecol 2001;108: 164–8.
2. Ingemarsson I, Arulkumaran S, Ratnam SS. Single injection of terbutaline in term labor. I Effect on fetal pH in cases with prolonged bradycardia. Am J Obstet Gynecol 1985;153:859–64.
3. Lamont RF. The development and introduction of anti-oxytocic tocolytics. Br J Obstet Gynaecol 2003;110: 108–12.
4. Afschar P, Schöll W, Bader A, Bauer M, Winter R. A prospective randomised trial of atosiban versus hexoprenaline for acute tocolysis and intrauterine resuscitation. Br J Obstet Gynaecol 2004;111:316–8.
5. National Collaborating Centre for Women's and Children's Health, National Institute for Health and Clinical Excellence. Induction of labour. Clinical Guideline. London: RCOG Press; 2008.
6. Ingemarsson I, Arulkumaran S, Ratnam SS. Single injection of terbutaline in term labor. II. Effect on uterine activity. Am J Obstet Gynecol 1985;153:865–9.
7. Palomaki O, Jansson M, Huhtala H, Kirkinen P. Severe cardiotocographic pathology at labor: effect of acute intravenous tocolysis. Am J Perinatol 2004;21:347–53.
8. Ezra Y, Wade C, Robin SH, Farine D. Uterine tocolysis at caesarean breech delivery with epidural anesthesia. J Reprod Med 2002;47:555–8.
9. Burgos J, Eguiguren N, Quintana E, Cobos P, Centeno M, Larrieta R, et al. Atosiban vs ritodrine as a tocolytic in external cephalic version at term: a prospective cohort study. J Perinat Med 2010;38:23–8.
10. Cluver C, Hofmeyr GJ, Gyte GM, Sinclair M. Interventions for helping to turn term breech babies to head first presentation when using external cephalic version. Cochrane Database Syst Rev 2012;1:CD000184.
11. DeSimone CA, Norris MC, Leighton DL. Intravenous nitroglycerine aids manual extraction of a retained placenta. Anesthesiology 1990;73:787–9.
12. Altabef KM, Spencer JT, Zinberg S. Intravenous nitroglycerin for uterine relaxation of an inverted uterus. Am J Obstet Gynecol 1992;166:1237–8.
13. Axemo P, Fu X, Lindberg B, Ulmsten U, Wessen A. Intravenous nitroglycerine for rapid uterine relaxation. Acta Obstet Gynecol Scand 1998;77:50–3.
14. O'Grady JP, Parker RK, Patel SS. Nitroglycerin for rapid tocolysis: development of a protocol and a literature review. J Perinatol 2001;20:27–33.
15. Chandraharan E, Arulkumaran S. Prevention of birth asphyxia: responding appropriately to cardiotocograph (CTG) traces. Best Pract Res Clin Obstet Gynaecol 2007;21:609–24.
16. de Heus R, Mulder EJ, Derks JB, Visser GH. Acute tocolysis for uterine activity reduction in term labor: a review. Obstet Gynecol Surv 2008;63:383–8.

VERSION

TF Baskett

Version refers to the procedure that changes the presenting part of the fetus. This may be carried out by *external* manipulation of the fetus, *internal* manipulation or *combined* (*bipolar*) internal and external manoeuvres. Bipolar version is discussed in the chapter on antepartum haemorrhage.

EXTERNAL CEPHALIC VERSION

External cephalic version (ECV) is used to alter the presentation of the fetus in the later weeks of pregnancy. Breech presentation, transverse or oblique lie may be converted to cephalic presentation.[1] This may also be achieved in early labour in some women, particularly the multiparous. Following delivery of the first twin, ECV may be undertaken for breech or oblique lie of the second twin.

EXTERNAL CEPHALIC VERSION

'In all cases, where, after eight months of gestation the head occupies either the iliac fossa or the superior uterine segment, we should perform cephalic version by external manoeuvres... The first stage of the operation consists in rendering the foetus moveable... To facilitate this displacement of the breech, we may at the same time exert slight pressure in an opposite direction over the cephalic extremity. The two fetal extremities being moveable and accessible, and the hands being applied over them, we should make slow and continued pressure in such a manner as to cause the breech to ascend and the head to descend by the shortest route.

Adolpe Pinard
A Treatise on Abdominal Palpation, as Applied to Obstetrics, and Version by External Manipulations. English Edition. New York: J. H. Vail & Co, 1885, p75–78

ASSESSMENT

- Potential associations with malpresentations such as placenta praevia should be considered and excluded.
- For antepartum cases it is usual to delay version until 36–37 weeks' gestation. From 37 weeks only 5–10% will revert to breech presentation after successful version. In addition, rare complications of version may necessitate immediate delivery, which is more acceptable if the fetus is mature. However, a randomized-controlled trial comparing early ECV at 34–36 weeks with ECV at 37–38 weeks showed more cephalic presentations at delivery in the early ECV group but no difference in caesarean delivery or preterm birth.[2]
- A detailed ultrasound examination is undertaken to confirm gestational age, exclude fetal anomalies, identify the type of breech presentation, locate the placenta and assess the amount of amniotic fluid.
- If the woman has a single previous transverse lower segment caesarean scar, and is planning labour and vaginal delivery, it is permissible to attempt gentle ECV in selected cases.

Technique

- Some obstetricians feel that these patients should be fasting because of the rare cases that require immediate delivery due to complications of the version. It is unpleasant for pregnant women to fast and, in addition, the fetus is often very quiet with maternal fasting. As it is helpful to have fetal movement to assist the version (see below) a reasonable compromise is to offer the woman a light snack 1–2 hours before the planned version.
- Ideally, a 20 minute pre-version cardiotocograph should show a reactive fetal heart rate.
- Perform an ultrasound scan to confirm the malpresentation, localize the placenta and determine the amount of amniotic fluid.
- The woman should be reasonably comfortable with slight elevation of the head of the bed and a minor left lateral tilt. After the ultrasound, remove the gel from the woman's abdomen and substitute talcum powder. This allows one's hands to move easily and smoothly over the abdomen and to avoid the use of excess force. It also facilitates the changing positions of the hands during the version. Others may use extra gel for the same purpose.
- It is usual to turn the fetus by promoting flexion, so that the fetus is moved in the direction it is 'looking'. This principle

should be explained to the woman. Tell her she will feel pressure from your hands and that this will be sustained but she should not feel pain.

- The essential first step, upon which success depends, is the displacement and elevation of the breech from the pelvis. This can require sustained, albeit gentle pressure from both hands (Fig 28-2). Once this has been achieved the right hand continues to elevate the breech while the left hand is moved behind the fetal head (Fig 28-3). With the hands working in unison, intermittent pressure is applied to both fetal poles. It is at this point that fetal movement may help propel the fetus in the right direction. Throughout the procedure, gentleness is the guiding rule. Discretion is the better part of valour and the procedure is either going to be achieved gently and without pain, or it should be abandoned. If these principles are followed it is extremely rare for there to be any maternal or fetal complications.

- Once the fetus has been turned ultrasound is again used to confirm the new presentation and assess the fetal heart rate. It is not uncommon for there to be transient bradycardia due to the manipulations. Some will use the ultrasound or doptone over the fetal thorax to monitor the fetal heart rate during version. After version the fetal heart rate should be monitored for about 30 minutes and, provided this is normal and the woman is clinically well and without abdominal pain or vaginal bleeding, she can be discharged.

- If the woman is Rh negative, blood should be drawn for Kleihauer testing and an appropriate dose of Rh immune globulin given.

- Although there are some studies that support the use of uterine tocolysis to aid ECV the results are mixed and most will not use routine tocolysis. However, if attempted version without tocolysis fails, and the failure is thought to be due to good uterine tone, it is rational to consider tocolysis.[1,3] The best tocolytics for this purpose are the β-adrenergic drugs and this is discussed in the section on acute tocolysis above.

- On rare occasions, if the need to achieve ECV is felt to be compelling, epidural or spinal anaesthesia may increase the chance of success.[4] Obviously the risks of the regional anaesthetic have to be balanced against the ultimate goal. In addition, with the removal of maternal pain sensation the obstetrician has to be very careful to avoid using excessive force in these circumstances.

- A reasonable compromise in cases of failed ECV for breech presentation is to assess the cervix on the morning of the booked elective caesarean section. If the cervix is

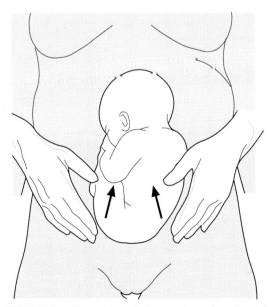

FIGURE 28-2 ■ External cephalic version: elevation of the breech from the pelvis.

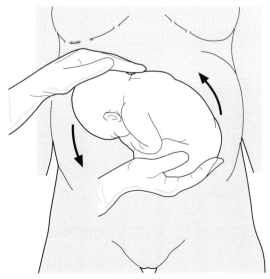

FIGURE 28-3 ■ External cephalic version: one hand elevates the breech and the other provides pressure behind the fetal head, neck and back.

favourable, epidural analgesia is established and ECV performed. If the fetus is successfully converted to a cephalic presentation, oxytocin and amniotomy induction of labour can be undertaken and caesarean delivery potentially avoided.

Predictive Factors

There are a number of factors which increase or diminish the chance of successful version:[1,5]

- *Parity* is the most important and success rates are higher in multiparous women, probably due to diminished abdominal and uterine muscle tone.
- *Gestational age:* the closer to term, the lower the success rate. This is particularly evident when version is attempted at 40 weeks' gestation or later, as the relative fetus to amniotic fluid volume ratio works against successful version.
- *Anterior placenta* may reduce the chances of success but this is not a major factor.
- *Obesity* reduces the chances of success.
- *Frank breech presentation* with the legs splinting the fetal body is less amenable to version compared with complete or footling breech.

Complications

- Abruptio placentae.
- Feto-maternal bleed which may initiate or worsen isoimmunization.
- Umbilical cord entanglement, which may cause abnormal fetal heart rate patterns with variable deceleration, prolonged deceleration or fetal bradycardia which, if sustained, may lead to fetal asphyxia. If this occurs one may have to turn the fetus back to the previous malpresentation in an attempt to alleviate the cord entanglement. On rare occasions this is the complication that leads to immediate caesarean delivery.
- With the appropriate safeguards as outlined, there should be no increased perinatal morbidity or mortality and a less than 1% need for emergency caesarean section.[1,6]

INTERNAL PODALIC VERSION

Internal podalic version involves the obstetrician placing one hand inside the uterus to turn the fetus from transverse or oblique lie to breech presentation. Probably the only justifiable indication for internal podalic version and breech extraction in modern obstetrics, when caesarean section is an available alternative, is in delivery of the second twin.[7,8] The risk of uterine rupture and fetal trauma with internal version associated with singleton pregnancy and neglected transverse lie or shoulder presentation in advanced labour is no longer acceptable.

A *sine qua non* for the performance of internal version is adequate analgesia and uterine relaxation. Epidural or spinal anaesthesia will provide good analgesia but no uterine relaxation. Thus, this procedure should either be carried out under general anaesthesia with halogenated agents for uterine relaxation or under regional anaesthesia with uterine tocolysis, usually in the form of intravenous nitroglycerine (see section on 'Acute tocolysis' above). The importance of good uterine relaxation for the safe performance of internal podalic version and breech extraction cannot be overemphasized. The ease of this procedure and the lack of trauma to the fetus and the uterus depend entirely upon adequate uterine relaxation.

INTERNAL PODALIC VERSION

'And then let him put his hands gently into the mouth of the womb, having first made it gentle and slippery with much oil; and when his hand is in let him find out the form and situation of the child...and so turn him that his feet may come forwards...and when he hath them both out, let him join them both together, and so by little and little let him draw the whole body from the womb.'
  Ambroise Paré
  The Works of Ambroise Paré (1549). Translated by T. H. Johnson. London: Clark, 1678

Recognition of Fetal Landmarks

Practice is required to become familiar with palpation of fetal anatomical landmarks to delineate the correct position and lie of the fetus. This familiarity can be gained by practising palpation of the newly delivered infant with one's eyes closed. The main landmarks and potential pitfalls are as follows:

- *Foot and hand:* The toes of the foot are roughly equal in length and the separation between the big toe and the others is less distinct. The fingers of the hand are not equal and the separation between the thumb and the remaining fingers is obvious. The heel of the foot is more prominent than the heel of the hand. It is possible to tell whether the hand is right or left by

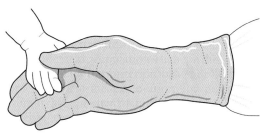

FIGURE 28-4 ■ Internal podalic version: distinguishing the particular hand by 'shaking hands with the fetus'.

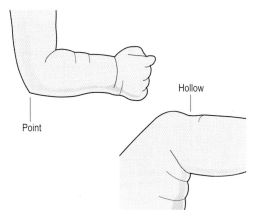

Point   Hollow

FIGURE 28-5 ■ Internal podalic version: distinguishing features between the elbow and the knee.

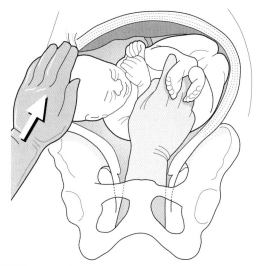

FIGURE 28-6 ■ Internal podalic version: the external hand manipulates the fetal head and trunk to the vertical position and the internal hand seeks the anterior fetal foot.

'shaking hands with the fetus' (Fig 28-4). To a degree the same can be said for 'shaking hands with the foot'.

- *The shoulder* can be recognized by the confluence of the humerus, scapula and clavicle. If in doubt the adjacent ribs can often be palpated.
- *Knee and elbow:* The flexed elbow has a prominent olecranon process, whereas the flexed knee has a dimple between the patella and tibia (Fig 28-5).
- *Mouth and anus:* Usually these can be easily distinguished but in an oedematous face presentation the mouth may be mistaken for the anus. The anus is smaller with greater tone and the adjacent ridges of the spines of the sacrum can usually be felt. In the case of the mouth the softer lips and adjacent gums and tongue should help make the distinction.

Technique

- With a long glove and the hand and forearm well lubricated the operator introduces the hand gently into the vagina and uterus. The external hand rests on the abdomen. Provided adequate uterine relaxation has been achieved the membranes should not be tense and one should be able to establish the lie and position of the fetus, with particular reference to the anatomical landmarks noted above.
- The anterior fetal foot should be identified, grasped and steady but gentle downward traction applied. The external hand helps by manipulating the fetal trunk and head to the vertical position (Fig 28-6). If it is possible to grasp both feet this is most desirable (Fig 28-7).
- At some point during this downward traction the membranes will rupture. However, by this time the fetus has been converted to a longitudinal lie and the breech will already be entering the pelvis. If it has only been possible to grasp the posterior leg, then during the downward traction there should be 180° rotation, such that the posterior leg becomes anterior. This prevents the anterior buttock from becoming impacted above the symphysis (Fig 28-8). The remainder of the delivery is accomplished by breech extraction as outlined in Chapter 16.
- At times the membranes rupture during the manipulations and the fetal hand and arm will prolapse. It is difficult and often traumatic to try and replace the hand and arm. Thus, one should just proceed and grasp the foot, or feet, and pull them down

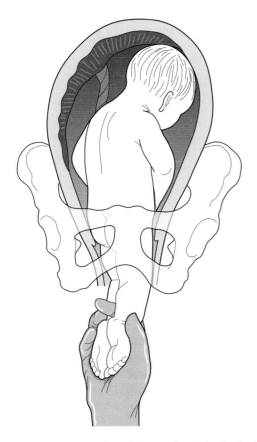

FIGURE 28-7 ■ Internal podalic version: ideally both feet are grasped and with steady downward traction the fetus is converted to a longitudinal lie.

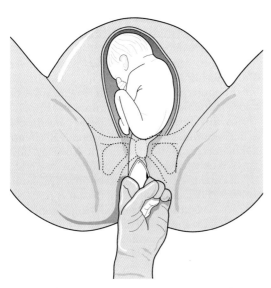

FIGURE 28-8 ■ Internal podalic version: if only the posterior leg is delivered the anterior buttock may straddle the symphysis and become obstructed.

through the introitus. As the fetal body turns the arm will automatically follow and can be delivered with the shoulders.

- Following delivery of the infant the uterus, cervix and upper vagina should be carefully explored for any lacerations.

Version, and its application, is one area of clinical care where the art of obstetrics remains relevant.

REFERENCES

1. Royal College of Obstetricians and Gynaecologists. External cephalic version and reducing the incidence of breech presentation. Guideline No. 20a. London: RCOG Press; 2010.
2. Hutton EK, Hannah ME, Ross SJ, Delisle MF, Carson GD, Windrim R, et al. The Early External Cephalic Version (ECV) 2 trial: an international multicentre randomised controlled trial of timing of ECV for breech pregnancies. Br J Obstet Gynaecol 2011;118:564–77.
3. Cluver C, Hofmeyer GJ, Gyte GM, Sinclair M. Interventions for helping to turn breech babies to head first presentation when using external cephalic version. Cochrane Database Syst Rev 2012;1:CD000184.
4. Goetzinger KR, Harper LM, Tuuli MG, Macones GA, Colditz GA. Effect of regional anaesthesia on the success rate of external cephalic version: a systematic review and meta-analysis. Obstet Gynecol 2011;118:1137–44 .
5. Burgos J, Cobos P, Rodriquez L, Pijoan J, Fernandez–Llebrez L, Martinez–Astorquiza T, et al. Clinical score for the outcome of external cephalic version: a two-phase prospective study. Aust NZ J Obstet Gynaecol 2012; 52:59–61.
6. Collaris RJ, Oei SG. External cephalic version: a safe procedure? A systematic review of version-related risks. Acta Obstet Gynecol Scand 2004;83:511–8.
7. Boggess KA, Chisholm CA. Delivery of the non-vertex second twin: a review of the literature. Obstet Gynecol Surv 1997;52:728–35.
8. Christopher D, Robinson BK, Peaceman AM. An evidence-based approach to determining route of delivery for twin gestations. Rev Obstet Gynecol 2011;4: 109–16.

UTERINE AND VAGINAL TAMPONADE

TF Baskett • S Arulkumaran

UTERINE TAMPONADE

When oxytocic agents fail to control postpartum haemorrhage, examination under anaesthesia is warranted. These cases may end in laparotomy and, if conservative surgical methods fail, hysterectomy may be necessary. A survey in the UK found that hysterectomy was the most common surgical procedure in women who did not respond to combinations of uterotonics, and that methods to reduce the need for hysterectomy were urgently needed.[1]

Uterine tamponade is a less invasive procedure which is simple, does not require major surgery, can be done within minutes, and will often immediately reduce or stop the bleeding. It can be tried as soon as uterotonics are found to be ineffective. If it stops the bleeding this will be apparent within minutes and the need for definitive surgery either averted or confirmed promptly. Thus, it may avoid the need for laparotomy and hysterectomy as well as reducing the need for blood transfusion with its inherent risks. It is ideal for postpartum haemorrhage due to non-traumatic causes and for those without any retained tissue in utero. It is important that conservative surgical procedures such as uterine tamponade or compression sutures are performed before coagulopathy sets in. It may be useful to consider clot stabilization with antifibrinolytic agents such as tranexamic acid 1–2 mg IV.

Rationale

A principle of first aid to stop bleeding is to apply pressure to the bleeding site sufficient to compress the blood vessels. This can be end-on or side-on compression and must be greater than the pressure of blood flow in that vessel. Once the applied pressure stops the bleeding, the blood can clot and form a permanent seal. Blood flows into the uterus with a mean arterial pressure of about 90 mmHg, although the spiral arteriolar arrangement in the uterus probably lowers the arterial pressure as the blood flows through the uterine muscle. After placental separation the venous sinuses and spiral arterioles are exposed, which results in bleeding from the placental bed if the uterus does not contract and retract efficiently enough to compress these vessels.

If, despite the appropriate use of oxytocic drugs, uterine atony continues, bimanual compression is undertaken after excluding any obvious lower genital tract trauma. If this does not stop the bleeding the uterus should be explored under anaesthesia to exclude retained products within the uterus and any uterine or lower genital tract trauma. If the bleeding is due to uterine atony a 'tamponade test' is useful to decide whether uterine tamponade itself would be therapeutic or whether laparotomy is needed to arrest the bleeding.[2]

Techniques

Uterine Packing

In the past, uterine tamponade could only be achieved by packing the uterus with cotton gauze. While this can be life-saving, there are a number of disadvantages; general, spinal or epidural anaesthesia is needed, the packing is done blindly, and it is hard to be sure that the entire uterine cavity is tightly packed. Incomplete and ineffectual packing can occur due to the fear of perforation (Fig 28-9). Packing the uterus in this manner requires several metres of 10 cm gauze tightly packed into the uterine cavity manually and with ring forceps. The vagina is also firmly packed and a Foley catheter placed in the bladder.[3] The gauze packing is removed in 12–24 hours.

Whether packing has been effective is not known for several minutes as the blood has to first soak through the pack before revealing itself at the cervix. To overcome some of these difficulties a sterile plastic bag may be introduced into the uterus first and the bag then packed with gauze. This facilitates more complete packing of the uterine cavity and makes for easier removal of the gauze. However, gauze packing can be cumbersome to place and remove, takes time, and is not always effective.[4] The use of balloon tamponade may overcome some of these drawbacks.

Balloon Tamponade

There are several reports in the literature describing success using hydrostatic balloon tamponade either alone or in combination with additional surgical methods. Different

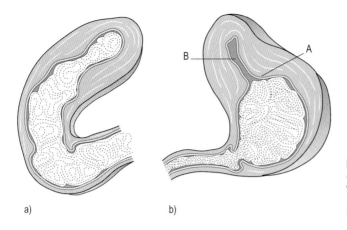

a)   b)

FIGURE 28-9 ■ Correct and incorrect method of uterine packing: (a) uterus carefully packed with gauze, (b) uterus with only the lower uterine segment packed. A = retraction ring, B = upper cavity of uterus unpacked.

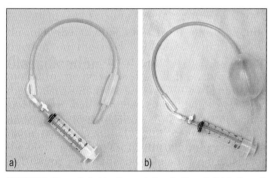

FIGURE 28-10 ■ Bakri balloon: (a) uninflated, (b) inflated.

types of balloons have been used, including the Sengstaken–Blakemore tube,[5] Rüsch urological balloon,[6] and the Bakri balloon[7] (Fig 28-10) filled with sterile water or saline at room or higher temperature. When uterotonics and uterine massage do not stop the bleeding, causes of local trauma or retained tissue in the uterus should be excluded. Balloon insertion may be achieved by performing a vaginal examination, identifying the cervix and manually passing the balloon into the uterine cavity without need for complex anaesthesia. Alternatively, under direct vision a vaginal speculum is passed and the anterior lip of the cervix is secured with sponge forceps. The balloon is held with another sponge forceps and inserted into the uterine cavity. The balloon is filled with about 200–500 ml of warm saline or sterile water. Care must be taken not to overfill the balloon, which may cause it to pass out through the cervix and to be expelled. Once the balloon is seen to bulge at the cervix it is adequately filled.

If the Sengstaken–Blakemore tube, Rüsch urological balloon or Bakri balloon are not available a simplified version can be fashioned as follows. Tie the cuff of a surgical glove or condom to a straight plastic urinary catheter with any suture material. Place the glove or condom and attached catheter into the uterus and fill via the catheter with a large syringe or intravenous fluid bag using the same principles outlined above.[8–11] For uterine bleeding following second trimester termination a simple Foley catheter balloon may provide adequate volume for intrauterine tamponade.

In the case reports available in the literature the volume used has been arbitrary (200–500 ml) and the practice has been to fill the balloon until part of it is visible via the cervix. At this stage, if there is no bleeding through the cervix and none through the drainage channel of the catheter the test of tamponade is pronounced successful and no further fluid is added.[2] When the intra-balloon pressure exceeds the arterial pressure of the patient no additional fluid need be added and the bleeding should stop.[12] If bleeding continues the test is a failure and further surgical treatment is needed, in the form of laparotomy, provided one is sure the bleeding is not from the lower genital tract.

Whether tamponade is going to be successful or not is known within minutes. Once found to be successful the uterine fundus is palpated abdominally and a mark is made with a pen to provide a reference line from which any enlargement or distension of the uterus would be judged during the period of observation.

Care after Uterine Tamponade

The woman should be kept fasting and under close surveillance after insertion of the balloon. Her pulse, blood pressure, uterine fundal height and signs of any vaginal bleeding or bleeding via the lumen of the catheter should be monitored. If there is doubt whether blood is oozing above the balloon, ultrasound may help to confirm or deny this. Her temperature should be recorded every 2 hours and urinary output measured hourly via an indwelling Foley catheter. The woman should receive broad-spectrum antibiotics from the time of insertion for up to 3 days. A low dose infusion of oxytocin, 40 units in 1 L of normal saline, is continued to keep the uterus contracted over the balloon. After 6 hours, if the uterine fundus remains at the same level and there is no active bleeding around the balloon via the cervix or via the central lumen of the catheter, it is safe to remove the catheter provided the woman is stable and adequate blood replacement has been given if required.

First the balloon is deflated but is not removed for 30 minutes. Provided there is no bleeding the oxytocin infusion is stopped for another 30 minutes and if there is still no bleeding the catheter is removed. These precautions are taken in case the woman starts bleeding when the balloon is deflated or the oxytocin is stopped, in which case the balloon can be re-inflated. In our experience there has not been an instance when the balloon needed to be refilled.[2] Six hours is usually sufficient for the placental bed to clot and stop bleeding. The reported success rate varies from 80 to 95%.[10,11,13]

Balloon tamponade and its associated 'tamponade test' can be used in cases of primary and secondary postpartum haemorrhage, and for cases of bleeding after second trimester miscarriage.[13,14] Both gauze packing and balloon tamponade may also be considered after caesarean section in cases without discrete bleeding points or retained tissue: for example, to provide tamponade of the poorly contracting lower uterine segment in placenta praevia.[14,15]

About 80–90% of cases of primary postpartum haemorrhage are due to uterine atony. In those cases unresponsive to the usual oxytocic drugs, laparotomy and surgical measures, such as uterine compression sutures, major vessel ligation and hysterectomy may be required. Another alternative is interventional radiological embolization of the internal iliac arteries. These procedures are covered elsewhere in this chapter but all require sophisticated facilities. If these facilities are not available, balloon tamponade and uterine packing can be used as an alternative or as a stop-gap measure until the woman can be transferred to an appropriate hospital or the equipment and personnel brought to her.

VAGINAL TAMPONADE

There are occasions when vaginal tamponade is necessary; for example with vaginal lacerations that continue to ooze despite suturing, or

paravaginal haematomas with no discrete bleeding points that can be oversewn. The options are:

- Vaginal packing with gauze. This may be facilitated (both insertion and removal) by packing into a plastic bag or lubricating the gauze pack itself. The vagina that has recently accommodated the passage of a term infant can be very capacious and require a lot of gauze.
- The Bakri, or similar balloon, can be used.[16]
- For the very capacious vagina a blood pressure cuff can be placed in the vagina inside a surgical glove or sterile plastic bag and inflated.[17,18]

REFERENCES

1. Mousa HA, Alfirevic Z. Major postpartum haemorrhage: survey of maternity units in the United Kingdom. Acta Obstet Gynecol Scand 2002;81:727–30.
2. Condous GS, Arulkumaran S, Symonds I, Chapman R, Sinha A, Razvi K. The 'Tamponade Test' in the management of massive postpartum hemorrhage. Obstet Gynecol 2003;101:767–72.
3. Maier RC. Control of postpartum hemorrhage with uterine packing. Am J Obstet Gynecol 1993;169:17–23.
4. Drucker M, Wallach RC. Uterine packing: a re-appraisal. Mount Sinai J Med 1979;46:191–4.
5. Katesmark M, Brown R, Raju KS. Successful use of a Sengstaken–Blakemore tube to control massive postpartum hemorrhage. Br J Obstet Gynaecol 1994;101:259–60.
6. Johanson R, Kumar M, Obhrai M, Young P. Management of massive postpartum haemorrhage: use of a hydrostatic balloon catheter to avoid laparotomy. Br J Obstet Gynaecol 2001;108:420–2.
7. Bakri YN, Amri A, Abdul Jabbar F. Tamponade-balloon for obstetrical bleeding. Int J Gynaecol Obstet 2001;74:139–42.
8. Baskett TF. Surgical management of severe obstetric haemorrhage: experience with an obstetric haemorrhage equipment tray. J Obstet Gynaecol Can 2004;26:805–8.
9. Akhter S, Begum MR, Kabir Z, Rashid M, Laila TR, Zabeau F. Use of a condom to control massive postpartum haemorrhage. Med Gen Med 2003;5:38.
10. Rathmore AM, Gupta S, Manaktala V, Gupta S, Dubey C, Khan M. Uterine tamponade using a condom catheter balloon in the management of non-traumatic postpartum haemorrhage. J Obstet Gynaecol Res 2012;38:1162–7.
11. Tindell K, Garfinkel R, Abu-Haydar E, Ahn R, Burke TF, Conn K. Uterine balloon tamponade for the treatment of postpartum haemorrhage in resource-poor settings: a systematic review. Br J Obstet Gynaecol 2012;120:5–14.
12. Belfort MA, Dildy GA, Garrido J, White GL. Intraluminal pressure in a uterine tamponade balloon is curvilinearly related to the volume of fluid infused. Am J Perinatal 2011;28:659–66.
13. Doumouchtsis SK, Papageorghiou AT, Vernier C, Arulkumaran S. Management of postpartum haemorrhage by uterine balloon tamponade: prospective evaluation of effectiveness. Acta Obstet Gynecol Scand 2008;87:849–55.

14. Vrachnis N, Iavazzo C, Salakos N, Papamargaritis E, Boutas I, Creatsas G. Uterine tamponade balloon for the management of massive haemorrhage during caesarean section due to placenta previa/increta. Clin Exp Obstet Gynecol 2012;39:255–7.

15. Ge J, Liao H, Duan L, Wei Q, Zeng W. Uterine packing during caesarean section in the management of intractable haemorrhage in central placenta previa. Arch Gynecol Obstet 2012;285:285–9.

16. Tattersall M, Braithwaite W. Balloon tamponade for vaginal lacerations causing severe postpartum haemorrhage. Br J Obstet Gynaecol 1994;101:259–60.

17. Pinborg A, Bodker B, Hogdall C. Postpartum hematoma and vaginal packing with a blood pressure cuff. Acta Obstet Gynecol Scand 2000;79:887–9.

18. Cameron A, Menticoglou S. Blood pressure cuff tamponade of vaginal lacerations causing significant postpartum haemorrhage. J Obstet Gynacol Can 2011;33:1207.

UTERINE COMPRESSION SUTURES

TF Baskett • S Arulkumaran

Uterine compression sutures of an improvised type have been used for decades: for example, figure-of-eight sutures in the lower uterine segment in cases of placenta praevia. In recent years more specific techniques for the application of compression sutures have been developed. In most cases these haemostatic sutures are used at the time of caesarean section, although they are occasionally used when all other methods of haemostasis have failed following vaginal delivery, and laparotomy is undertaken with a view to definitive arrest of haemorrhage by hysterectomy. In such cases major vessel ligation and/or uterine compression sutures may be used as a last-ditch attempt before resorting to hysterectomy. As with uterine tamponade, major vessel ligation and other rarely performed procedures, it is wise for each labour unit to have the equipment and instruments readily available in an identifiable pack so that it can be made rapidly available when needed.[1,2] Diagrams of the various techniques of compression sutures can be added to the obstetric haemorrhage pack.[2]

Strong suture material is required for compression sutures, such as No. 1 polyglactin 910 (Vicryl), polyglycolic acid (Dexon) or *poliglec-aprone* (Monocryl). If available, No. 2 chromic catgut is also suitable. For most compression sutures a curved needle of at least 70–80 mm and sometimes larger is required; straight needles should be 8–10 cm long. In many of the standard packaged suture materials the needles are not of adequate dimension. It may therefore be advisable to have larger eyed needles available in the haemorrhage equipment pack.

With all of the techniques for uterine compression sutures it is important to assess the efficacy of the technique. To this end the patient should be placed in the Lloyd Davies (frog-legged) position so that an assistant can remove any clots from the vagina. With both hands providing compression of the uterus it can be seen whether or not this will stop the bleeding. If it does, the compression suture is applied and, upon its completion, a careful appraisal will confirm whether the bleeding has been controlled – the 'test of tamponade'.[3]

B-LYNCH SUTURE

The first standardized technique of uterine compression sutures was described and named after himself by B-Lynch in 1997.[4] This type of suture is performed following low transverse caesarean section and is usually done for uterine atony unresponsive to oxytocic agents. With the uterus out of the abdominal incision and using a large (≥70 mm) round bodied, preferably blunt needle the first suture is placed from outside in to the uterine cavity approximately 3 cm below the lateral margin of the lower transverse caesarean incision and guided through the uterine cavity and out 3 cm above the caesarean incision. The suture material is then looped over the fundus of the uterus down to the posterior wall of the uterus opposite the caesarean incision. The suture is carried through the posterior wall into the uterine cavity and out on the other side roughly opposite the lateral margins of the caesarean incision. This suture is then looped over the posterior wall of the uterus down the anterior wall and placed through the uterus 3 cm above the other lateral margin of the caesarean incision and out 3 cm below (Fig 28-11a). Each of the suture insertion points is placed about 4 cm from the lateral border of the uterus. The two ends of the suture are then progressively tightened, with an assistant applying continuous anteroposterior compression to the uterus with both hands. The loops of the sutures over the fundus of the uterus are placed approximately 4 cm from each lateral border of the uterus. It is very important that there be progressive compression and tightening of the suture which may take 1–2 minutes to be completely effective. Once it is achieved the two ends of the suture are tied across the midline below the transverse caesarean incision (Fig 28-11b). At this point the assistant carefully checks the blood loss from the vagina to ensure that the suture has arrested the bleeding. If so, the low transverse incision is closed in the routine fashion, followed by closure of the abdomen. The placement of the suture is further illustrated in Figure 28-11c.

Modified B-Lynch Suture

A simplified adaptation of the B-Lynch suture has been proposed by Bhal et al.[5] This retains the same principles but uses two separate sutures, one for each side. Figure 28-12a shows the entry and exit points of both sutures. As in the B-Lynch technique, progressive manual compression and tying down of the suture is vital. As shown in

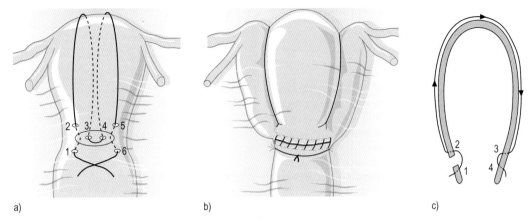

a)   b)   c)

FIGURE 28-11 ■ B-Lynch compression suture.

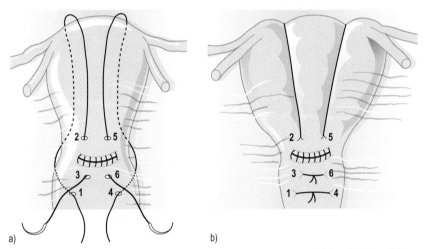

a)   b)

FIGURE 28-12 ■ Modification of B-Lynch compression suture (After Bhal et al[5]).

Figure 28-12b each of the sutures is tied across in the midline. The advantages of this technique are that it is a little easier to remember and by using one suture on each side the standard length (70 cm) of a polyglactin 910 suture is adequate on each side. With the B-Lynch technique one may have to tie two suture lengths together to achieve the entire suture placement.

VERTICAL UTERINE SUTURE

This is an even simpler modification proposed by Hayman et al.[6] Using a straight needle and ensuring that the bladder is well reflected the individual vertical sutures are passed from anterior to posterior approximately 3 cm below the site of a transverse caesarean incision. Depending on the width of the uterus, anything from 2 to 5 of these sutures may be placed. The usual

manual compression is carried out and the sutures are tied at the fundus (Fig 28-13). The advantages of this technique are its simplicity, the fact that it can be done with or without a caesarean incision and the variable number of sutures which can be placed depending upon the width of the uterine fundus.

SQUARE COMPRESSION SUTURES

In this technique the anterior and posterior walls of the uterus are compressed together using a straight needle passing from front to back through the entire uterine wall and moving laterally approximately 3 cm coming back through the uterine wall from back to front. From this exit point the needle is placed 3 cm below from front to back and then laterally 3 cm to a final pass of the needle from back to front to

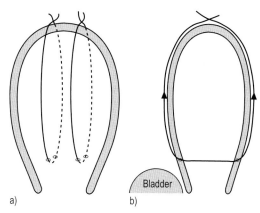

FIGURE 28-13 ■ Vertical compression sutures.

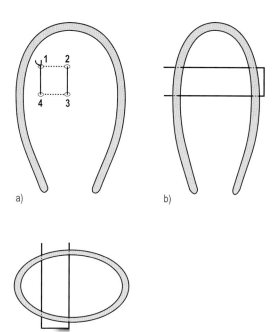

FIGURE 28-14 ■ Square compression sutures.

complete the square (Fig 28-14). The anterior and posterior walls are then compressed together and the suture snugly tied down.[7] This technique can be repeated at a number of sites, if necessary, to cover the entire uterine cavity.

In cases of bleeding from the lower uterine segment in placenta praevia, with or without partial accreta, this technique may be used in the lower segment alone, assuming the upper uterine segment is well contracted.

Many technical variations of compression sutures have been described and the potential number may be limited only by the available variety of embroidery stitches.[8–11] In many cases the application of an individual compression suture technique will be adequate. In others more than one type of suture may be necessary. For example, the B-Lynch technique may leave 'shoulders' of a very broad uterine fundus that are not compressed. In such cases additional square sutures may be useful. Others have found a combination of intrauterine balloon tamponade and compression sutures to be effective; the so-called 'uterine sandwich'.[12,13]

In all of the techniques it is important to ensure that the lower uterine segment is not completely obliterated and that there is egress for blood and lochia. This is particularly so with the use of square compression sutures in the lower segment associated with placenta praevia.

Complications of compression sutures are relatively few, although long-term follow up is limited. With all techniques it is important to ensure that the bladder is reflected inferiorly to avoid inclusion in the suture. Theoretically, as the uterus involutes, long-lasting suture material may remain and loops and bowel could potentially become entangled and obstructed. For this reason, at least on theoretical grounds, long-acting sutures such as PDS (Polydioxanone – S) should be avoided. Isolated cases of pyometra and myometrial necrosis have been described.[14,15]

The information on longer term menstrual and fertility sequelae is limited, but intrauterine synechia have been described.[16] There are, however, reassuring reports of subsequent uneventful pregnancies.[17,18] In some cases at caesarean section in a subsequent pregnancy a slight grooving of the uterine muscle from the compression suture can be seen, confirming that a degree of ischaemic necrosis occurs in some cases.[18]

The complications of these techniques must be put in the context of a procedure that is usually being done as a last resort before moving to hysterectomy. In the reported series, uterine compression sutures have been successful in arresting haemorrhage and avoiding hysterectomy in 75–90% of cases, and it is with this perspective that subsequent effects on fertility should be judged.[18–22]

REFERENCES

1. Anderson ER, Black R, Brocklehurst P. Acute obstetric emergency drill in England and Wales: a survey of practice. Br J Obstet Gynaecol 2005;112:372–5.
2. Baskett TF. Surgical management of severe obstetric haemorrhage: experience with an obstetric equipment tray. J Obstet Gynaecol Can 2004;26:805–8.
3. Condous GS, Arulkumaran S, Symonds I, Chapman R, Sinha A, Razvi K. The 'tamponade test' in the management of massive postpartum hemorrhage. Obstet Gynecol 2003;101:767–72.
4. B-Lynch C, Cocker A, Lowell AH, Abu J, Cowan MJ. The B-Lynch surgical technique for control of massive

postpartum haemorrhage: an alternative to hysterectomy? Five cases reported. Br J Obstet Gynaecol 1997; 104:372–5.

5. Bhal K, Bhal N, Mullik V, Shankar L. The uterine compression suture – a valuable approach to control major haemorrhage with lower segment caesarean section. J Obstet Gynaecol 2005;25:10–4.

6. Hayman RC, Arulkumaran S, Steer PJ. Uterine compression sutures: surgical management of postpartum hemorrhage. Obstet Gynecol 2002;99:502–6.

7. Cho JH, Jun SH, Lee CN. Hemostatic suturing technique for uterine bleeding during cesarean delivery. Obstet Gynecol 2000;96:129–31.

8. Hackethal A, Brueggmann D, Oehmke F, Tinneberg HR, Zygmunt MT, Muenstedt K. Uterine compression U-sutures in primary postpartum haemorrhage after caesarean section: fertility preservation with a simple and effective technique. Hum Reprod 2008;23:74–8.

9. Stanojevic D, Stanojevic M, Zamurovic M. Uterine compression suture technique in the management of severe postpartum haemorrhage as an alternative to hysterectomy. Serb Arch Med 2009;137:638–40.

10. Mostfa AA, Zaitoun MM. Safety pin suture for management of atonic postpartum haemorrhage. ISRN Obstet Gynecol 2012. doi:10.5402/2012/405795.

11. Shazly SA, Badee YA, Ali MK. The use of multiple 8 compression suturing as a novel procedure to preserve fertility in patients with placenta accreta: case series. Aust NZ J Obstet Gynaecol 2012;52:395–9.

12. Danso D, Reginald P. Combined B-Lynch suture with intrauterine balloon catheter triumphs over massive postpartum haemorrhage. Br J Obstet Gynaecol 2002; 109:963.

13. Yoong W, Ridout A, Memtsa M, Stavroulis A, Adib MA, Marcelle ZR. Application of uterine compression suture in association with intrauterine balloon tamponade ('uterine sandwich') for postpartum haemorrhage. Acta Obstet Gynecol Scand 2011;91:147–51.

14. Ochoa M, Allaire AD, Stitely MI. Pyometria after hemostatic square suture technique. Obstet Gynecol 2002; 99:506–9.

15. Treloar EJ, Anderson RS, Andrews HS, Bailey JI. Uterine necrosis following B-Lynch suture for primary postpartum haemorrhage. Br J Obstet Gynaecol 2006; 113:486–8.

16. Rathat G, Trinh PD, Mercier G, Reyftmann D, Dechanet C, Boulot P. Synechia after uterine compression sutures. Fertil Steril 2011;95:405–9.

17. Allahdin S, Aird C, Danielian P. B-Lynch sutures for major primary postpartum haemorrhage at caesarean section. J Obstet Gynaecol 2006;26:638–42.

18. Baskett TF. Uterine compression sutures for postpartum haemorrhage: efficacy, morbidity, and subsequent pregnancy. Obstet Gynecol 2007;110:68–71.

19. Wohlmuth CT, Gumbs J, Quebral-Ivie J. B-Lynch suture: A case series. Int J Fertil 2005;50:164–73.

20. Price N, B-Lynch C. Technical description of the B-Lynch brace suture for treatment of massive postpartum hemorrhage and review of published cases. Int J Fertil Womens Med 2005;50:148–63.

21. Mallappa CS, Nankani A, El-Hamany E. Uterine compression sutures, an update: review of efficacy, safety and complications of B-Lynch suture and other uterine compression techniques for postpartum haemorrhage. Arch Gynecol Obstet 2010;281:581–8.

22. Kayem G, Kuinczuk J, Alfirevic Z, Spark P, Brocklehurst P, Knight M. Uterine compression sutures for the management of severe postpartum haemorrhage. Obstet Gynecol 2011;117:14–20.

PELVIC VESSEL LIGATION AND EMBOLIZATION

TF Baskett

In other parts of this book, measures to deal with life-threatening obstetric haemorrhage have been outlined including: the use of oxytocic agents, uterine tamponade, uterine compression sutures and hysterectomy. In this section we are concerned with the role of major pelvic vessel ligation or embolization when other methods to control bleeding have failed. The main indications for pelvic vessel ligation or embolization are bleeding of uterine origin in which preservation of the uterus is sought, and in vaginal and paravaginal trauma when local measures fail to achieve haemostasis. These indications may include haemorrhage from placenta praevia, placenta accreta, abruptio placentae with Couvelaire uterus, uterine atony unresponsive to oxytocics, extension of lower segment caesarean incision into the broad ligament or vagina, uterine rupture, paravaginal haematoma, and extensive cervical and/or vaginal lacerations.

For cases of haemorrhage occurring at the time of caesarean section, or at laparotomy for uterine rupture, recourse to major vessel ligation at an early stage in an attempt to preserve the uterus is logical. For cases delivered vaginally other efforts to control haemorrhage without moving to laparotomy and pelvic vessel ligation should be tried. If these are unsuccessful one has the option of either resorting to laparotomy and pelvic vessel ligation or, if facilities are available, interventional radiology and pelvic vessel embolization.

ANATOMY AND HAEMODYNAMICS

The common iliac artery bifurcates at the level of the lumbo-sacral junction in front of the sacro-iliac joint. The external iliac artery runs lateral and superior, while the internal iliac (hypogastric) artery descends medially and inferiorly towards the sacral hollow. The ureter runs antero-laterally to the internal iliac artery just below the bifurcation. Posterior to the internal iliac artery lies the internal iliac vein, which is very close and vulnerable to trauma during attempts to ligate the artery. The internal iliac artery runs for 3–4 cm before dividing into anterior and posterior divisions. The posterior division divides into three branches: the ilio-lumbar, lateral sacral and the superior gluteal arteries – the latter leaves the pelvis through the greater sciatic foramen to supply the gluteal muscles. The anterior division usually has eight branches: the superior and inferior vesical, obturator, middle haemorrhoidal, uterine, vaginal and the terminal internal pudendal and inferior gluteal arteries (Fig 28-15). There are, however,

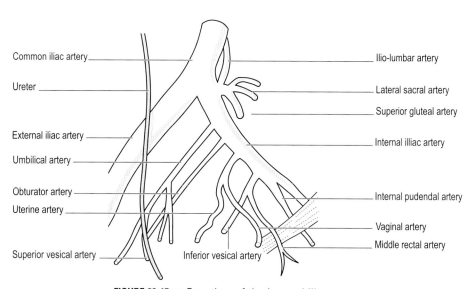

FIGURE 28-15 ■ Branches of the internal iliac artery.

variations and the internal pudendal and obturator arteries can arise from the posterior division.

There are a number of collateral anastomoses, the three main ones being:[1]

- the lumbar artery arises from the aorta and anastomoses with the ilio-lumbar artery from the internal iliac artery
- the middle sacral artery from the aorta anastomoses with the lateral sacral artery of the internal iliac artery
- the superior haemorrhoidal artery, which is the terminal branch of the inferior mesenteric artery from the aorta, joins the middle haemorrhoidal artery of the internal iliac artery (Fig 28-16).

Other collaterals that may link the aorta with branches of the internal iliac artery include: the ovarian artery and the uterine artery; the femoral artery with the internal pudendal artery via the profunda femoris and femoral circumflex vessels; and the circumflex iliac arteries from the common iliac with the superior gluteal artery of the internal iliac artery.

The haemodynamics of pelvic blood flow after internal artery ligation were demonstrated by Burchell in the 1960s.[2] He showed that unilateral ligation reduced the pulse pressure by about 75% on that side, and with bilateral ligation the reduction was 85%. The mean arterial pressure was reduced by 25% but the blood flow by almost 50%. Thus, bilateral internal iliac artery ligation almost reduces the pulse pressure to that of a venous system and allows clotting to occur. Blood flow does not stop completely, due to the presence of the previously outlined collateral anastomoses. These collateral channels

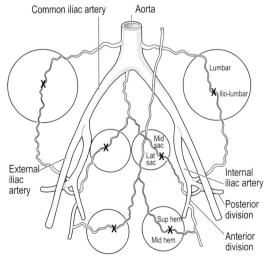

FIGURE 28-16 ■ The three main anastomoses between branches of the internal iliac artery and the aorta.

open immediately after ligation of the internal iliac artery and flow is reversed so that all branches of the iliac artery are again filled with flowing blood, but at the reduced pressures noted above. This collateral system opens immediately and is so efficient that even bilateral internal iliac artery ligation does not result in tissue necrosis or interfere with subsequent menstrual or reproductive function.[3]

The uterine artery carries the majority of the blood supply to the body of the uterus. The ovarian artery arises directly from the aorta just below the renal arteries and passes down to the pelvis in the infundibulo-pelvic ligament to the mesovarium and mesosalpinx. It passes superior to the ovary, provides branches to the ovary and tube, and ends by anastomosing with the ascending uterine artery about the level of the utero-ovarian ligament. It thus contributes to the blood supply of the uterine fundus.

UTERINE ARTERY LIGATION

Uterine artery ligation is the simplest major vessel ligation and may be effective for uterine haemorrhage.[4] It is usually carried out in association with the equally simple ovarian artery ligation. It is only likely to be effective for haemorrhage from the body of the uterus as the technique described involves ligation of the ascending branch of the uterine artery. Haemorrhage from the lower uterine segment, cervix and paracolpos will not be effectively treated by this technique.

The uterus should be elevated out of the abdominal incision and the fundus tilted away from the side to be ligated. Using a large curved tapered needle with No. 0 or 1 absorbable suture the needle is passed through the myometrium from anterior to posterior, about 2 cm medial to the lateral edge of the uterus (Fig 28-17). The suture is then brought back through an avascular space in the broad ligament and tied. Including a good 'cushion' of myometrium ensures inclusion of all branches of the uterine vessels and helps stabilize the ligature (Fig 28-18). The level at which one places the suture is approximately 2–3 cm below a low transverse caesarean incision.

It is important to ensure that the bladder is well away from the placement of the suture to avoid ureteric or bladder injury. The procedure is repeated on the other side. Uterine artery ligation has been reported to have 80–95% success rate in dealing with postpartum haemorrhage unresponsive to oxytocics at the time of caesarean section.[4-6] Not all of us have this high level

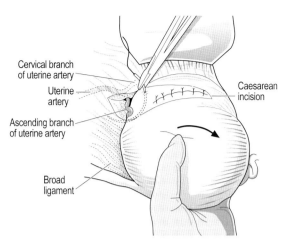

FIGURE 28-17 ■ Uterine artery ligation: tilt fundus of uterus to opposite side; place suture 2–3 cm below the caesarean incision and include 2–3 cm of the lateral myometrium.

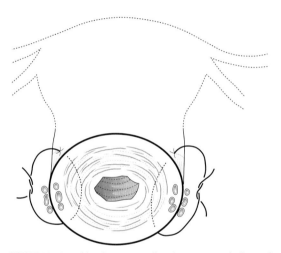

FIGURE 28-18 ■ Uterine artery ligation: coronal view of lower segment and placement of suture to include adjacent myometrium and all branches of the uterine vessels.

of success, but uterine artery ligation is very simple, safe, can be rapidly performed and has no detrimental effect on subsequent menstrual and reproductive function.

OVARIAN ARTERY LIGATION

Because of the previously mentioned anastomosis of the ovarian artery with the ascending branch of the uterine artery it is logical to include ovarian artery ligation when performing ligation of the uterine artery. The technique is identical to ligation of the uterine artery except that the suture is placed just below the utero-ovarian

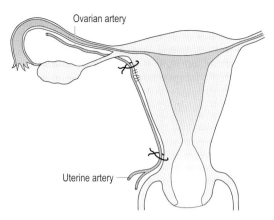

FIGURE 28-19 ■ Uterine and ovarian artery ligation sites.

ligament. Ligation at this point does not interfere with the blood supply to the tube or ovary (Fig 28-19).

INTERNAL ILIAC ARTERY LIGATION

Uterine and ovarian ligation can only reduce or stop bleeding from the body of the uterus. Bleeding from the lower uterine segment, cervix, broad ligament and vaginal and paravaginal areas may require internal iliac artery ligation. This is a more intimidating procedure for the general obstetrician and gynaecologist, but the principles are straightforward. The key is to familiarize oneself with the anatomy of the retroperitoneal space, which is best done when performing elective abdominal hysterectomy in gynaecology.

The uterus is elevated out of the abdominal incision and the fundus tilted away from the side to be ligated. The mid-portion of the round ligament is clamped and divided between two forceps. This permits entry to the retroperitoneal space and the avascular posterior leaf of the broad ligament is further opened with sharp dissection. Using a moistened gauze on a sponge forceps the retroperitoneal space is opened with gentle blunt dissection. If not immediately visible the common iliac artery and its bifurcation can be located by palpation. At this point the ureter should be identified and retracted medially with the attached peritoneum. Either using a gentle suction cannula or a moistened 'peanut' sponge, identify the bifurcation of the common iliac and clear the areola tissue around the internal branch. It is also wise to identify the external iliac artery and be in a position to palpate the femoral pulse. The main hazard is trauma to the adjacent external iliac veins or to the internal iliac vein, which lies just beneath the internal iliac artery.

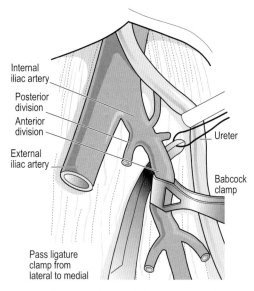

Internal
iliac artery

Posterior
division

Anterior
division

External
iliac artery

Ureter

Babcock
clamp

Pass ligature
clamp from
lateral to medial

FIGURE 28-20 ■ Internal iliac artery ligation.

There is a theoretical advantage to ligation of only the anterior division of the internal iliac artery. By ligating the artery distal to the posterior division its terminal superior gluteal artery is preserved and the risk of subsequent ischaemic buttock pain is avoided – although the latter is rare. However, it is not always easy to identify the anterior and posterior divisions and attempts to do so may risk damage to adjacent veins. Thus, it is best to ligate the internal iliac artery about 3 cm from the bifurcation, which should avoid the posterior division. It may be helpful to elevate the artery gently with a Babcock clamp and pass a double strand of No. 1 absorbable suture behind the artery with a right angle forceps. Pass the forceps from lateral to medial to reduce the risk of trauma to adjacent veins. The artery is then doubly ligated but not divided (Fig 28-20). The same procedure is carried out on the other side. Success rates with internal iliac ligation are variable, between 40 and 90%.[7–12]

PELVIC VESSEL EMBOLIZATION

In the past 30 years numerous reports have confirmed the value of angiographic embolization of pelvic vessels in the control of obstetric haemorrhage.[13–17] Success rates are in the 95% range.[18] The main limitation is the immediate availability of interventional radiologists and the relatively sophisticated equipment required. This technique is particularly valuable in women who have delivered vaginally but have intractable postpartum haemorrhage from uterine atony,

cervical and vaginal lacerations, or paravaginal haematoma. Sometimes temporary measures such as uterine and/or vaginal tamponade will allow one to transfer the patient to a hospital with facilities for angiographic embolization.

The procedure is done under local anaesthesia and, via a femoral artery puncture, under angiographic control a vascular catheter is guided to the aortic bifurcation and an aortogram performed to define the vascular anatomy and locate extravasation of contrast material from bleeding vessels. Angiography will detect flow rates of 1–2 ml per minute, which is usually present in cases of severe postpartum haemorrhage. However, in some cases of uterine atony there may be no discrete extravasation of contrast but just a general picture of uterine hypervascularization. If discrete bleeding points are seen, the cannula is advanced to that vessel which is embolized using either gelatin sponge pieces (Gelfoam) or polyvinyl alcohol particles (PVA). It is usual to embolize the contralateral vessel, even if no collateral circulation is identified. If no discrete bleeding points are found the anterior divisions of both internal iliac arteries are usually embolized.[19,20]

As with vessel ligation, subsequent menstrual and reproductive functions are usually unaffected, although uterine necrosis can occur on rare occasions.[21,22]

Both surgical ligation and embolization of pelvic vessels have a role in the management of severe postpartum haemorrhage. Each technique aims to stop bleeding and preserve the uterus. For women who deliver vaginally with extensive cervical and/or vaginal lacerations, and/or vulvovaginal haematomas unresponsive to local treatment, vascular embolization saves the woman a laparotomy and is usually more effective in dealing with the bleeding vessels than internal iliac artery ligation. Similarly, in cases of uterine atony that are unresponsive to uterine tamponade, embolization, provided the woman can be sustained until the procedure is undertaken, is advisable. In women delivered by caesarean section with uterine haemorrhage there is much to recommend the simple and safe combination of uterine and ovarian artery ligation. If the bleeding is from the lower uterine segment and paracolpos, bilateral internal iliac artery ligation may be successful. The problem with this is that it may not be within the general obstetrician's competence and, if it is performed and fails to control the haemorrhage, subsequent vascular embolization is rendered more difficult and in some cases impossible, with no access for the vascular catheter to the internal iliac artery.[19,20]

REFERENCES

1. Burchell RC, Olsen G. Internal iliac ligation: aortograms. Am J Obstet Gynecol 1966;94:117–24.
2. Burchell RC. Physiology of internal iliac artery ligation. J Obstet Gynaecol Br Commonw 1968;75:642–51.
3. Likeman RK. The boldest procedure possible for checking the bleeding – a new look at an old operation, and a series of 13 cases from an Australian hospital. Aust NZ J Obstet Gynaecol 1992;32:256–62.
4. O'Leary JL, O'Leary JA. Uterine artery ligation for control of postcesarean hemorrhage. Obstet Gynecol 1974;43:849–52.
5. Fahmy K. Uterine artery ligation to control postpartum hemorrhage. Int J Gynaecol Obstet 1987;25:363–7.
6. O'Leary JA. Uterine artery ligation in the control of post-cesarean hemorrhage. J Reprod Med 1995;40:189–93.
7. Clark SL, Phelan JP, Bruce SR, Paul RH. Hypogastric artery ligation for obstetric hemorrhage. Obstet Gynecol 1985;66:353–6.
8. Evans S, McShane P. The efficacy of internal iliac ligation. Surg Gynecol Obstet 1985;160:250–3.
9. Chattopadhyay SK, Deb RB, Edress YB. Surgical control of obstetric hemorrhage; hypogastric artery ligation or hysterectomy. Int J Gynaecol Obstet 1990;32:345–51.
10. Thavarasah AS, Sivolingam N, Almohdzar SA. Internal iliac and ovarian artery ligation in the control of pelvic haemorrhage. Aust NZ J Obstet Gynaecol 1989;29:22–5.
11. Joshi VM, Otiv SR, Majumder R, Nikam YA, Shirivastava M. Internal iliac artery ligation for arresting postpartum haemorrhage. Br J Obstet Gynaecol 2007;114:356–61.
12. Morel O, Malartic C, Muhlstein J, Gavat E, Judlin P, Soyer P, et al. Pelvic arterial ligations for severe postpartum haemorrhage: indications and techniques. J Vasc Surg 2011;148:e95–102.
13. Vedantham S, Goodwin SC, McLucas B. Uterine artery embolization: An underused method of controlling pelvic haemorrhage. Am J Obstet Gynecol 1997;176:938–48.
14. Hansch E, Chitkara V, McAlpine J. Pelvic arterial embolisation for control of obstetric haemorrhage: a five-year experience. Am J Obstet Gynecol 1999;180:1454–60.
15. Winograd RH. Uterine artery embolization for postpartum haemorrhage. Best Pract Res Clin Obstet Gynaecol 2008;111:1119–32.
16. Royal College of Obstetricians and Gynaecologists, Royal College of Radiologists and British Society of Interventional Radiology. The role of emergency and elective interventional radiology in postpartum haemorrhage. Good practice No. 6. London: RCOG; 2007.
17. Ganguli S, Stecker MS, Pyne D, Baum RA, Fan CM. Uterine artery embolization in the treatment of postpartum uterine hemorrhage. J Vasc Interv Radiol 2011;22:169–76.
18. Sentilhes L, Gromez A, Clavier E, Resch B, Verspyck E, Marpeau L. Predictors of failed pelvic arterial embolization for severe postpartum haemorrhage. Obstet Gynecol 2009;113:992–9.
19. Boulleret C, Chahid T, Gallot D, Mofid R, Hi RT, Raval A, et al. Hypogastric arterial selective and superselective embolisation for severe postpartum haemorrhage: a retrospective review of 36 cases. Cardiovasc Intervent Radiol 2004;27:344–8.
20. Hong TM, Tseng HS, Lee RC, Wang JH, Chang CY. Uterine artery embolisation: an effective treatment for intractable obstetrical haemorrhage. Clin Radiol 2004;59:96–101.
21. Cottier JP, Fignon A, Tranquart F, Herbreteau D. Uterine necrosis after arterial embolisation for postpartum hemorrhage. Obstet Gynecol 2002;100:1074–7.
22. Sentilhes L, Trichot C, Resch B, Sergent F, Roman H, Marpeau L, et al. Fertility and pregnancy outcomes following uterine devascularisation for severe postpartum haemorrhage. Hum Reprod 2008;23:1087–92.

OBSTETRIC HYSTERECTOMY

TF Baskett

We are concerned here with emergency hysterectomy carried out following caesarean section or vaginal delivery.

In a recent 10-year review (2001–2010) of 32 reports of emergency obstetric hysterectomy a pattern of indications and maternal morbidity emerged.[1] The incidence varied from 1 in 5000 to 1 in 200 deliveries and there was a strong association with caesarean delivery in both the index and previous pregnancies. Maternal death ranged from 0 to 24% and severe maternal morbidity was common, with mean rates of blood transfusion (90%), need for intensive care (40%), re-operation (24%) and bladder or ureteric injury (10%). The higher rates of hysterectomy and associated maternal mortality are more often found in low-resource settings, but severe maternal morbidity is common even in well-equipped hospitals. Indeed, emergency obstetric hysterectomy is a universal marker of severe maternal morbidity.[2,3] Multiple pregnancy has been shown to have a two- to eightfold increased risk of hysterectomy, compared with singletons.[4–6] Because of the increasing rates of both caesarean delivery and assisted reproductive technology induced multiple pregnancy, the incidence of emergency obstetric hysterectomy is likely to rise worldwide.[7,8]

Described elsewhere in this book are a number of alternative techniques and procedures that can be undertaken for the control of haemorrhage, which is the main reason for obstetric hysterectomy. These include the appropriate use of oxytocic drugs; uterine tamponade; uterine compression sutures; and major vessel ligation and embolization. The obstetrician should be familiar with these alternatives and be prepared to perform them as both life-saving and uterus-preserving alternatives to hysterectomy.

INDICATIONS

Emergency obstetric hysterectomy is usually required for complications of delivery associated with haemorrhage. In most cases it is a last resort life-saving procedure, undertaken when other more conservative measures to control haemorrhage have failed. There is a fine balance between premature recourse to hysterectomy and excessive delay associated with repeated ineffectual application of conservative measures and descent into irreversible disseminated intravascular coagulation (DIC). Included in this equation will be the woman's age, parity and desire for future child-bearing. The main reasons for emergency hysterectomy are as follows.[8–15]

Abnormal Placentation

With the rising caesarean section rate the number of pregnant women with a previous caesarean delivery has increased, leading to a higher incidence of placenta praevia and/or placenta praevia accreta in subsequent pregnancies. In developed countries these two conditions are now the commonest reason for emergency obstetric hysterectomy.

Under exceptional circumstances abruptio placentae may be so severe as to cause extensive extravasation of blood into the myometrium (Couvelaire uterus). Usually the myometrium will still respond to oxytocics but on occasion atony may prevail and hysterectomy is necessary.

Uterine Atony

The range of modern oxytocic drugs has improved the management of uterine atony (see Chapter 20). However, on rare occasions the uterus may be refractory to all of the available oxytocic agents. This is most commonly found in prolonged labour with chorioamnionitis – the exhausted and infected uterus may not respond to oxytocic drugs. Other structural abnormalities of the uterus, such as congenital anomalies and uterine fibroids, are slightly more prone to uterine atony.

Uterine Rupture

This is most commonly associated with a previous uterine scar – the majority of which are caesarean section scars (see Chapter 15). In multiparous women, the intact uterus may rupture in response to inappropriate use of oxytocic drugs during the first or second stage of labour. In areas with limited resources uterine rupture can occur in obstructed multiparous labour; in some African districts uterine rupture is the commonest indication for obstetric hysterectomy.[16,17]

Traumatic uterine rupture can be caused by obstetric manipulation, such as internal version and breech extraction in obstructed labour, or instrumental manipulation such as the classical application of the anterior blade of Kielland's forceps or uterine exploration for postpartum haemorrhage, either manually or with a curette. External trauma, such as a fall, domestic violence or motor vehicle accident may rarely cause uterine rupture.

Sepsis

This is an uncommon indication for obstetric hysterectomy but can occur when postpartum intrauterine sepsis does not respond to appropriate antibiotics. This is more common with clostridial infections in which there may be myometrial abscesses refractory to antibiotic treatment. Uterine scar infection, necrosis and dehiscence ('rotting scar') usually manifest 1–3 weeks after caesarean delivery and may cause unstoppable haemorrhage.[18] Some cases of secondary postpartum haemorrhage, with or without overt infection, may not respond to curettage or other supportive treatment and require hysterectomy for a combination of bleeding and infection. Another rare cause of intractable, delayed postpartum haemorrhage is arteriovenous fistula formation secondary to uterine trauma and/or infection.[19]

Chronic Recurrent Uterine Inversion

In most instances acute uterine inversion responds to replacement and does not recur (see Chapter 22). Rarely, however, despite successful manual replacement, uterine inversion may recur in the days immediately following delivery, necessitating hysterectomy.

Ectopic Pregnancy

Rare varieties of ectopic pregnancy, including cornual and cervical pregnancies, may require hysterectomy to control haemorrhage.

SURGICAL CONSIDERATIONS

While many of the surgical principles of emergency obstetric hysterectomy are similar to hysterectomy in the gynaecological patient there are a number of anatomical and physiological changes in the pregnant uterus and pelvis that create potential difficulties.[1] The uterus is greatly enlarged and all the adjacent pelvic tissues are oedematous and friable. The uterine and collateral vessels are enlarged (up to five times normal calibre), engorged and tortuous.

The choice of abdominal incision will depend upon the circumstances. If the hysterectomy is being done following caesarean section then the incision is likely to have been of the Pfannenstiel variety. If laparotomy is being performed with a view to hysterectomy following vaginal delivery a lower midline incision is preferable, due to speed and greater pelvic access. With either type of incision it is advisable to manually eventrate the uterus and, if there was a caesarean section, this can be easily achieved by hooking the fingers in the uterine incision.

The choice between total and subtotal hysterectomy will depend upon the indications for the procedure. If the trauma and/or bleeding is confined to the upper uterine segment there is much to recommend subtotal hysterectomy – which can be performed more rapidly and with less risk of trauma to the ureters and bladder. If the cervix and paracolpos are involved then total hysterectomy will be needed to achieve haemostasis. Be careful in women with prolonged labour and dystocia at full cervical dilatation that are delivered by caesarean section. In these cases, in addition to bleeding from the upper uterine segment associated with the uterine atony, there may be cervical trauma from the prolonged pressure and distension of the cervix – so that bleeding may continue from this area after the body of the uterus has been removed. Thus, in cases of subtotal hysterectomy it is advisable to clean out the vagina and check for continued blood loss before closing the abdomen.

In cases of haemorrhagic urgency, initial steps will have to be taken to reduce or stop the bleeding before definitive hysterectomy is performed. In cases of uterine trauma this will involve the use of Green–Armytage clamps and/or sponge forceps to the bleeding edges of uterine muscle. On each side, adjacent to the uterus, a large straight clamp is applied to include the base of all adnexal structures: round ligament, utero-ovarian ligament and fallopian tube. This will control the collateral flow from the ovarian vessels. The uterus is elevated and the broad ligament transilluminated on each side to find an avascular space opposite the level of a lower uterine segment caesarean incision. Through these two spaces in the broad ligament a catheter, penrose drain, or intravenous tubing can be passed and tightly twisted and held with a straight clamp around the lower segment, just above the cervix, to occlude the uterine arteries. These measures should stem the bleeding so that hysterectomy can then be systematically performed.

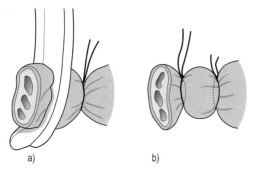

FIGURE 28-21 ■ Double clamp technique: (a) the proximal clamp is replaced by a free tie, (b) the distal clamp is replaced with a transfixing suture.

The main vascular pedicles are often thick and oedematous. These should be double clamped. The proximal clamp is removed first and replaced by a free tie. The distal clamp is then replaced by a transfixing suture (Fig 28-21). In this way haematoma formation in the pedicle is prevented. Avoid taking too much tissue in each clamp – the proximal one-third of a pedicle within a clamp is not secure. Thus, substantial pedicles should only be grasped to fill the distal two-thirds of the clamp to ensure security. Pedicles should be held in the normal anatomical plane while clamping and tying. Untwisting of the pedicle, especially if it had too much tissue, is one reason for suture slippage and subsequent haemorrhage.

SURGICAL TECHNIQUE

The uterus is lifted out through the incision and the adnexal structures placed on tension by the assistant. On each side a long straight clamp is applied close to the uterine body and across the uterine origin of the adnexal structures – round ligament, utero-ovarian ligament and fallopian tube. The round ligament is grasped with a short straight clamp about 3 cm from its attachment to the uterus and is incised just medial to this clamp, allowing access to the broad ligament between the two leaves of peritoneum. The areolar tissue within the broad ligament is gently separated using the index finger. The anterior leaf of the broad ligament is now incised infero-medially. If a lower segment caesarean section has been performed this incision of the anterior leaf joins up with the lateral aspect of the incision of the utero-vesical peritoneum. When ligating the round ligament it is important to ensure that the small artery (Sampson's artery) that consistently runs beneath the round ligament is included.

The posterior leaf of the broad ligament is now transilluminated and incised either with scissors or a finger. The now-exposed pedicle containing the utero-ovarian ligament and fallopian tube is isolated medial to the ovary and secured with a curved clamp. The posterior leaf of the broad ligament can now be transilluminated and incised down to the level of the utero-sacral ligaments. Further dissection of the areolar tissue in the base of the broad ligament with the index finger and, if necessary, by gentle sharp dissection should allow exposure of the uterine vessels. The above technique is used on each side.

It is important to identify and dissect the bladder free of the operative field. With a previous caesarean section it is common for the posterior wall of the bladder to be adherent to the lower uterine segment. Precise sharp dissection is required to free this adherence. Blunt dissection with gauze is not recommended as this may cause more bleeding, tearing and perforation of the friable adherent posterior bladder wall. When dissecting the bladder down limit the lateral dissection to avoid the vascular bladder pillars. At this stage, dissection of the bladder is only required sufficient to safely place curved clamps across the uterine vessels. This vascular bundle is doubly clamped and ligated. The level of placement of the uterine clamps is at the junction of the cervix with the isthmus of the uterus. This can be hard or impossible to appreciate at full cervical dilation, but is usually about 2 cm below the transverse incision of a caesarean section. From now on all clamps are placed medially to the uterine clamps to avoid ureteric damage.

Large curved clamps can now be placed across the lower uterine segment at the junction of the cervix on each side, allowing excision of the body of the uterus. If the bleeding is due to uterine atony or trauma in the upper uterine segment, the haemorrhage should now be controlled and, if there is no bleeding from the cervix, then this subtotal hysterectomy should suffice. If the bleeding involves the cervix this will now be more readily accessible – although it can be hard to distinguish the level of the cervix if the hysterectomy was performed at full cervical dilatation. At this point a finger placed through the uterine incision should allow one to identify the rim of the cervix (Fig 28-22). The cervical angle clamps are ligated with a transfixing suture and held. The rim of cervix is carefully identified to ensure that the entire body of the uterus has been excised – if not, the edges can be trimmed to achieve this. In the case of the cervix that is fully dilated the area to be stitched is quite broad.

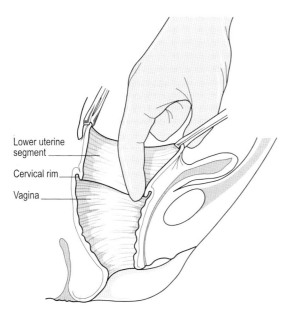

Lower uterine
segment

Cervical rim

Vagina

FIGURE 28-22 ■ The body of the uterus has been excised and the finger can more readily identify the rim of the cervix.

This is achieved with figure-of-eight haemostatic sutures or a continuous locking suture in one or two layers as required.

If removal of the cervix is deemed necessary the bladder may have to be further dissected from the anterior part of the cervix. Here again, careful identification of the rim of cervix is necessary. The utero-sacral and cardinal ligaments are taken with curved clamps and the angle of the vagina is incorporated into the cardinal ligament suture ligation. The vaginal cuff can either be closed with a continuous locking suture or interrupted figure-of-eight sutures. If drainage is deemed necessary the vaginal vault can be kept open by a continuous locking suture of the edges of both the anterior and posterior walls of the vagina.

Even with good technique bladder injuries may occur; the important thing is to recognize the injury, repair it at the time, and obviate the risk of vesico-vaginal fistula. It is therefore essential to test the integrity of the bladder in all cases once the hysterectomy has been achieved. This may be done by manipulating the bulb of the Foley catheter through the bladder wall, so that a hole in the bladder becomes obvious if the bulb of the catheter is seen. Alternatively, the bladder can be filled with a marking medium such as methylene blue or sterile milk taken from the nursery. Milk is preferable as it does not cause permanent staining of the tissues – so that after repair, or in dealing with continued haemorrhage, further use of milk installation in the

bladder can be seen more easily than the permanently methylene blue-stained tissues.

If there is a tear in the bladder it should be closed in two layers using continuous running sutures of 3/0 Vicryl or its equivalent. Ensure that the ureteric orifices are not involved in the repair, which is especially likely in posterior tears of the bladder wall adherent to a previous caesarean scar.

Identification of the ureter is advisable and it is particularly vulnerable at three sites. If bleeding has necessitated removal of the ovary and tube on one side, the ureter may be caught when clamping the infundibulo-pelvic ligament lateral to the tube and ovary. During clamping of the uterine vessels the ureter is very close as it runs about 2 cm beneath the vessels. It is best to identify the ureter at the pelvic brim on the medial leaf of the broad ligament and follow its course down beneath the uterine vessels. Provided all subsequent clamps are placed medially to the uterine vessel clamps, and the bladder is dissected from the front of the cervix, the ureter as it enters the bladder (the third vulnerable site) should be avoided. From a medico-legal point of view it is wise to include a description of the identification of the bladder and ureters in the operation record. If there is any doubt about the integrity of the ureters, cystoscopy should be performed postoperatively, facilitated by giving intravenous indigo carmine 10–15 minutes before to highlight the efflux of dye-stained urine from the ureters. If no cystoscope is available a diagnostic laparoscope or hysteroscope can be used. Provided the condition of the patient allows it, and the resources are available, it is preferable to identify and treat ureteric obstruction or damage at the time of the initial operation, which reduces both the postoperative morbidity and litigation vulnerability.[20] Once the operation is complete the pelvis can be filled with water or saline to check that all pedicles are intact and that there are no additional bleeding sites. It is not necessary to re-peritonize the pelvis.

In rare cases after hysterectomy the traumatized tissues of the pelvic basin continue to ooze, despite careful ligation of obvious bleeding points. Many, but not all of these cases are associated with DIC. Local haemostatic agents over bleeding points and the use of anti-fibrinolytic agents can help to control generalized oozing. The application of a pelvic pressure pack can be life-saving, either by providing permanent haemostasis or limiting the bleeding until other resources can be mustered – such as major vessel embolization.[21] A plastic bag is filled with gauze roll and the narrow neck of the bag placed

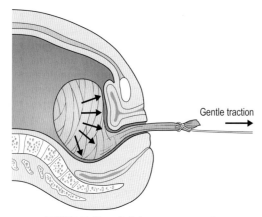

FIGURE 28-23 ■ Pelvic pressure pack.

through the vaginal vault from above. Gentle traction on the neck of the bag from below allows the gauze-filled portion of the bag to mould to the pelvic basin and apply pressure to the oozing soft tissues. (Fig 28-23). The gauze and plastic bag can be removed the next day, under conscious sedation if necessary, provided the patient is stable.

POSTOPERATIVE CONSIDERATIONS

Perioperative antibiotic prophylaxis is given and, depending on the duration of labour or potential chorioamniontitis, this may be continued for 24–48 hours. Thromboprophylaxis can also be instituted once haemostasis is secure.

Detailed perioperative notes should be recorded and a debriefing session with involved staff is advisable.

Once the woman's initial postoperative recovery is secure the whole sequence of events should be reviewed and discussed with her by an experienced obstetrician. In hospital reviews of obstetric hysterectomy, with its potentially devastating fertility-ending implications,[10,22] up to 25% may be in primiparous women. The woman may be psychologically traumatized by a sequence of events that started with an expectation of normal labour and delivery only to spiral out of control with blood transfusion, general anaesthesia, intensive care and loss of her uterus and fertility. Gentle explanation, listening and sympathy for her and her partner, with appropriate follow up, are essential.

Cases involving emergency obstetric hysterectomy demand from the obstetrician a decisive blend of the art and science of obstetrics under the most trying circumstances.

REFERENCES

1. Baskett TF. Peripartum hysterectomy. In: Arulkumaran S, Karoshi M, Keith LG, Lalonde AB, B-Lynch C, editors. A comprehensive textbook of postpartum haemorrhage. Duncow: Sapiens Publishing; 2012. p. 462–5.
2. Baskett TF. Epidemiology of obstetric critical care. Best Pract Res Clin Obstet Gynaecol 2008;22:763–74.
3. Baskett TF, O'Connell CM. Severe obstetric maternal morbidity: a 15-year population-based study. J Obstet Gynaecol 2005;25:7–9.
4. Walker MC, Murphy KE, Pan S, Yang Q, Wen SW. Adverse maternal outcomes in multifetal pregnancies. Br J Obstet Gynaecol 2004;111:1294–6.
5. Francois K, Ortiz J, Harris C, Foley MR, Elliott JP. Is peripartum hysterectomy more common in multiple gestations? Obstet Gynecol 2005;105:1369–72.
6. Baskett TF, O'Connell CM. Maternal critical care in obstetrics. J Obstet Gynaecol Can 2009;31:48–53.
7. Wen SW, Huang L, Liston RM, Heaman M, Baskett TF, Rusen ID. Severe maternal morbidity in Canada, 1991–2001. Can Med Assoc J 2005;173:759–63.
8. Kwee A, Bots ML, Visser GHA, Bruinse HW. Emergency peripartum hysterectomy: a prospective study in the Netherlands. Eur J Obstet Gynecol Reprod Biol 2006;124:187–92.
9. Englesen IB, Albrechtsen S, Iverson OE. Peripartum hysterectomy – incidence and maternal morbidity. Acta Obstet Gynecol Scand 2001;80:409–12.
10. Baskett TF. Emergency obstetric hysterectomy. J Obstet Gynaecol 2003;23:353–5.
11. Knight M, Kuriuczuk JJ, Spark P, Brocklehurst P. Cesarean delivery and peripartum hysterectomy. Obstet Gynecol 2008;111:97–105.
12. Glaze S, Ekwalanga P, Roberts G, Lange I, Birch C, Rosengarten A, et al. Peripartum hysterectomy, 1999 to 2006. Obstet Gynecol 2008;111:732–8.
13. Lone F, Sultan AH, Thakar R, Beggs A. Risk factors and management patterns for emergency obstetric hysterectomy over 2 decades. Int J Gynaecol Obstet 2010;109:12–5.
14. Awan N, Bennett MJ, Walters WA. Emergency peripartum hysterectomy: A 10-year review at the Royal Hospital for Women, Sydney. Aust NZ J Obstet Gynaecol 2011;51:210–5.
15. Orbach A, Levy A, Wignitzer A. Peripartum caesarean hysterectomy: critical analysis of risk factors and trends over the years. J Mat Fet Med 2011;24:480–4.
16. Moodley J. Emergency peripartum hysterectomy. East African Med J 2001;78:70–4.
17. Rabiu KA, Akinlusi FM, Adewunmi AA, Akinola OI. Emergency peripartum hysterectomy in a tertiary hospital in Lagos, Nigeria: a five-year review. Trop Doct 2010;40:1–4.
18. Rivlin ME, Carroll CS, Morrison JC. Conservative surgery for uterine incisional necrosis complicating cesarean delivery. Obstet Gynecol 2004;103:1105–8.
19. Aziz N, Lenzi TA, Jeffrey RB, Lyell DJ. Postpartum uterine arteriovenous fistula. Obstet Gynecol 2004;103:1076–8.
20. Gilmour DT, Baskett TF. Disability and litigation from urinary tract injuries at benign gynaecological surgery in Canada. Obstet Gynecol 2005;105:109–14.
21. Dildy GA, Scott JR, Saffer CS, Belfort MA. An effective pressure pack for severe pelvic hemorrhage. Obstet Gynecol 2006;108:1222–6.
22. Seffah JD, Kwane-Aryee RA. Emergency peripartum hysterectomy in the nulliparous patient. Int J Gynaecol Obstet. 2007;97:45–6.

SYMPHYSIOTOMY

TF Baskett • RC Pattinson

'I believe the operation fills a most useful place in practice, and that is the opinion of many others, and if everyone would deliberately struggle against taking up an extensive extreme position with regard to the operation, that place could be more exactly determined'.

MUNRO KERR, 1908

The operation of symphysiotomy has had a rather chequered history. It was originally performed upon the dead as an alternative to postmortem caesarean section by Claude Dela Courveé in 1665. It was performed on the living by Jean René Sigault in 1777. The patient was a rachitic dwarf, said to have an obstetric conjugate of 6.5 cm. She had four previous stillborn infants and Sigault performed a symphysiotomy and produced a live child: although the patient developed a vesico-vaginal fistula and was unable to walk for 2 months. Symphysiotomy enjoyed some popularity on the continent but this was short-lived due to the postoperative urological and orthopaedic morbidity. It enjoyed a resurgence on the continent, in Ireland and in South America in the late 19th and early 20th centuries.

In modern obstetrics the use of symphysiotomy is almost completely confined to the developing world, although a plea has been made for its occasional use in specific rare situations in countries with well-developed health services.[1,2]

Symphysiotomy is the surgical division of the fibrocartilaginous symphysis pubis. A 2–3 cm separation of the pubic symphysis increases the area of the pelvic brim by 15–20% and increases all the pelvic transverse diameters by about 1 cm. This increase is permanent and carries over into subsequent pregnancies. About 85% of women with cephalopelvic disproportion treated by symphysiotomy will deliver vaginally in a subsequent pregnancy.[3]

Second stage caesarean section has a high morbidity and mortality in developing countries[4] and even in developed countries.[5] Symphysiotomy has several advantages over second stage caesarean section in that it is rapid, simple – only local anaesthesia with no operating theatre, anaesthetist or sophisticated equipment[6] – and has minimal postoperative complications.[6,7] The main role for symphysiotomy, therefore, is in those countries where clinical and cultural factors mitigate against caesarean section for cases of mild-to-moderate cephalopelvic disproportion. This is especially so in some African communities in which caesarean section may be seen as a 'failure' of maternal achievement. Furthermore, in a subsequent pregnancy the woman previously delivered by caesarean section may avoid hospital confinement and rupture of her uterus in a remote community. If contraceptive services are not available or unacceptable to the woman she may have to endure the risks of multiple repeat caesarean sections. This was one of the reasons for the popularity of symphysiotomy in predominately Catholic countries in the late 19th and early 20th centuries.

INDICATIONS

Cephalopelvic Disproportion

As discussed above, women with obstructed labour and mild-to-moderate cephalopelvic disproportion may, for clinical and cultural reasons, be managed with symphysiotomy. It is not appropriate to expect symphysiotomy to safely overcome severe disproportion. Thus, only two-fifths or less of the fetal head should be palpable above the maternal pelvic brim and the degree of moulding of the fetal head should not show an irreducible overlap of the cranial bones.[7]

Breech Presentation

A rare but dreaded complication of vaginal breech delivery is entrapment of the after-coming head due to disproportion. This should be rare in a properly conducted labour for vaginal breech delivery. However, it can occur and one option for dealing with this is rapid symphysiotomy. A number of case series have shown that this will save about 80% of such infants.[8,9]

Shoulder Dystocia

Symphysiotomy has been put forward as a solution to severe cases of shoulder dystocia that do not resolve with the usual manoeuvres (see Chapter 12). Although this treatment has been suggested, and in theory may have some logic if symphysiotomy can be rapidly performed, there are very few cases reported and some of those show poor outcome for both mother and infant.[10,11]

TECHNIQUE

The main advantages of the procedure are that it can be done under local anaesthesia by a doctor or a nurse trained to do symphysiotomy but who may not have the training or the facilities to perform caesarean section. In some settings it may be performed more rapidly than caesarean section and may thus be life-saving in some cases of obstructed labour with fetal distress or with entrapment of the after-coming head in vaginal breech delivery. The operative principles of symphysiotomy are as follows:[7,12–15]

- The operator should be familiar with the anatomy of the symphysis pubis (Fig 28-24).
- The woman is placed in the lithotomy position with her legs supported by two assistants. The angle between the legs should not exceed 80° (Fig 28-25). This restricted degree of abduction is necessary to avoid excessive separation of the symphysis with damage to the underlying urethra and bladder neck and to avoid excessive traction on the sacro-iliac joints.

- Local anaesthesia in the form of 1% lidocaine is infiltrated into the skin over the symphysis pubis and into the subcutaneous tissues as well as into the joint space. The local anaesthetic needle may be helpful to identify the space and can be left in place as a guide to the subsequent incision site. In addition, local anaesthetic should be infiltrated into the site of the proposed episiotomy.
- A number 14 Foley catheter is inserted into the bladder and the bulb inflated with 5 ml saline or sterile water. If the fetal head is

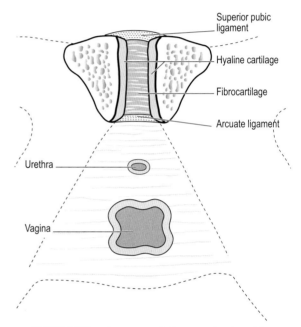

FIGURE 28-24 ■ Anatomy of the symphysis pubis.

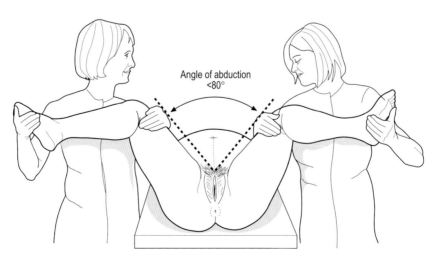

FIGURE 28-25 ■ Assistants support the legs.

firmly lodged in the pelvis a firmer silastic catheter may be necessary. It is essential to ensure that the bladder is completely drained. The index and middle fingers of the left hand are inserted vaginally and placed alongside the catheter in the urethra. These fingers push the catheter and the urethra to the side so that the middle finger lies underneath the symphysis pubis joint space – a firmer catheter may facilitate this lateral movement (Fig 28-26).

• Incision of the symphysis pubis is best done with a solid-bladed scalpel if available. A small incision is made through the overlying skin, just enough to allow the scalpel to gain access to the deeper tissues. The symphysis pubis joint should be incised in the midline starting at the junction of the upper and middle thirds. Using the left middle finger as a guide the scalpel blade is pushed through the joint until the tip is felt and, using a levering action, incises the lower two-thirds of the symphysis. The scalpel blade is then withdrawn from the joint, rotated 180°, re-inserted and used to incise the upper third of the symphysis (Fig 28-27). During this time constant vigilance is kept by means of the vaginal finger lest there should be any intrusion of the blade into the tissues underneath the symphysis. The thumb of the left hand held in front of the symphysis will detect the onset of separation. This separation should not exceed the width of the thumb, approximately 2.5 cm (Fig 28-27).

• At this point the anterior vaginal wall and underlying urethra and bladder neck are unsupported and vulnerable, so it is essential that the assistants maintain the support of the legs and do not allow separation beyond 80°.

• At the time of delivery a generous mediolateral episiotomy is performed to reduce the tension and pressure on the anterior

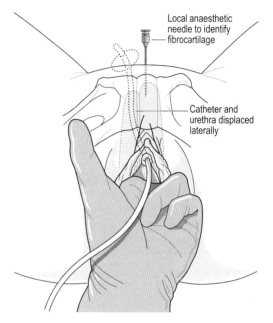

FIGURE 28-26 ■ Catheter and urethra pushed to one side by the index and middle fingers of the operator's hand.

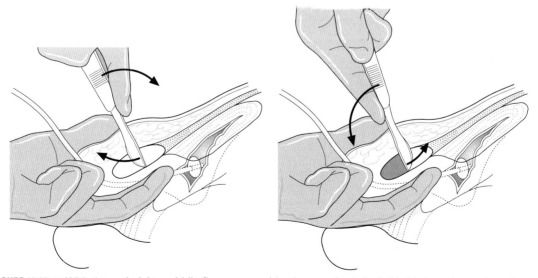

FIGURE 28-27 ■ With the underlying middle finger as a guide, the symphysis is divided in two steps using a levering action of the scalpel.

vaginal wall. Often, delivery of the head will be spontaneous, but if assistance is required the vacuum is preferred over forceps. To further reduce trauma to the tissues under the symphysis pubis the assistants are instructed to adduct the legs at the point of delivery of the fetal head.

- After delivery of the infant and the placenta, the symphysis and underlying soft tissues are compressed between the thumb above and the index and middle fingers below for 3–5 minutes. This should reduce the risk of bleeding from the very vascular inferior vesical plexus of veins around the upper urethra and bladder neck. The episiotomy and any vaginal lacerations should be sutured in addition to the stab wound over the symphysis.

POST-DELIVERY CARE

- Bladder drainage should be continued for 4–7 days. If there is haematuria then drainage should be continued until the urine has been clear for at least 3 days.
- A broad-spectrum antibiotic is given for 1 week to reduce the risk of urinary tract infection and infection of the tissues of the symphysis.
- Depending on other risk factors thromboprophylaxis may be given.
- The patient should be nursed mostly on her side with her knees strapped loosely together to avoid inadvertent and excessive abduction. She should remain mostly at rest in this position for the first 3 days. Thereafter ambulation should be encouraged and, if necessary, assisted by walking-aids.
- The patient is discharged once she is confident with her walking but is advised against excessive physical activity for 3 months until the fibrous healing of the joint has occurred. Although the benefits of symphysiotomy will extend to her next pregnancy and likely result in uncomplicated vaginal delivery she is advised that subsequent deliveries should be in hospital.

COMPLICATIONS

Haemorrhage

Initial bleeding from the symphysis pubis can be brisk. However, this is usually venous in origin and responds to the pressure applied by the thumb and vaginal fingers outlined previously.

The bleeding is likely to be more if the incision has been made away from the midline or too deep. Careful identification of the middle of the symphysis with the local anaesthetic needle and the guidance of the underlying finger should reduce this risk. A retropubic haematoma can occur postoperatively but is usually self-limiting. Obviously, there is an increased risk of postpartum haemorrhage for which the clinician should be prepared.

Urinary Complications

Infection of the urinary tract is common but reduced by prophylactic antibiotics. Inadvertent incision of the bladder can occur and if identified and small it should heal with 10–14 days of continuous bladder drainage. If a vesico-vaginal fistula is suspected this should be confirmed as soon as possible with urethrocystoscopy as it will often respond to 6 weeks of continuous bladder drainage without the need for subsequent surgery. The incidence of stress incontinence is likely to be increased but there are no good studies to confirm or deny this.

Orthopaedic

Osteitis pubis can occur but this complication is reported in less than 1% of cases. Instability of the sacro-iliac joints and pubic symphysis can cause significant ambulatory difficulties but the reported incidence is 1–2%. Overall, in large series of symphysiotomy conducted by appropriately trained personnel the incidence of serious long-term orthopaedic and urinary complications is around 2%.[7]

Symphysiotomy has little or no role in countries with well-developed, hospital-based obstetric services. It does, however, have a significant and potentially life-saving role for both mother and infant for the obstructed after-coming head of the breech and as an alternative to second stage caesarean section for obstructed labour in regions with less-developed medical services.

Unfortunately the controversy around symphysiotomy being either an outdated and even unacceptable procedure, against that of being a life-saving procedure in certain clinical situations still exists.[6,7] Until a randomized trial can be performed, the evidence of case series should be used as a guide and in this case there is a clear place for symphysiotomy in situations described above.

REFERENCES

1. Wykes CB, Johnston TA, Paterson-Brown S, Johansen RB. Symphysiotomy: a life saving procedure. Br J Obstet Gynaecol 2003;110:219–21.

2. Johanson R, Wykes CB. Symphysiotomy. In: Johanson R, Cox C, Grady K, Howell C, editors. Managing obstetric emergencies and trauma – the MOET course manual. London: RCOG Press; 2003. p. 237–9.

3. VanRoosmalen J. Safe motherhood: cesarean section or symphysiotomy? Am J Obstet Gynecol 1990;163:1–4.

4. Cebekulu L, Buchmann EJ. Complications associated with caesarean section in the second stage. Int J Gynecol Obstet 2006;96:110–11.

5. Allen VM, O'Connell CM, Baskett TF. Maternal and perinatal morbidity of caesarean delivery at full cervical dilatation compared with caesarean delivery in the first stage of labour. Br J Obstet Gynaecol 2005;112:986–90.

6. Hofmeyer GJ, Shweni PM. Symphysiotomy for feto-pelvic disproportion. Cochrane Database Syst Rev 2010;10:CD005299.

7. Bjorklund K. Minimally invasive surgery for obstructed labour: a review of symphysiotomy during the twentieth century (including 5000 cases). Br J Obstet Gynaecol 2002;109:236–8.

8. Spencer JA. Symphysiotomy for vaginal breech delivery: two case reports. Br J Obstet Gynaecol 1987;94:16–8.

9. Menticoglu SM. Symphysiotomy for the trapped after-coming parts of the breech: a review of the literature and a plea for its use. Aust NZ J Obstet Gynaecol 1990;30:1–9.

10. Goodwin TM, Banks E, Millar L, Phelan J. Catastrophic shoulder dystocia and emergency symphysiotomy. Am J Obstet Gynecol 1997;177:463–4.

11. Hofmyer GJ. Obstructed labor: using better technologies to reduce mortality. Int J Gynecol Obstet 2004;85(Supp 1):S62–S72.

12. Hartfield VJ. Subcutaneous symphysiotomy: time for a reappraisal? Aust NZ J Obstet Gynaecol 1973;13:147–52.

13. Seedat EK, Crichton D. Symphysiotomy: technique, indications and limitations. Lancet 1962;1:154–8.

14. Crichton D, Seedat EK. The technique of symphysiotomy. South Afr Med J 1963;37:227–31.

15. Gebbie D. Symphysiotomy. Clin Obstet Gynaecol 1982;9:663–83.

DESTRUCTIVE OPERATIONS ON THE FETUS

TF Baskett • RC Pattinson

When caesarean section was still a lethal operation and serious degrees of pelvic contraction were commonplace throughout the world, obstructed labour frequently dragged on until the infant died. When it proved impossible to deliver the infant the man-midwife was called in to perform a destructive operation on the fetus to reduce its size and allow vaginal delivery in the hope that the mother's life could be saved.

The procedures to be considered here have for their objective the diminution of the bulk of the fetus, in order to permit of its more easy passage through the birth canal. Such procedures are only performed on the fetus with a lethal anomaly or in the fetus already dead. Other than the special case of drainage of the hydrocephalic fetal head these procedures have no place in modern obstetrics in regions with developed health services. However, similar to the arguments in favour of symphysiotomy, there are occasions, for cultural and clinical reasons, in regions with poorly developed health services, when destructive operations on the fetus may be necessary to save the life of the mother. When training and facilities for caesarean section are absent or unsafe these procedures may allow safe delivery of the mother, in addition to avoiding a uterine scar that may rupture if she is unable or unwilling to find suitable hospital-based obstetric care in a future pregnancy.

Even in developing countries the incidence of destructive operations is decreasing and is usually well under 1%.[1-2] In the vast majority of cases the indication is obstructed labour with a dead fetus.[3] When hospital facilities are limited, caesarean section for obstructed labour, particularly with a shoulder presentation in an over-distended and infected uterus, probably has a higher risk of maternal death than a fetal destructive procedure. In addition, the caesarean incision may have to be of the classical type with the implications for uterine rupture in subsequent pregnancy.

The role of these operations will depend upon the clinical circumstances and the level of obstetric services available – particularly safe caesarean section. In cases of obstructed labour with mild-to-moderate cephalopelvic disproportion and a live fetus, symphysiotomy may be chosen. If there is gross disproportion and the fetus is alive then caesarean section should be performed. Similarly, if obstructed labour is due to a transverse lie, shoulder or compound presentation and the fetus is alive, caesarean section will be less risky to both mother and infant than internal version and breech extraction – which are fraught with the risk of uterine rupture and a potentially fatal outcome for both infant and mother. However, when the fetus is dead and facilities for safe caesarean section are absent or marginal, craniotomy may be necessary for cases of cephalopelvic disproportion and decapitation may be indicated for transverse lie.[4] In addition, the social and cultural context in which the woman lives may lead her to refuse caesarean delivery under all circumstances.

GENERAL PRINCIPLES

In the majority of cases with obstructed labour the woman has been through a prolonged, painful and harrowing experience. She is likely to be exhausted, demoralized, dehydrated, septic and in pain.

- Initial first aid management should involve resuscitation with intravenous crystalloids and placement of a Foley catheter to monitor and guide fluid management.
- Blood should be taken for full blood count, cross-match and coagulation screen if possible. Many of these women are already anaemic and, with prolonged obstructed labour, atonic postpartum haemorrhage is more likely. In addition, trauma to the genital tract during the destructive procedure may increase blood loss.
- Infection is likely and, indeed, may be assumed, so that intravenous broad-spectrum antibiotics should be administered.
- In addition to her physical condition the woman may be so exhausted and demoralized as to be barely able to comprehend her situation. She may not even know yet that the fetus is dead. After the initial resuscitation manoeuvres have been undertaken and analgesia provided the woman and her husband and, if appropriate, a senior relative should be involved in the discussion and plan for delivery. Fully informed consent in these situations is

difficult but every effort must be made to obtain this to the extent feasible under the circumstances.

- The choice of anaesthesia will depend on what is available and the patient's condition. General anaesthesia has some advantages for both the patient and operator under these trying circumstances. However, spinal anaesthesia combined with sedation may be a safer option. If these are not available local anaesthesia with pudendal block, paracervical block and intravenous sedation may be adequate.
- Ideally, the cervix should be fully dilated for the performance of these procedures, although an experienced operator may be able to work within a cervix of 7 cm or more dilatation. The true conjugate of the pelvic brim should be at least 8 cm.
- In all cases of neglected obstructed labour the possibility of uterine rupture should be considered before embarking upon the procedure.

OPERATIVE PROCEDURES

Craniotomy

This is the most commonly performed destructive operation and is used for a neglected obstructed labour with a dead fetus in cephalic presentation. The ease and safety of this procedure depend upon the degree of pelvic contraction, the size of the fetal head and the experience of the operator. In general, if the fetal head is palpable more than three-fifths above the pelvic brim or is mobile at the pelvic brim then the procedure is difficult, dangerous and can be impossible. In such cases, even with a dead fetus, caesarean section is usually less hazardous for the mother.

In addition to adequate anaesthesia it is essential to confirm that the Foley catheter is properly placed and that the bladder is empty. The ideal instrument for perforation of the fetal head is Simpson's perforator (Fig 28-28). The depth of the two cutting blades is limited by the instrument's shoulders beneath them. The handles are held together by a hinged-crossbar and are wide apart when the cutting blades are in apposition. By pressing the handles together the cutting blades are separated. The head of the infant is steadied by the assistant using suprapubic pressure. The fingers of one hand are used to protect the maternal tissues and guide the points of the perforator to the anterior or posterior fontanelle, whichever is more accessible. The

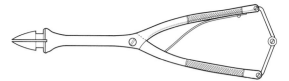

FIGURE 28-28 ■ Simpson's perforator.

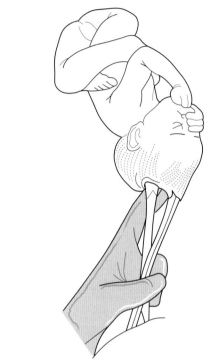

FIGURE 28-29 ■ Perforation of the skull. The perforator is pushed into the skull in the neighbourhood of the anterior fontanelle, the ideal site for perforation. The blades are separated by pressing the handles together and the opening of the skull is enlarged.

perforator should be at right angles to the surface of the skull as the instrument is pushed into the head up to the shoulders of the blades and opened as widely as possible to make a longitudinal incision on the scalp and the bone below, usually by separation of the sutures. This is followed by closing the blades and turning the perforator through 90° and repeating the procedure to produce a cruciate incision in the skull (Fig 28-29).

Keeping the perforator inside the cranium, it should be opened and closed, and the points of the instrument pushed into the skull and the brain broken up in all directions. Provided the perforator is kept in the skull up to the instrument's shoulders, and this is monitored by the fingers of the other hand, there should be no risk of trauma to the maternal soft tissues. The perforator is now withdrawn under protection of the other hand. Brain matter will usually ooze out of the incision and this evacuation can be assisted digitally.

If Simpson's perforator is not available, sharp Mayo's or similar scissors can be used to make a cruciate incision on the fetal scalp followed by introduction of the scissors into the fetal head via the most accessible fontanelle or suture line. The scissors are retained in the fetal skull and opened repeatedly in all directions to facilitate evacuation of the brain tissue.[5]

Once the head has been reduced in size, delivery can be assisted by traction on the edges of the cranium by Kocher's forceps or vulsella. If the cervix is not yet fully dilated, a bandage can be tied through the handles of these forceps and a weight applied to the end to facilitate complete cervical dilatation and delivery of the head during subsequent uterine contractions. If the degree of pelvic contraction is slight and the decompressed head is low in the pelvic cavity then ordinary obstetric forceps such as Simpson's or Neville–Barnes may be used to effect delivery of the fetal head. In cases of face presentation the most convenient site for perforation is the palate.

Craniotomy of the After-Coming Head

This may be required for the dead fetus with the breech delivered and an obstructed after-coming head. Once the arms of the infant have been brought down the assistant ensures that the fetal back is anterior and applies traction to the legs in a direction that facilitates access of the operator to the occipital region. Protecting the maternal tissues with the fingers of one hand, Simpson's perforator is pushed through the skull in the neighbourhood of the posterior lateral fontanelle (Fig 28-30). In some cases of contracted pelvis this may be difficult to reach, in which case the occipital bone is perforated in the midline. The manoeuvres to enlarge the incision and evacuate the contents of the skull are the same as with the forecoming head. Once the size of the head has been reduced it may be delivered by the Mauriceau–Smellie–Veit manoeuvre or forceps to the after-coming head.

Craniocentesis

Minor degrees of hydrocephalus that are diagnosed in the antenatal period by ultrasound and in which the infant is felt to have a reasonable chance of survival and good quality of life are likely to be delivered by caesarean section. We are concerned here with cases of severe

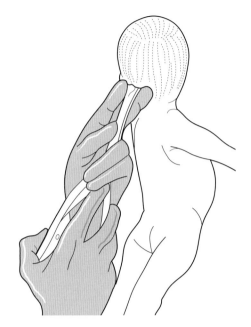

FIGURE 28-30 ■ Perforating the after-coming head through the posterolateral fontanelle.

hydrocephalus in which the infant is either dead or because of the degree of hydrocephalus, and perhaps other associated anomalies, the chance of infant survival after birth is remote. Of all the procedures under consideration in this chapter, craniocentesis – the drainage of the excess cerebrospinal fluid (CSF) is the easiest. The fetus almost invariably presents by the head or breech – transverse lie or shoulder presentation is extremely rare with severe hydrocephalus.

If the fetus presents by the head, the CSF can be drained transabdominally using a spinal needle, preferably under ultrasound guidance. As labour progresses it may be necessary to drain additional fluid transvaginally. Once the cervix has dilated, transvaginal drainage can be carried out using a spinal needle or pudendal block needle – the latter has the advantage of a guard which can be introduced through the vagina and cervix en route to the fetal head. If the fetus is already dead or severely malformed, the head may also be drained transvaginally using a Drew–Smythe catheter or Simpson's perforator or a pair of sharp scissors. These more comprehensive methods of drainage are more likely to result in the infant being stillborn.

If the fetus presents by the breech, labour can be allowed to progress until the body of the infant is delivered. If, as is not uncommon, there is an associated spina bifida, a catheter is passed through this opening up to the cranium and the CSF will drain effectively. If there is

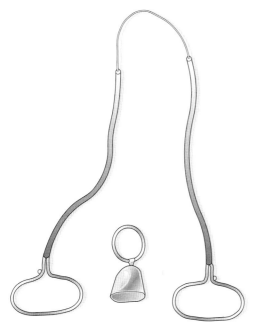

FIGURE 28-31 ■ The Blond–Heidler and thimble decapitating wire. The ends of the wire (saw) are protected with rubber tubing. The traction handles are detachable.

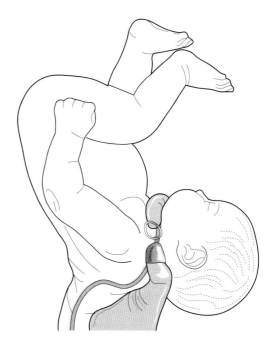

FIGURE 28-32 ■ Method of passing the decapitating wire around the fetal neck using the Blond–Heidler thimble.

no spina bifida it is possible to transect the thoracic spine (spondylotomy) and pass a catheter up the canal into the head to drain the CSF. Alternatively, the base of the fetal skull can be entered with Simpson's perforator as for craniotomy of the after-coming head (Fig 28-30). With all these methods of drainage the delivery of the head is usually spontaneous or easily assisted.

Decapitation

Of all the procedures outlined in this chapter decapitation is the most distressing for all involved. It is indicated in cases of neglected labour with a dead fetus in transverse lie with a prolapsed arm or shoulder presentation. In this situation the alternative of internal version or breech extraction carries such a high risk of uterine rupture that it is contraindicated. The safest and most simple technique is to use a Blond–Heidler saw (Fig 28-31). The operator mounts the thimble on one thumb and attaches the wire to the slot in the thimble. If there is a prolapsed arm, counter traction is put on this to make the fetal neck accessible. The thumb with the thimble is passed in front of the fetal neck and the fingers behind. The middle finger feels for the metal loop that projects from the thimble and, having secured it, pulls the thimble with the

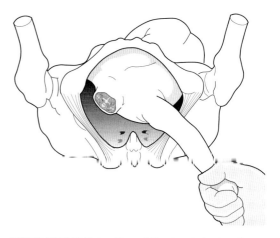

FIGURE 28-33 ■ Extraction of the trunk by traction on the fetal arm.

attached wire off the thumb and round the fetal neck (Fig 28-32).

The ends of the wire are now mounted on the handles shown in Figure 28-31 and by a to-and-fro motion the neck is severed. This technique is much safer, simpler and less traumatic to the maternal tissues than the previously used decapitation hooks. After the head is completely severed the trunk is removed by traction on the arm (Fig 28-33). The head is steadied by applying suprapubic pressure and can usually be delivered by finger traction through the baby's mouth, or by the application of forceps, or by using vulsellum or other toothed forceps on the fetal scalp. Care must be taken during delivery of the head that sharp bony protrusions of the cervical spine do not injure the maternal tissues.

Evisceration

The operation of evisceration consists in the removal of the abdominal and/or thorax contents, with the object of diminishing the bulk of the child so it can be extracted vaginally. Obviously this is only considered in the case of a dead fetus. It is occasionally necessary in the fetus with a distended abdomen or thorax due to fluid or a tumour. Using a perforator or embryotomy scissors the abdomen or thorax, whichever is accessible, is opened. The organs are removed manually or by traction with sponge forceps. Entry from the thorax to the abdomen and vice versa can be gained via the diaphragm.

Paracentesis

If there is fetal hydrops of a degree that obstructs labour, and if the fetus is dead or not viable, this can be drained by passing a spinal needle through the maternal abdomen and into the fetal peritoneal cavity. If the fetus is in breech presentation and the legs and breech are delivered with the distended fetal abdomen causing obstruction, this can be drained by a spinal or pudendal block needle guided vaginally. If necessary, scissors, a perforator, or a Drew–Smythe catheter can be used to enter the abdomen and drain the fluid.

Cleidotomy

This is considered in cases where the head is delivered, large shoulders are obstructing delivery and the fetus is dead. If delivery of the shoulders cannot be achieved by the usual manoeuvres used to overcome shoulder dystocia (see Chapter 12) the operation of cleidotomy – division of one or both clavicles to reduce the bulk of the shoulder girdle – is performed. One hand is placed vaginally along the ventral aspect of the fetus and under this protection strong straight embryotomy scissors are introduced to cut the clavicle. It is best to cut the skin over the clavicle first and push the scissors round the bone. Considerable strength is often required to break the bone at about its mid-point.

POST-DELIVERY CARE

Post-delivery complications are common, with postpartum haemorrhage, puerperal sepsis and urinary tract infection being the most frequent.[6]

- Active management of the third stage of labour should be carried out and an oxytocin infusion continued for 6–8 hours as the risk of atonic postpartum haemorrhage following prolonged obstructed labour is high.
- The genital tract should be carefully inspected for any signs of trauma, including uterine exploration to rule out rupture. Lacerations of the cervix and vagina should be carefully repaired.
- The bladder in many cases has been distended for a prolonged period of time and an indwelling catheter should be left for 5–7 days to allow bladder tone to be regained.
- Broad-spectrum antibiotics should be continued for several days.
- Thromboprophylaxis should be instituted.
- As much as possible the infant should be restored anatomically with suturing. This, along with careful and tasteful placement of blankets should help reduce the trauma to the parents when they view their newborn dead infant.
- In addition to attention to the physical welfare of the mother her psychological wellbeing and that of her husband/partner and close family members should be considered. The most knowledgeable and senior member of the staff involved should review all of the events with the woman and the implications and plans for subsequent pregnancy care.

It bears re-emphasis that in all cases when destructive operations are considered the operator should consider the alternative of delivery by caesarean section, even if the fetus is dead. This decision will be guided by the availability of safe caesarean section, the operator's experience in destructive operations, and other clinical, social, and cultural aspects, which may include the woman's refusal to have a caesarean delivery and the implications of a caesarean section scar in future pregnancies should she agree to caesarean delivery.

REFERENCES

1. Sikka P, Chopra S, Kalpdev A, Jain V, Dhaliwal I. Destructive operations – a vanishing art in modern

obstetrics: 25 year experience at a tertiary center in India. Arch Gynecol Obstet 2011;283:929–33.

2. Biswas A, Chakraborty PS, Das HS, Bose A, Kalsar PK. Role of destructive operations in modern day obstetrics. J Indian Med Assoc 2001;99:248, 250–1.

3. Gupta D, Chitra S. Destructive operations still have a place in developing countries. Int J Gynaecol Obstet 1994;44:15–9.

4. Lawson J. Delivery of the dead or malformed fetus. Clin Obstet Gynaecol 1982;9:745–55.

5. St. George J. A simple and safe method of vaginal delivery of cases of prolonged obstructed labour with head presentation. West Afr Med J 1975;23:34–40.

6. Singhai SR, Chaudhry P, Sangwan K, Shighai SK. Destructive operations in modern obstetrics. Arch Gynecol Obstet 2005;273:107–9.

INDEX

NB: Page numbers in *italics* refer to boxes, figures and tables.

A

Abdominal examination, 95–96
Aberdeen knot, *219*, 220
Abruptio placentae *see* Placental abruption
Accelerations, fetal heart rate (FHR), 42, 51
Acidosis *see* Fetal asphyxia
Action Medical Research (UK), 85–86
Active Management of Labour (O'Driscoll), 33, *35*
Active Management of Labour, philosophy, 40
Acupuncture, 237
Acute tocolysis, 245–247, *245*
  administration, tocolytics, 246–247
  atosiban, 245, 247
  beta-adrenergic drugs, 245
  indications, 245–246
  nitroglycerine, 245–246
Acute uterine inversion, 211–216
  acute tocolysis, 246
  causes, 211–212
  clinical presentation, 212
  management, 212–214, *213–215*
  recurrent, 214–215
  types, 211, *212*
Adrenaline (epinephrine), 241, 245
Advanced Cardiac Life Support, 25
All-fours position, 128–129, *128*
Allis forceps, 213–214
ALSO (Advanced Learning Support in Obstetrics) training, 26
American College of Obstetricians and Gynecologists, 8–9, *39*, *97*, 124–125
Amnioinfusion, 50
Amniotic fluid
  assessment, *38*
  cord prolapse, 174
  meconium-stained, 50
Amniotic fluid embolism (AFE), 234–235
  diagnosis, 234–235
  management, 235
  pathophysiology, 234
Amniotomy, 40
  complications, 75–76
  cord prolapse, 174
  induction of labour, 74, *74*
  outcomes, 77
Anaesthesia *see* Analgesia and anaesthesia
Anal sphincter trauma, obstetric, 220–221
Anal triangle, 217
Analgesia and anaesthesia, 236–241
  acute uterine inversion, 213
  assisted vaginal delivery, 98
  breech delivery, 158–159
  caesarean hysterectomy, 195
  caesarean section (CS), 136, 241
  destructive operations, 277

Analgesia and anaesthesia (*cont'd*)
  local anaesthesia, 239, 241, 272
  pain pathways, 236
  pain relief, methods, 236–241
    local infiltration, 239–240, *239*
    non-pharmacological, 236–237, *237*
    paracervical block, 240–241, *241*
    pharmacological, 237–239, *238*
    pudendal block, 240, *240*
  twins, 170
Anatomy of the Human Gravid Uterus (Hunter), 1
Anderson, Anne, *71*
Annular detachment of cervix, 222–223
Antenatal preparation, 31–32
Antepartum haemorrhage (APH), causes, 178, *178*, *179*
  see also Placenta praevia; Placental abruption; Vasa praevia
Anterior placenta, 250
Antibiotics, 84–85, 137, 280
Anti-Duff antibodies, 48
Anti-Kell antibodies, 48
Antithrombin, 232
Aorta, 262, *262*
'Apt test', 192
Arabin pessary, 83
Arnott, Neil, 90–91
Asherman's syndrome, 193
Asphyxia *see* Fetal asphyxia
Assisted vaginal delivery, 88–115
  analgesia, 98
  assessment, 95–98, *95*, *96*
  classification, *97*, 98
  complications, 111–113
    fetal, 111–113
    maternal, 111
  error, types, 10, *10–11*
  forceps *see* Forceps delivery
  historical perspective, *88–91*
  indications, 97–98
    fetal, 97
    maternal, 97
    poor progress/dystocia, 97
  informed consent, 98
  with rotation, 104–108
    digital, 104, *104*
    manual, 104–105, *105*
  shoulder dystocia, 124
  training, 98
    simulation, 25
  trial, 98–99
  utero-fetal-pelvic relationships, 92–95
    bony pelvis, 94–95, *94*, *95*
    fetal head, 93–94, *94*
    maternal effort, 92–93, *93*
    uterine work, 92
  vacuum extractor *see* Vacuum assisted delivery

Asynclitism, fetal head, *94*
Atosiban, 245, 247
Audit, 13, 15–21, 69
  defined, 15
Aviation model of training, 26–27
Axis-traction devices, 89–90

B

Bakri balloon, 253–255, *254*
Bandl's ring, *153*
Barnes, Fancourt, *245*
Barnes, Robert, *71*
Barton, Lyman, 90
Bart's hydrops, 48
Baseline, fetal heart rate, 42
  variability, 42
Bell, William Blair, *71*
Bergstrom, Sune, *71*, *203*
Beta-adrenergic drugs, 245
Betke–Kliehauer (BK) test, 183–184
Bimanual uterine compression, 204, *204*
Bipolar podalic version, 186, *187*
Bird, Geoffrey, *91*, 108
Birth *see* Labour and delivery; Preterm birth
Bishop's cervical scoring system, 74, *74*, 77
Bladder injuries, 269
Blond–Heidler saw, 121–122, 172, 279, *279*
Blond–Heidler thimble, *279*, *279*
Blood group antibodies, 48
Blood testing, 137
Blood transfusion, 189, 196, 226, *228*
  feto-maternal, 48–49, *48*
Blundell, James, *225*, *228*
B-Lynch suture, 258–259, *258*
  modified, 257–258, *258*
Bolam's Principle, 66
Bolitho's Principle, 66
Bony pelvis, 94–95, *95*
  pelvic diagonal conjugate, *94*, *95*
Brachial plexus injury (BPI) *see* Obstetric brachial plexus
  injury (OBPI)
Brain injury, 65
Braxton Hicks
  bipolar podalic version method, 186, *186*
  contractions, 180
Breech delivery, 25, 157–168
  acute tocolysis, 246
  anaesthesia, 158–159
  complications, 163–166
    extended arms, 163
    head entrapment, 165–166
    Løvset's manoeuvre, 163–164, *163*, *164*
    nuchal arm, 164–165, *165*
    posterior arm, bringing down, 164, *164*
    trunk and head, posterior rotation, 165
  extraction, 166–168, *166–167*
  first stage, labour, 159, *159*
  intrapartum fetal risks, 158
  procedure, 159–163
    breech and legs, 159–161, *160*
    head, 161–163, *161*
    shoulders and arms, 161, *161*
  symphysiotomy, 271
  version, 250
Breech presentation, caesarean section (CS), 135, 142,
  157–158
Broad ligament haematomas, 223
Brow presentation, *118*, 119
  diagnosis, 119
  management, 119

C

Caesarean hysterectomy
  major risks, *196*
Caesarean section (CS), 132–144
  anaesthesia, 136, 241
  audit, 17–18, 21
  classification, 20–21, *20*
  complicated, 140–141
    breech presentation, 135, 142, 157–158
    classical, 140–141, *141*
    fetal head, deeply engaged, 141–142, *142*
    low vertical, 141
    obesity, 97
    transverse lie, 142
  costs, 148
  vs destructive operations, 276, 280
  documentation, 97
  electronic fetal heart rate monitoring (EFM), 37
  historical perspective, *132–134*
  indications, 17–19, *18*, 135–136
    generally accepted, 135–136
    indisputable, 135
    malpresentation, 121
    marginal, 136
  NICE guidelines, 67
  'once a caesarean always a caesarean', 145, *145*,
    154–155
  perimortem, 26, 143, *143*
  perioperative care, 137
  placenta praevia, 186–189
  popularity, rise in, 132–134, *133*
  postmortem, 25, 143, *143*
  preoperative considerations, 136–137
  previous, 77, 135
  shoulder dystocia, 124–125
  surgical techniques, 138–140, *139–140*
  vs symphysiotomy, 271
  transverse/oblique lie, 121
  twins, 172
  types, 137–138
    classical, 137–138, 140–141, *141*
    low transverse, 137
    low vertical, 137, 141
  urgency, classification, 136
  vaginal birth *see* Vaginal birth after caesarean section
    (VBAC)
Cameron, Murdoch, 133
Caput succedaneum, 94, *95*, 112, *112*
Carbetocin, 200, *201*, 202
Cardiopulmonary resuscitation (CPR), 143,
  235
Cardiotocographs (CTGs)
  archives, 68
  brain injury, 65
  categorization, 45–49
  classification, 45
  contractions, annotation, 49–50
  'cycling', 44–45, *47*
  electrocardiography (ECG) and, 53, *53*
  fetal asphyxia, 57–59, 65, 67
  high-risk pregnancy, 42
  hypoxia *see* Hypoxia
  interpretation, 9, 23–24, *24*, 53–54, 57,
    67
    basic principles, 54
  medicolegal implications, 65–66
  pathological, 50–51, 53
  vs pulse oximetry, 51
  technical errors, 67–68
  training, 69
  vascular ischaemic injury (VII), 64

Care
  bundle, 9
  intrapartum *see* Intrapartum care
  standards, 15–30
Carlisle, Sir Anthony, 113
Causation, 65–66
Centre for Maternal and Child Enquiries (CMACE),
    22
Cephalhaematoma, 112, *112*
Cephalic malpresentations, 36
Cephalic traction, 186, *188*
Cephalopelvic disproportion, 37, 135, 271
Cerebrospinal fluid (CSF), 278–279
Cervical cerclage, 83, 242–244
  materials/management, 243
  risks, 243
  surgical procedure, 242, *243*
  timing, 242–243
Cervix
  annular detachment, 222–223
  assessment, *38*
  cervical ripening, 2–5, *2–5*, 77
  cervical spine dislocation, 158
  incompletely dilated, 165–166
  lacerations, 222, *222*
  purpose, 36–37
  removal, 269
  scoring system, 74, *74*
  size/shape, 32, *32*
Chamberlen family, 88–89, *89*
Chapman, Edmund, 89, 99
Chloroform, *239*
Chronic recurrent uterine inversion, 267
Cleidotomy, 280
Clinical Negligence Scheme for Trusts (CNST), 23, 68,
    130
Clinical practice guidelines, 8–9
Coagulation *see* Disseminated intravascular coagulation
    (DIC)
Coagulopathy, dilutional, 228
Cochrane systematic reviews
  corticosteroids, 84
  episiotomy, 219
  fetal surveillance, 50–51, 53
  induction of labour, 72–73
  intraumbilical vein injection, oxytocics,
      210
  vacuum extractor, 92
Collect and Analyze patient safety data (RADICAL
    framework), 12–13
Colloids, 204, 227
Communication, training, 27
Competence, 22–30
Complete breech, 159, *159*
Compound presentation, 122
Computer software programmes, 16
Confidential Enquiry into Maternal and Child Health
    (CEMACH), 198
Confidential Enquiry into Stillbirths and Deaths in Infancy
    (CESDI), 22–23, 57, 68, 130
Conjoined twins, 172
Connective tissue disorders, 212
Contractions *see* Uterine contractions
Cord
  clamping, 207
  entanglement, 158
  traction, controlled, 207
Cord prolapse, 174–177
  acute tocolysis, 246
  breech presentation, 158
  diagnosis, 175, *175*

Cord prolapse (*cont'd*)
  management, 175–177
    compression relief, 175–176, *176*
    cord replacement, 177
    delivery, 177
    fetal assessment, 176
    patient transfer delay, 176
  predisposing factors, 174–175
    amniotic fluid, 174
    cord length, 175
    fetal, 174
    maternal, 174
    obstetric manipulation, 175
    placental, 174
Corticosteroids, 84
Cortisol, 4–5
Costs, 23, 148
Courveé, Claude De la, 271
Couvelaire uterus, 190, *191*
Craniocentesis, 278–279
Craniotomy, 277–278, *277*
  after-coming head, 278, *278*
Cryoprecipitate, 232
Crystalloid, intravenous, 204, 227, 245, 276
CTG *see* Cardiotocographs (CTGs)

D
Dale, Sir Henry, 71, *203*
Darwin, Erasmus, 207
De Ribes, Camille Champetier, *71*
Decapitation, 121–122, 172, 279–280, *279*
Decelerations, fetal heart rate (FHR), 42–44
  early, 43, *43*
  late, 44, *46*
  variable, 43, *44*
    atypical, 43, *45*
Dehiscence, defined, 152
Dehydro-epiandrosterone sulphate, 5
Delivery units, safety, 7–8
  see also Labour and delivery
Denman, Thomas, *71*, 169, 177
Descent phase, defined, 111
Design for safety (RADICAL framework), 8–12
Destructive operations, fetus, 276–281
  general principles, 276–277
  procedures, 277–280
Diabetes mellitus, maternal, 72, 123–124
Diamorphine, 137
Digital rotation, 104, *104*
DIGITAT trial, 73
Dilutional coagulopathy, 228
Dislocation of limbs, 158
Disseminated intravascular coagulation (DIC), 230–233
  causes, 230
  clinical presentation, 231
  diagnosis, 231
  hysterectomy, 266, 269–270
  management, 231–233
    maintain circulation, 232
    procoagulants, replacement, 232–233
    treat the cause, 232
  pathophysiology, 230–231, *231*
Documentation, 49–50, 97, 130
Donald, Ian, 99
Doppelnaht technique, 133
Double clamp technique, 268, *268*
Double layer technique, 133
Doyen retractor, 138, 140, 189
Drew–Smythe catheter, 278, 280
du Coudray, Madam Angélique, 22

du Vigneaud, Vincent, *203*
Dudley, Harold, *203*
Dystocia, 36, 97, 135
   audit, 18–19, *18*
   shoulder *see* Shoulder dystocia

E

Eclampsia, simulation, 25
Ectopic pregnancy, 267
Elective caesarean section (CS), 18
Elective induction of labour, 73
Electrocardiography (ECG), 67–68
   waveform analysis, 52–53, *52, 53*
Electronic fetal heart rate monitoring (EFM), 33, 37
   continuous, 41–44, *42*
   training, 23–24, *24*
   twins, 170
Emergency situations
   caesarean section (CS), 18
   training, 27
Encephalopathy, neonatal, 54
EPICURE study, 82
Epidemiological data, 16–17
Epinephrine (adrenaline), 241, 245
Episiotomy, 126–127, 217–220, *218*
   dehiscence, 220
   mediolateral, 219
   midline, 218–219
   second degree tears, 219
   technique, 219–220, *219*
Erb's palsy, 130
Erb's Palsy Group, 130
Ergometrine®, 200, 204, 207
   characteristics/side effects, 201–202, *201, 202*
Ether, *239*
Evisceration, 280
External anal sphincter (EAS), 217, *218*
External aortic compression, 204–205
External cephalic version (ECV), 147, 248, *248*
   acute tocolysis, 246
   assessment, 248–250
   complications, 250
   predictive factors, 250
   technique, 248–250, *249*
   twins, 171, *171*
External tocography, 49
Eye injuries, 113

F

Face presentation, 116–119
   causes, 116
   diagnosis, 116–117
   management, 117–119, *118–119*
Facial palsy, 113
Facial skin trauma, fetal, 112
Ferguson, Haig, 90, 99–100
Ferguson's reflex, 92
Fetal asphyxia, 57–70
   adverse outcomes, reducing, 66–69
      CTG interpretation, 67
      education/training, 68–69
      inappropriate action, 67
      incident reporting/audit, 69
      record keeping, 68
      technical errors, 67–68, *68*
   brain injury, 65
   definitions, 57–58
   fetal heart rate (FHR), patterns, 58–65
   medicolegal implications, 65–66

Fetal death
   intrauterine, 77–78, 155
   see also Destructive operations, fetus
Fetal disorders
   distress, 136
   facial skin trauma, 112, *112*
   hypoxia, 135
   immaturity, 75
   scalp trauma, 112, *112*
Fetal fibronectin (fFN), 82–83
Fetal head, 93–94
   assessment, *38*
   attitude, 93
   caput succedaneum, 94, *95*, 112, *112*
   moulding, 94, *95*
   position, 93
   rotation, 90
   station, 93–94
   synclitism, 93, *94*
Fetal heart rate (FHR)
   accelerations, 42, 51
   asphyxia, 58–65
   auscultation, 41
   baseline, 42
      variability, 42
   decelerations, 42–44
   electronic monitoring (EFM), 23, 33, 41
   features, classification, *47*
   high-risk pregnancy, 42
   pathological, 50
   pseudo-sinusoidal pattern, 48–49, *48*
   records, 68
   sinusoidal pattern, 45–49, *47*
   stimulation tests, 51
   technical errors, 67–68
   twins, *171*
   uterine contractions, 49–50, *49*
Fetal landmarks, 116, *117*, 250–251
Fetal movements (FM), 41
Fetal position, utero-fetal-pelvic relationships, 92–95
Fetal pulse oximetry, 51
Fetal scalp blood sampling (FBS), 45, 50–51, *51*, 59
Fetal skull, diameters/landmarks, 116, *117*
Fetal surveillance, 41–56
   alternative methods, 51–53
   behavioural state, 44–45, *47*
   CTG categorization, 45–49
   fetal scalp blood sampling (FBS), 45, 50–51, *51*, 59
   high-risk pregnancy, 42–44, *42*
   intermittent auscultation (IA), 41–42
   maternal pyrexia/neonatal encephalopathy, 54
   meconium-stained amniotic fluid, 50
   position, 36
   uterine contractions, 49–50, *49*
Fetal trunk, traction, 158
Fibrin degradation products (FDP), 230–233
Foley catheter, transcervical, 75
Footling breech, 159, *159*
Forceps
   invention, 88–89, *89*
   pelvic curve, 89
   straight, 90
   use of, 25
Forceps delivery, 99–100, *99*
   after-coming head, 162, *162*
   classical, 100–103, *100–103*
   occipito-posterior, 103–104, *103*
   with rotation, 105–108
      classical (inversion) technique, 106, *107*
      direct technique, 106, *107*
      wandering technique, 106, *107*

Forceps delivery (*cont'd*)
   sequential instrumental delivery, 111
   vs vacuum extractor, 91–92
Fractures, 158
Frank, Fritz, 15, 133
Frank breech, 159–160, *159–160*
Fresh frozen plasma (FFP), 232
Freud, Sigmund, 65
Friedman, Emmanuel, 33

G
Galileo, 15
Gates Foundation, 85–86
Genital tract trauma *see* Lower genital tract trauma
Gestational age, 250
Gestational hypertension, 72
Giffard, William, 163, 211
Global Alliance to Prevent Prematurity and Stillbirth, 81
Glyceryl trinitrate, 203, 210
Green–Armytage clamps, 139, 189, 195, 267
Growth Restriction Intervention trial (GRIT), 73
Guidelines, clinical practice, 8–9

H
Haematomas, 223
   classification, 223
   clinical presentation, 223
   management, 223
Haematuria, 153
Haemoglobinopathy, 48
Haemorrhage
   antepartum *see* Antepartum haemorrhage (APH)
   intracranial, 113
   massive, 10–12
   postpartum *see* Postpartum haemorrhage (PPH)
   subgaleal, 112, *112*
   symphysiotomy, 274
   uterine rupture, 153
Haemorrhagic shock, 225–229
   clinical features, 226
   haemorrhage arrest, 229
   management, 226–228
   monitoring, 228
   pathophysiological response, 225–226
   physiological changes, pregnancy, 225
Haemostasis, mechanisms, 199, *199*
Haggard, Howard Wilcox, 236
Harm, preventable, 22–23
Haultain's operation, 214, *215*
HELLP syndrome, 230–232, 235
Helping Babies Breathe program, 26
Hermann of Berne, 90
Hexoprenaline, 247
High parity, 78
High-risk pregnancy, 42–44, *42*
Hippocrates, 1, 7
Hospital facilities, 148
Hubert's traction bar, 90
Hunter, William, 1, *3*, 80, 99, 178, 211
Huntington's operation, 213–214, *214*
Hyperstimulation, defined, 39
Hypertension, gestational, 72
Hypertonus, defined, 39
Hypnosis, 237
Hypoperfusion, 226
Hypothermia, 228
Hypovolaemia, treatment, 204, 227, 245
Hypovolaemic shock, 226
   classification, 226

Hypoxaemia, defined, 57–58
Hypoxia, 226
   acute, 58–59
   defined, 57–58
   gradually developing, 59–62, *62–63*
   longstanding, 62–64, *64*
   subacute, 59, *60–62*
Hypoxic ischaemic encephalopathy (HIE), 65–66
Hysterectomy *see* Obstetric hysterectomy
Hysterotomy, 146

I
Incident reporting, 12–13
Induction of labour, 71–79
   classification, *20*, 21
   complications, 75–76
   elective, 73
   historical perspective, *71*
   indications, 17, 19, *19*, 71–73, *72*
   methods, 74–75, *74*
   shoulder dystocia, 124
   special situations, 77–78
   systematic approach, 76–77
      phase I, *74*, 76
      phase II, 76–77
      phase III, *74*, 77, *77*
   unsuccessful, 76
   vaginal birth after caesarean section (VBAC), trial, 148
INFANT Trial, 54, 67
Infection
   fetal, 48
   obstructed labour, 276
   postoperative, 147
   reducing, 83
   susceptibility, 5, *6*
Information
   classification, 19
   collection, 12–13, 15–16
   labour events/outcomes, 16–17, *17*
   management interpretation, 21
   Multidisciplinary Quality Assurance Programme (MDQAP), 15, *16*, 19, 21
   retrieval/presentation/dissemination, 16
   10-group classification system (TGCS), 19–21, *20*
Informed consent
   assisted vaginal delivery, 98
   caesarean hysterectomy, 195
   caesarean section (CS), 136–137
   destructive operations, 276–277
Inhalation analgesia, 237–238, *238*
In-house training, 27
Instrumental delivery *see* Assisted vaginal delivery
Intermittent auscultation (IA), 41–42
Internal anal sphincter (IAS), 217, *218*
Internal iliac artery, 262, *262*
   branches, *261*
   ligation, 263–264, *264*
Internal manoeuvres, shoulder dystocia, 127
Internal podalic version, 250–252, *250*
   fetal landmarks, 250–251
   technique, 251–252, *251–252*
International Statistical Classification of Disease and Related Health Problems, 10th Revision (ICD-10) (WHO), 80
Interventions, 16–17, 33–34, 36
Intra-abdominal organs, damage, 158
Intracranial haemorrhage, 113, 158
Intrapartum care, 33
   improved training, 22
   personal attention, 35–36, 237

Intrapartum care (*cont'd*)
  standards, 15–21
  teamwork, 27
  twins, *171*
Intrauterine fetal death
  late, 77–78
  and stillbirth (IUFD), 155
Intrauterine growth restriction (IUGR), *42*, 58–59, 67, 73
Involve users (RADICAL framework), 12

J
Jehovah's Witness patients, 189, 196
Joel–Cohen transverse skin incision, 140
Joint Commission on Accreditation of Healthcare
  Organizations (JCAHO), 23

K
Kehrer, Ferdinand, 133
Kennedy, Evory, 45, 50
Kergaradec, Jacques Alexandre, 41
Kerr, Munro, 1, 176, 181, 211–212, 271
  caesarean section (CS), 133–134, 138
Kielland, Christian
  forceps, 90, 99–100, *99*, 105–108, *107*
  malpresentation, 117–119, *118*
Kings Fund, 22–23
Kleihauer–Betke test, 48–49
Klikovich, Stanislav, *238*
Knee-chest position, 175–176, *176*
Kobayashi Silastic cup, 108
Kocher's forceps, 278

L
Labour and delivery, 1–6
  amniotic fluid embolism (AFE), 234–235
  anaesthesia *see* Analgesia and anaesthesia
  assessment, 32
    normal and abnormal, 36–37
    poor progress, 37–40, *38*, 97
  assisted *see* Assisted vaginal delivery
  audit, 15–21
  biological control, 4–5, *4–6*
  caesarean section *see* Caesarean section (CS); Vaginal
    birth after caesarean section (VBAC)
  cervical ripening, 2–5, *2–5*, 77
  contentious issues, 40
  duration, 39–40
  fetus *see* Fetal surveillance
  induction *see* Induction of labour
  lower genital tract trauma, 217–224
  malpresentation *see* Breech delivery; Malpresentations
  management, 31–40
    antenatal preparation, 31–32
    care *see* Intrapartum care
    diagnosis, 32–33, *32*
    general principles, 31–36
    labour ward, 32
    partogram, 33, *34–35*
    spontaneous onset, 33–34
    stages of labour, 33, 97
  myometrial function, 1–2, *2–3*
  obstructed, 37
  safety *see* Risk management
  standards of care, 15–30
  third stage labour
    management, 207–208
    physiology, 198–199

Labour and delivery (*cont'd*)
    see also Acute uterine inversion; Postpartum
      haemorrhage (PPH); Retained placenta
    triplets, 169, 172
    twins *see* Twins, delivery
Lacerations, 221–223
  annular detachment of cervix, 222–223
  cervical, 222, *222*
  periurethral/periclitoral, 221
  vaginal, 221–222, *222*
Lactate measurements, fetal scalp, 53
Lamaze, Dr Fernand, 236–237
Laparotomy, 154
Latent pathogens, 13
Latent phase, prolonged, 37
Le Boyer, Frederick, 236–237
Leadership, roles/responsibilities, 27
Learn from experience (RADICAL framework), 13
Lectures on Midwifery (Simpson, 1860), 1
Levret, André, 89
Liability, 65–66
Lidocaine, 239, 241, 272
Limbs, dislocation, 158
Little, William John, 57
'Living ligatures', 199
Lloyd Davies position (frog-legged), 257
Local anaesthesia, 239, 241, 272
Locked twins, 172, *172*
London Protocol System Analyses, 13
Løvset, Jørgen, 163
Lower genital tract trauma, 217–224
  anatomy, 217, *218*
  episiotomy *see* Episiotomy
  haematoma *see* Haematomas
  laceration *see* Lacerations
  obstetric anal sphincter trauma, 220–221, *221*
  perineal trauma, 217, *219*
  postpartum haemorrhage (PPH), 203
Lower uterine segment (LUS)
  physiology, 180, *181*
  placental 'migration', 180, *181*
  thickness, 147
Low-resource settings, skills training, 26
Lumbar artery, 262
Lushbaugh, P.E., 234

M
McRoberts' position, 126, *126–127*
Macrosomia, 123
Magnesium sulphate, 84
Magnetic resonance imaging (MRI), 57, 64–66
Malmström, Tage, 91, 108
Malpresentations, 116–122, *118*
  cephalic, 36
  cord prolapse, 174
  intrapartum version, 246
  placenta praevia, 185–186
  twins, 169
  see also Breech delivery
Management
  information, interpretation, 21
  modification, 21
March of Dimes (US), 85–86
Maternal disorders, 136
  assessment, shoulder dystocia, 129
  collapse, training, 25–26
  diabetes mellitus, 72, 123–124
  obesity, 12, 124
  pyrexia, 54
Maternal Mortality Report (UK, 1924), 22

Maternity services, failures, 8
Mauriceau, Francois, 88–89, 174, 208, *219*
Mauriceau–Smellie–Veit manoeuvre, 162–163, *163*, 165, 278
Mayor, François, 41
Mayo's scissors, 278
Meconium-stained amniotic fluid, 50
Medical Research Committee (UK, 1917), 22
Medicolegal implications, fetal asphyxia, 65–66
Membranes
    assessment, *38*
    preterm rupture *see* Preterm premature membrane rupture (pPROM)
    sweeping, 74–75
Meperidine, 238–239
15-Methyl prostaglandin F2α, 204
    characteristics/side effects, *201*, 202
Middle sacral artery, 262
Millennium Development Goals, 22–23
Misgav Ladach method, 140
Misoprostol, 9–10, 78, 207
    characteristics/side effects, *201*, 202
Moir, Chassar, 96, 98–99, 117, *203*, 222
Monoamniotic twins, 170
Moolgaoker, Arvind, 90
Morphine, 137
Morris, W., 123
Moulding, fetal head, 94, *95*
Multidisciplinary Quality Assurance Programme (MDQAP), 15, *16*, 19, 21
Multiparous women, 38–39
Multiple pregnancy, 73
Murphy, Edward W., 212
Murray, Milne, 90
Myerscough, P.R., 7, 134
Myomectomy, 146, 153
Myometrial architecture, 199, *199*

N
Narcotic analgesia, 238–239, *239*
National Health Service Litigation Authority (NHSLA), 23, 130
    cardiotocographs (CTGs), 54, 57, 68
    legal claims, 7–8, 57
    substandard care, 23, 54
National Health Service (NHS), 67
National Institute for Health and Clinical Excellence (NICE), 8–9, 42, 67, 73, 77–78
    cardiotocograph (CTG) guidelines, 45, *47*
    diabetic pregnancy, 72, 124
    intrapartum guidelines, 23, *24*
National Maternity Hospital, 40
Natural childbirth, 236–237, *237*
Neonatal assessment, shoulder dystocia, 129
Neonatal encephalopathy, 54
Neville–Barnes forceps, 99–100, 278
Nitabuch's zone, 193
Nitric oxide donors, 75
Nitroglycerine, 245–246
Nitrous oxide, 237–238, *238*
    administration technique, 238
Non-steroidal anti-inflammatory drugs (NSAIDs), 137
Nuchal arm, 164–165, *165*
Nulliparous women, 38

O
Obesity, maternal, 124, 250
    additional considerations, 12
    caesarean section (CS), 97

Obstetric anal sphincter injuries (OASIS), 217, 220–221, *221*
Obstetric balance, 71–72, *72*
Obstetric brachial plexus injury (OBPI), 113, 129–130
    breech delivery, 158
    classification, 130
    total, 130
Obstetric hysterectomy, 266–270
    indications, 266–267
    postoperative considerations, 270
    surgical considerations, 267–268, *268*
    surgical technique, 268–270, *269–270*
Obstructed labour, 37, 276–277
Occipito-posterior position, 36
Occipito-transverse position, 36
O'Driscoll, Kieran, 33, 39
OmniCup, 110
On Generation (Hippocrates), 1
Operative Midwifery (Kerr), 1
OPPTIMUM study, 83
Orthopaedic complications, symphysiotomy, 274
O'Sullivan's hydrostatic replacement technique, 213, *214*
Ould, Fielding, 170–171, *218*
Outlet phase, defined, 111
Ovarian artery ligation, 263, *263*
Oxytocic drugs
    characteristics/side effects, 201–202, *201*
    historical perspective, *203*
    intraumbilical vein injection, 210
    postpartum haemorrhage (PPH), 204–205
    third stage labour, 207
Oxytocin, 159, 170, 210, 245
    audit, 18–19
    characteristics/side effects, 201, *201*
    dosage, 40, *78*
    guidelines for use, 9–10
    induction of labour, *71*, 74, *74*, 76, 77
    postpartum haemorrhage (PPH), 203–204
    potential risks, 39
    third stage labour, 200, 207

P
Pain pathways, 236
Pain relief, methods, 236–241
Pajot, Charles, 89–90, 100
Pajot's manoeuvre, 89–90, *90*, 107–100
Paracentesis, 280
Paracervical block, 240–241, *241*
Paravaginal haematomas, 223
Paré, Ambroise, *250*
Parity, 250
Partogram, 33, *34–35*
Partus conduplicato corpore (spontaneous delivery), 120
Pelvic curve, forceps, 89
Pelvic floor muscles, *218*
Pelvic pressure pack, 269–270, *270*
Pelvic vessel embolization, 264
Pelvic vessel ligation, 261–265
    anatomy/haemodynamics, 261–262, *261–262*
    internal iliac artery, 263–264, *264*
    ovarian artery, 263, *263*
    uterine artery, 261, 262–263, *263*
Pelvis, 36–37
    pelvic diagonal conjugate, *94, 95*
    utero-fetal-pelvic relationships, 92–95
Periclitoral lacerations, 221
Perimortem caesarean section (CS), 26, 143, *143*
Perineal trauma, recognition, 10
Perineum muscles, *218*
Periurethral lacerations, 221

Personal attention, 35–36, 237
Pfannenstiel incision, 140
Philpott, Hugh, 33
Physiological reserve, fetal, 58
'Physiological sutures', 199
Pinard, Adolphe, *248*
Pinard's manoeuvre, 165, *167*
Piper's forceps, 162
Placenta
  abnormal, 266
  anterior, *250*
  antibodies crossing, 48
  retained *see* Retained placenta
  separation, 198–199
    clinical signs, 199, *204*
    twins, 169
Placenta accreta, 208
Placenta adherens, 208
Placenta praevia, 135, 178–189, *178*
  antepartum management, 182–184
    asymptomatic, 182–184
    care reassessment, 183
    fetal well-being, 184
    follow-up, 184
    major haemorrhage, 183
    minor haemorrhage, 183
    subsequent expectant, 183
  caesarean section (CS), 186–189
    delivery, 188–189
    preoperative preparation, 186–188
    skin incision, 188
    third stage, management, 189
    uterine incision, 188
  classification, 178–180, *179*
  cord prolapse, 174
  differential diagnosis, *182*
  hysterectomy, 266
  invasive, 193–196, *193*
    classification, 193
  Jehovah's Witness patients, 189
  lower uterine segment (LUS), physiology, 180, *181*
  placental 'migration', 180, *181*
  risk factors, 178, *179*
  vaginal bleeding, assessment, 180–182, *181*, *194*
  vaginal delivery, 184–185
    major haemorrhage, 185
    malpresentation, 185–186
    minor haemorrhage, 185–186
Placenta praevia accreta, 193
  hysterectomy, 266
Placenta praevia increta, 193
  risk factors, *193*
  screening, 193–194
  surgical strategies, 194–196, *196*
Placenta praevia percreta, 193
Placental abruption, 178, 189–191
  classification, 190, *190*
  diagnosis/management, 191
  differential diagnosis, *182*
  hysterectomy, 266
  pathophysiology, 190
Platelet transfusion, 232
Polyhydramnios, 174
Pomeroy's manoeuvre, 104–105
Poor progress, 97
Porro, Eduardo, 132–133
Portal, Paul, 119, 157, 178, *178*
Posterior arm delivery, 127, *127*
Postmortem caesarean section (CS), 25, 143, *143*
Postoperative analgesia, 137
Postoperative infection, 147

Postpartum haemorrhage (PPH), 24, 198–206
  disseminated intravascular coagulation (DIC), 231–232
  oxytocic drugs, 201–202, *201*, *203*
  primary, 153, 198–200
    causes, 203
    management, 204–205, *204*
    prevention, 203–204
  secondary, 205
    causes, 205
    management, 205
  third stage labour
    management, 198–199, *200*
    physiology, 198–199
    placental separation, 198–199, *200*
  training, 205
Poullet, J., 90
PPROMEXIL trial, 73
Prague manoeuvre, reverse, 165, *165*
Pre-eclampsia, 72
Pregnancy
  ectopic, 267
  high-risk, 42–44, *42*
  inter-pregnancy interval, 147
  multiple, 73, 174
    see also Twins, delivery
  physiological changes, *225*
  prolonged, 72
Prematurity, 174
Prescott, Oliver, 200
Presentation, assessment, *38*
Preterm birth, 81
  complications, 84–85
  incidence, 81
  mode of delivery, 85
Preterm labour, 80–87
  aetiology/mechanisms, 81
  definition, 80–81
  diagnosis, 83
  management, 83
  prediction, 82–83, *82*
  vs preterm birth, 81
  prevention, 83
  risk factors, *82*
  tocolysis, 84
Preterm premature membrane rupture (pPROM), 73, 78, *78*, 85, 174
  diagnosis, 85
  prognosis/management, 85
Preventable harm, 22–23
Primary dysfunctional labour, 37
Primary postpartum haemorrhage *see under* Postpartum haemorrhage (PPH)
PROBAAT trial, 75
Progesterone, 5, 83
Prolonged pregnancy, 72
Prostaglandins, 9–10, 71, 200, 210
  dosage, *78*
  induction of labour, 74–75, *74*
Pseudo-sinusoidal pattern, fetal heart rate (FHR), 48–49, *48*
Pudendal block, 240, *240*
Pugh, Benjamin, 89
Pulse oximetry, fetal, 51
Pyrexia, maternal, 54

R
RADICAL framework *see under* Risk management
Raising Awareness (RADICAL framework), 7–8
Recombinant activated factor VIIa, 232
Record keeping, CTG traces, 68

Reid, Grantly Dick, 236–237, *237*
Remifentanil, 239, 241
Reporting, incident, 69
Resuscitation
    maternal collapse, 25–26
    neonatal, 26
Retained placenta, 207–210
    acute tocolysis, 246
    management, 209
    oxytocic drugs, intraumbilical vein injection,
        210
    predisposing factors, 208
    removal, timing, 208–210, *208*
    technique, removal, 209, *209–210*
    tocolysis, 210
    types, 208
Retroperitoneal haematomas, 223
Rhesus antibodies, 48
Rigby, Edward, 178, 193
Risk management, 7–14
    patient safety, tools, 9
    RADICAL framework, 7
        Raising Awareness, 7–8
        Design for safety, 8–12
        Involve users, 12
        Collect and Analyze patient safety data,
            12–13
        Learn from experience, 13
Risk Management standards (CNST), 23
Risk register, 13
Ritgen, Ferdinand, 133
Ritodrine, 247
Robson 10-group method, 135
Root cause analysis, 13
Rosenheim, Max, 22
Rotational manoeuvres
    assisted vaginal delivery, 104–108
        forceps, 105–108
    bipolar version, *187*
    Løvset's manoeuvre, 163–164, *163*, *164*
    nuchal arm, 164–165, *165*
    shoulder dystocia, 128, *128*
    trunk and head, posterior, 165, *165*
Royal Australia and New Zealand College of Obstetricians
        and Gynaecologists, 8–9
Royal College of Midwives (RCM), 23, 54, 67, 69, 130
Royal College of Obstetricians and Gynaecologists
        (RCOG), 8–9, 23, 54, 67, 69, 84, 155, 232
    shoulder dystocia guidelines, 124–125, 130
'Rule of 30s', 226
Rüsch urological balloon, 253–254

S

Sacral hand wedge, 110
Safe Births: everybody's business (Kings Fund report), 22
Safety incidents, reporting, 13
    see also Risk management
Sanger, Max, 133
Saving Mothers' Lives (CMACE, 2011), 22
Saxtorph, Mathias, 89–90
Scalp trauma, fetal, 112
Secondary arrest, 37
Secondary postpartum haemorrhage *see under* Postpartum
        haemorrhage (PPH)
Sengsten–Blakemore tube, 253–254
Sepsis, 267
Sequential instrumental delivery, 111
*Sett of Anatomical Tables with Explanations and an
    Abridgement of the Practice of Midwifery* (Smellie), 1
'Shock index', 226

Shoulder dystocia, 123–131
    acute tocolysis, 246
    anticipation, 12
    definition, 123
    documentation, 130
    incidence, 123
    management, 125–129
        actions to avoid, 129
        all-fours position, 128–129, *128*
        assistance, 125
        episiotomy, 126–127
        follow-up, 129
        internal manoeuvres, 127
        last resort manoeuvres, 129
        McRoberts' position, 126, *126–127*
        posterior arm delivery, 127, *127*
        recognition, 125
        rotational manoeuvres, 128, *128*
        stating the problem, 125–126
        suprapubic pressure, 126, *127*
    obstetric brachial plexus injury (OBPI), 113, 129–130
    pathophysiology, 123, *124*
    prediction, 124
    prevention, 124–125
    previous, 124
    risk factors, 123–124
        intrapartum, 124
    symphysiotomy, 272
    training recommendations, 130–131
Shoulder presentation, *120*
Sigault, Jean René, 271
Simpson, James Young, 1, 91, *91*, 99–100, *99*, *239*
Simpson's forceps, 278
Simpson's perforator, 277–279, *277*
Sims' lateral position, 175–176, *176*
Simulation-based medical education (SMBE), 24–25
    assisted vaginal delivery, 25
    cord prolapse, 177
    eclampsia, 25
    postpartum haemorrhage (PPH), 205
    vaginal breech delivery, 25
Sinusoidal pattern, fetal heart rate (FHR), 45–49, *47*
Skills training, 23
    low-resource settings, 26
    maternal collapse, 25–26
    neonatal resuscitation, 26
    'Skill Drills', 23
    teamwork, 26–27
    see also Simulation-based medical education (SMBE)
Skull fracture, 113
Smart pulse tocograph, 67–68, *68*
Smellie, William, 1, 198, 207
    assisted vaginal delivery, 89–90
    malpresentations, 117, 162
    management of labour, *31*, 32
    Mauriceau–Smellie–Veit manoeuvre, 163
Society of Obstetricians and Gynaecologists of Canada,
        8–9
Spinal cord injury, 113
Spontaneous evolution, 120, *120*, *121*
STAN waveform analyzer, 52–53
    guidelines, 53, *53*
Standards of care
    audit, 15–21
    competence, 22–30
Stark, Michael, 140
Stearns, John, 200
Steiner, C.C., 234
Stimulation tests, fetal, 51
Structured multidisciplinary intershift handover (SMITH)
        protocol, 9

Subgaleal haemorrhage, 112, *112*
Superior haemorrhoidal artery, 262
Supervision, 12
Suprapubic pressure, 126, *127*
Surgical safety checklist, 9
Sutures *see* Uterine compression sutures
Symphysiotomy, 129, 271–275
   complications, 274
   indications, 271–272
   post-delivery care, 274
   technique, 272–274, *272–273*
Symphysis pubis, 271–273, *272*
Synclitism, 93, *94*
Syntometrine®, 200, 207
   characteristics/side effects, *201*, 202
Systems Analysis, 13

T

Tachysystole, defined, 39
Tarnier, Etienne Stéphane, 89–90
Teamwork, 12, 16
   leadership, roles/responsibilities, 27
   training, 26–27
10-group classification system (TGCS), 19–21, *20*
Tentorial tear, 158
Terbutaline, 67, 203, 247
Term Breech Trial, 25, 157, 159, 169
Theobald, Geoffrey, *71*
'Three Delays', 198
Thromboprophylaxis, 12, 137, 270, 280
Tocography
   external, 49
   see also Cardiotocographs (CTGs)
Tocolysis
   preterm labour, 84
   retained placenta, 210
   see also Acute tocolysis
Tocolytic drugs, 203
Tommy's the Baby Charity (UK), 85–86
Traction, fetal trunk, 158
Training, 12
   fetal asphyxia, 68–69
   programme effectiveness, 28
   shoulder dystocia, 130–131
   see also Skills training
Transcervical Foley catheter, 75
Transcutaneous electrical nerve stimulation (TENS), 237
Transperineal pudendal block, 240, *240*
Transvaginal pudendal block, 240
Transverse lie, 119–122, *120*
   caesarean section (CS), 142
   causes, 119–120
   diagnosis, 120
   labour, course of, 120, *120*
   management, 121–122
      during labour, dead fetus, 121–122
      during labour, live fetus, 121
      late pregnancy before onset of labour, 121
Trap-door effect, 138–139
Trapped placenta, 208
Treatise of Midwifery (Pugh), 89
Treatise on the Theory and Practice of Midwifery (Smellie), 1, *31*
Trial of labour, 155
   defined, 146
Trial of scar, defined, 146
Triplets, 169, 172
Tucker–MacLean forceps, 99–100

Turnbull, Alec, 71, *71*
Turtle-neck sign, 125
Twin Birth Study, 169, 171
Twins, delivery, 73, 169–173
   first stage, labour, 170
   second stage, labour, 170
   third stage, labour, 171
   anaesthetic factors, 170
   conjoined twins, 172
   locked twins, 172, *172*
   obstetric factors, 169–170
      individual considerations, 169–170
      malpresentations, 169
      maternal risks, 170
   second twin, 169–171, *171*
   vaginal birth after caesarean section (VBAC), 25–26

U

Umbilical cord *see* Cord; Cord prolapse
Ureter, 269
Urinary complications, symphysiotomy, 274
Urogenital triangle, 217
Uterine artery, *261*, 262
   ligation, 262–263, *263*
Uterine atony, 203, 266
Uterine compression sutures, 257–260
   B-Lynch suture, 258–259, *258*
      modified, 257–258, *258*
   square compression suture, 258–259, *259*
   vertical uterine suture, 258, *259*
Uterine contractions
   assessment, 39
   excessive, 245–246
   fetal surveillance, 49–50, *49*
   inefficient, 36
Uterine hyperstimulation, 75
Uterine incision closure, 147
Uterine inversion
   chronic recurrent, 267
   see also Acute uterine inversion
Uterine massage, 207–208
Uterine relaxation *see* Acute tocolysis
Uterine rupture, 152–156, 266–267
   Bandl's ring, *153*
   causes, 152–153
   classification, 152
   clinical presentation, 153–154
   delivery after, 154
   fetal outcomes, 155
   management, 154
   maternal outcomes, 155
   prevention, 154–155
   risks, 92–93
'Uterine sandwich', 259
Uterine scars
   classical, 146
   hysterotomy, 146
   low vertical, 146
   myomectomy, 146
   rupture, 146
   transverse lower segment, 146
Uterine tamponade, 253 255
   aftercare, 254–255
   rationale, 253
   techniques, 253
      balloon tamponade, 253–254, *254*
      uterine packing, 253, *254*
Utero-fetal-pelvic relationships, 92–95

V

Vacuum assisted delivery, 108–111, *108–110, 109*
  sequential instrumental delivery, 111
Vacuum extractor
  vs forceps, 91–92
  historical perspective, 90–91
  use of, 25
Vaginal birth after caesarean section (VBAC), 145–151
  Edwin Craigin, 145, *145*
  selection criteria, 146–148
    adverse outcome prediction, 148
    costs, 148
    decision aids, 148
    external cephalic version (ECV), 147
    hospital facilities, 148
    inter-pregnancy interval, 147
    lower uterine segment thickness, 147
    postoperative infection, 147
    previous caesarean section (CS), 146–147
    previous vaginal delivery, 147
    twins, 25–26
    uterine incision closure, 147
    uterine scar, type, 146
  trial, management, 148–150
    adverse outcomes, prediction, 148
    antenatal care, 148
    induction of labour, 148, 155
    labour, 148–150
Vaginal delivery
  breech, simulation, 25
  see also Assisted vaginal delivery; Labour and delivery;
    Vacuum assisted delivery; Vaginal birth after
    caesarean section (VBAC)

Vaginal examination, 37, *38*, 40, 95–96
  episiotomy, 220
Vaginal lacerations, 221–222, *222*
Vaginal tamponade, 255
van Rymsdyk, Jan, 1
Vasa praevia, 191–193, *192*
Vascular ischaemic injury (VII), 64–65
Velvoski technique, 236–237
Version, 248–252
  external *see* External cephalic version (ECV)
  internal *see* Internal podalic version
Vibroacoustic stimulus, 51
Voorhees, James, *71*
Vulval haematomas, 223

W

Waiter's tip position, 130
Waller, Dr C., 228
Water, intradermal injection, 237
Willet scalp forceps, 186, *186, 188*
World Health Organization (WHO), 22–23, 80, 210
  Essential Newborn Care course, 26
  partogram, 33, *34*

Y

Yonge, James, 90–91

Z

Zananelli manoeuvre, 129